M. Kaltenbach, R. Hopf,
B. Kunkel (Eds.)

New Aspects of Hypertrophic Cardiomyopathy

Morphology, Mechanisms and Therapie

Steinkopff Verlag Darmstadt
Springer-Verlag New York

Prof. Dr. M. Kaltenbach
P.-D. Dr. R. Hopf
Zentrum Innere Medizin
Abteilung Kardiologie
Theodor-Stern-Kai 7
6000 Frankfurt 70

Prof. Dr. B. Kunkel
Medizinische Poliklinik
der Universität Erlangen
Östliche Stadtmauerstraße 29
8520 Erlangen

CIP-Titelaufnahme der Deutschen Bibliothek

New aspects of hypertrophic cardiomyopathy: morphology,
mechanisms and therapy / M. Kaltenbach ... (eds.). —
Darmstadt: Steinkopff; New York: Springer, 1988
  ISBN 3-7985-0747-3 (Steinkopff) Gb.
  ISBN 0-387-91317-3 (Springer) Gb.
NE: Kaltenbach, Martin [Hrsg.]

Medical editor: Juliane K. Weller — Copy editing: Deborah Marston — Production: Heinz J. Schäfer

Printed in Germany

Type-Setting und Printing: Vereinigte Buchdruckereien, Bad Buchau

Overview

A myocardial disease with concentric hypertrophy was first described in 1907 by the pathologist Schmincke. The disease was clinically first diagnosed in the 1950s. In subsequent years the diagnosis became routine, mainly due to the widespread use of echocardiography. Today a considerable number of cardiac patients are diagnosed and have to be treated.

Besides the practical importance, hypertrophic cardiomyopathy has remained a challenge for scientists. The pathophysiological concept has shown astonishing changes and was subject to many controversies over the last decades. This is reflected not only in more than 50 different names of the disease but also in fundamental differences in understanding. One example are the different views on the importance of ventricular obstruction. Some investigators have considered this to be the primary disorder, others think that obstruction is a secondary phenomenon and consider the gradient merely the consequence of overcontraction.

The clinical manifestations of hypertrophic cardiomyopathy can usually be clearly separated in the obstructive and non-obstructive form. Despite these different manifestations, the disease is regarded as one nosological entity. The primary disorder appears to be hypercontractility rather than hypertrophy. Hypercontraction goes along with or leads to myocardial hypertrophy and might be related to increased calcium ion availability linked by an increased amount of calcium channels. Myocardial disarray is a common finding but is unspecific and can be found in many other disorders with ventricular hypertrophy.

Myocardial hypertrophy is characterized by an increased myocardial muscle mass. It involves the total myocardium but usually is predominant in either the proximal part of the interventricular septum or around the apex of the heart. Even in patients with remarkable increases in septal and left ventricular free wall diameters, the average myocardial cell diameter has often been found to be normal (Kunkel). Thus, an increased number of myocardial fibers, i.e., myocardial hyperplasia, may be responsible for hypertrophy (Frenzel). Hyperplasia which normally only exists during prenatal life seems to persist after birth in patients with this disorder (Ferrans).

Hypercontractility and concentric hypertrophy is present in both manifestations of hypertrophic cardiomyopathy, a left ventricular and/or, in a minority of patients, a right ventricular gradient is found only in the obstructive form. Today the gradient is mostly considered to be the consequence of two factors, namely hypercontractility and thickening of the proximal intraventricular septum. These two factors together produce a high blood stream velocity along the proximal septum. By this, the mitral valve, in particular its anterior leaflet, is sucked towards the septum by the Venturi effect (Wigle, Lemke). Systolic anterior movement of the mitral valve, systolic obstruction and mitral insufficiency is the consequence.

Clinical symptoms can mainly be attributed to ventricular outflow tract obstruction on one hand, and to impaired diastolic filling on the other. In a considerable number of patients arrhythmias are also the predominant problem. Another important factor, particularly in late stage disease not responding to therapy is extensive myocardial fibrosis.

Low cardiac output can be caused by severe outflow tract obstruction, by impaired ventricular filling or by a combination of both. It is well known that ventricular or supraventricular arrhythmias in combination with the above factors can create dramatic clinical situations. The loss of late diastolic filling by atrial fibrillation often causes severe deterioration.

Angina pectoris is a common symptom, its precise origin is not yet known. Small vessel disease can be found in some patients (Maron, Cannon); however, no convincing evidence that this is the cause of symptoms has been demonstrated. The genesis of myocardial ischemia is most probably similar to that in severe aortic valve stenosis, i.e., the consequence of increased ventricular wall thickness, high oxygen demand and reduced diastolic perfusion by elevation of filling pressure.

Medical therapy with beta blockade has been the answer to the pathophysiological concept with outflow tract obstruction being the main disorder. Calcium blockers of the verapamil type have also a beneficial effect on systolic overcontraction by their negative inotropic activity. Unlike beta blockade, this negative inotropic effect can be overcome by beta adrenergic activity. In contrast to beta blockade, they have an additional favourable influence on diastolic abnormalities, brought about by improved myocardial relaxation.

Long-term effects of verapamil therapy over 10 years have been documented (Hopf). Comparison of propranolol and verapamil demonstrates the superiority of calcium blocker treatment (Kober). Combined therapy with beta blockade and calcium blockade is inferior to treatment with verapamil alone in individually adjusted doses from 360—640 mg/day (Hopf).

Surgical therapy today usually consists of left ventricular septal myectomy. The procedure is aimed at reducing outflow tract obstruction. Desobstruction leads to reduced local blood-flow velocity and may eliminate the Venturi mechanism. It is possible that myectomy also has a beneficial influence on diastolic ventricular filling characteristics by reducing myocardial stiffness (Wigle, Schulte).

Verapamil therapy and surgery thus might both operate on systolic as well as on diastolic abnormalities and are the most effective forms of treatment available today and perhaps in some patients only the combination of both measures can achieve the best result.

This volume contains contributions on anatomy, pathology and pathophysiology of hypertrophic cardiomyopathy and related disorders. Clinical diagnosis and therapy is described, including long-term results with calcium blockers and surgery. Results of a multicenter trial comparing propranolol and verapamil treatment are published for the first time, as well as of a study about the combination of betablockade with calcium blockade. Among the authors are international experts in the field. All contributions were written after an extensive discussion among all contributors. Thus, the book as an entity provides an updated overview on this fascinating disorder.

November 1987   M. Kaltenbach, R. Hopf, B. Kunkel

Contents

Development and regression of right heart ventricular hypertrophy: Biochemical and morphological aspects

M. Schneider[1], S. Wiese[1], B. Kunkel[2], H. Hauk[1], B. Pfeiffer[1]

Senckenbergisches Zentrum der Pathologie, Universitätsklinik Frankfurt/M ([1])
and Zentrum der Inneren Medizin, Abteilung für Kardiologie, Universitätsklinik Erlangen ([2]), F.R.G.

Introduction

Since the introduction of myocardial biopsy in the diagnostic management of human
heart disease, by Konno (31), morphologic myocardial research has received a fresh im-
petus, as documented by many monographs (3, 24, 25, 36, 39, 63).

But even now, myocardial hypertrophy remains one of the central unresolved problems
in cardiology. The two most important questions in this regard are:
1. Does a "physiologic" myocardial hypertrophy exist and can it be distinguished from
   a "pathologic" hypertrophy (8, 32, 40, 43, 44, 60)?
2. Is myocardial hypertrophy reversible or not (11, 12, 21–23, 30, 40, 44, 45, 48, 53)?
   These questions will be the main topic of this investigation.

As an experimental model, we chose the hypobaric right heart hypertrophy in rats,
which is in our opinion, a physiologic model imitating human cor pulmonale (6, 16, 26,
49, 57–59).

Materials and Methods

Experimental Design

All experiments animals were male white Wistar rats with a body weight ranging from
200–250 g. Three investigations were carried out.
1. Development of myocardial hypertrophy:
   40 animals were exposed in a hypobaric chamber to a pressure degree of 345 Torr,
   corresponding to 6000 meters in altitude, where they remained permanently. At
   weekly intervals for up to 4 weeks' duration, ten animals were investigated, five with
   biochemical techniques and five with morphological methods.
2. Regression of myocardial hypertrophy after 2 weeks of hypobaric conditions:
   40 animals were exposed for 2 weeks to the above pressure. After this, they were
   brought to normobaric conditions and also were investigated at weekly intervals.

Dedicated to Prof. Dr. K. Hübner on the occasion of his 60th birthday.

3. Regression of myocardial hypertrophy after 4 weeks of hypobaric conditions:
   50 animals were exposed to high altitude conditions for 4 weeks. They were sacrificed 1, 2, 3, 4 or 8 weeks after cessation.
   Ten animals were used as untreated controls.

Morphological investigations

All animals received 1 µCi 3H-Thymidine by i.p. injection 1 h before sacrificing. Under deep ether narcosis the abdomen was opened. The abdominal aorta was cannulated with a transfusion set (Venofix) and the heart was perfused and fixed, by retrograde perfusion, with a solution of 3 % glutaraldehyde (in 0.1 M cacodylate buffer, at a pressure of 200 cmH_2O). During the 1 h interval, the titriated thymidine is incorporated into all DNA-synthesizing nuclei which can be easily detected as black grains in paraffin sections which had been covered with a photoemulsion (Kodak G5). Thus, labeled nuclei can be counted. Small pieces of lung and heart were preserved for this procedure. From this paraffin-embedded material, sections were also obtained for the usual histological stains (H.-E., van Gieson).

The remaining parts of the heart (right and left ventricle separately) were sliced into small cubes, dehydrated in acetone and embedded in Araldite for electron microscope investigations.

Using the stereologic point-counting method of Weibel and Gomez (1, 46, 56) in randomized semi-thin sections (light microscope, mangification × 1,000) the amount of heart interstitium was determined. In randomized ultra-thin sections (electron microscope, EM 101, Siemens, magnification × 10,000) the amount of myofibrils and mitochondria of heart muscle cells were determined (point-rasters with 100 points each).

The wall thickness of the pulmonary arteries was determined on paraffin embedded lung sections by direct morphometry (ELAS, Leitz, Program UNI 2000).

Biochemical investigations

For this investigation, the still-beating heart of the animal was removed from the thorax under deep ether narcosis. The ventricles were dissected along the ventricular septum and weighed separately. A small cube of about 0.5 mm³ was removed from the right ventricle and put into 3 % phosphotungstic acid and the usual negative staining method for mitochondrial F1 ATPase (technical details: Refs. 7, 42) was performed. The remaining parts of both ventricles were lyophilized and pulverized separately. The protein content, according to Lowry (35), and the DNA content, according to Dische (13) and Burton (10), were subsequently determined from this material.

In all figures, the mean values and the standard deviations of the measurements are marked (from five animals each). Comparable values of age-matched untreated controls are indicated by the dotted bands. In all figures "U" indicates the start and "F" the end of hypobaric conditions.

Results

Development of myocardial hypertrophy

Under the hypobaric conditions mentioned above, equivalent to an altitude of 6000 m, the animals promptly developed pulmonary hypertension which was easily proved in

Table 1. Main data of developing myocardial hypertrophy in male Wistar rats, under hypobaric conditions, simulating an altitude of 6,000 m.

	Lung Small pulmorary arteries wallthickness (μm)	Right ventricle				Left ventricle			
		wet weight (mg)	dry weight (mg)	protein content (mg)	DNA content (mg)	wet weight (mg)	dry weight (mg)	protein content (mg)	DNA content (mg)
Untreated control animals	1.8±0.2	130±10	29±2.0	18±1.2	2.9±0.2	470±38	102±9.4	65±6.3	10.0±1.1
1st week	2.5±0.4	225±18	38±3.1	30±2.4	3.0±0.2	500±47	120±10	74±6.8	9.8±1.2
2nd week	3.1±0.5	312±27	58±4.9	42±3.5	4.0±0.3	510±50	130±12	79±6.7	9.8±1.0
3rd week	3.8±0.4	320±28	68±5.2	44±3.8	4.9±0.4	588±52	142±12	85±7.1	10.1±1.2
4th week	3.9±0.5	350±28	72±6.0	49±3.6	4.9±0.4	602±51	145±12	84±7.3	10.2±1.0

histologic sections of the lung. The width of the media of small pulmonary arteries increased from 1.8 to 3.9 μm (Table 1), as can also be appreciated in the illustration (Fig. 1). Consequently, the animals developed severe hypertrophy of the right ventricle. The wet-weight and the dry weight of the right ventricle increased markedly (Table 1). Therefore, this phenomenon can be called cor pulmonale, according to the WHO definition (62).

Corresponding to the increasing ventricular weight, the protein and DNA content increased almost in parallel (Table 1).

The time courses of the changes in DNA and protein concentration in relation to dry weight of the ventricle were different, as shown in Fig. 2. The protein concentration increased markedly in the first week and reached subnormal values in the fourth week. The protein can be considered to represent the amount of heart muscle cells and their myofibrils. The amount of interstitium in this biochemical determination is negligible.

The DNA concentration increased to a minor degree, but in the fourth week subnormal values were also found (Fig. 2). In contrast to the protein measurements, the biochemical estimation of DNA included nuclei of the heart muscle cells and of interstitial cells.

By the autoradiography method, DNA synthesizing nuclei of cardiomyocytes and interstitial cells could be distinguished. The results are compiled in Fig. 3. Most DNA producing cells were located in the interstitium, in which the labeling index increased about six fold, due to expansion of the interstitium by proliferation. Here, mitoses were frequent. Unfortunately, because of the chosen method (paraffin sections), it was not

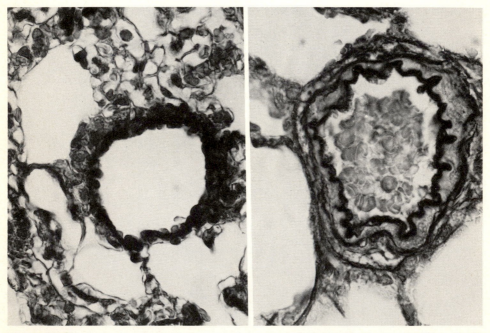

Fig. 1. Small pulmonary arteries. Left: untreated control animal, normobaric conditions. Right: animal from the 4th week of hypobaric conditions (Light microscope, Mag.: × 450, van Gieson).

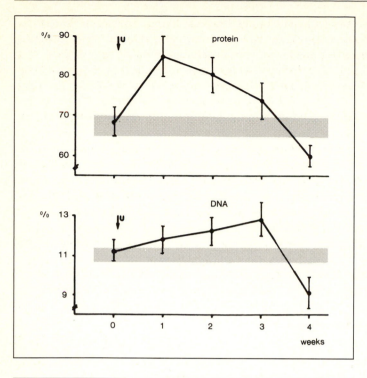

Fig. 2. Time course of changes in protein and DNA concentration in the hypertrophying right ventricle, related to dry weight of myocardium.

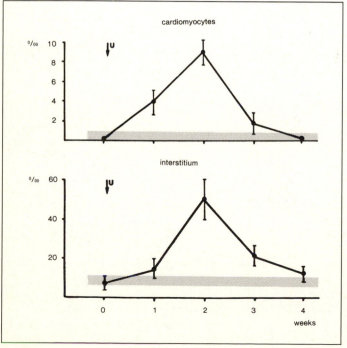

Fig. 3. Variations in the amount of labeled nuclei of cardiomyocytes (above) and nuclei of interstitial cells (below) of hypertrophying rat myocardium (autoradiographic method).

possible to distinguish clearly between endothelial nuclei and nuclei of other interstitial cells. Thus, the real amount of proliferating endothelial cells could not be determined. But heart muscle cells were also involved in DNA synthesis, although they made a much smaller contribution (Fig. 3). This may have been due to hyperplasia of cardiomyocytes, although mitoses of these cells were never observed.

The amount of interstitium, measured by the method of point counting, increased from 11% to almost 20% of total myocardium (Fig. 4).

The composition of the heart muscle cells was studied by electron microscopy. An example of the characteristics of hypertrophying cardiomyocytes is given in Fig. 5. As compared to a control animal (left), under hypobaric conditions the muscle cells of the right ventricle show focally increased mitochondria of varying shapes and focal loss of myofibrils. In Fig. 6, these observations are confirmed morphometrically. Indeed, there is a loss of myofibrils in the fourth week of observation and an increase in total mitochondrial mass in the third and fourth week.

The functions of mitochondria were investigated by a negative staining method to demonstrate F1 ATPase. An example of these investigations is demonstrated in Fig. 7, as indicated in the legend. The differences in the appearance of the mitochondrial ATPase complexes during the process of myocardial hypertrophy are highly impressive.

Regression of myocardial hypertrophy

Complete resolution of all determined morphological and biochemical parameters of right heart ventricle could be observed in all animals that spent only 2 weeks in the hypobaric chamber. A separate illustration for this seems unnecessary. All animals that spent 4 weeks under hypobaric conditions did not show a complete regression of right ventricular hypertrophy. The wet and the dry weight of the right ventricle did not decrease to normal values (Table 2). Of more importance seem to be the changes in protein

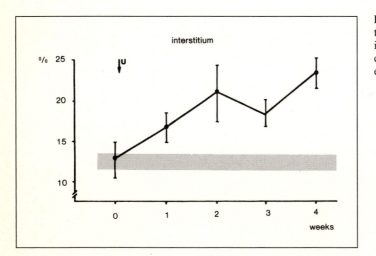

Fig. 4. Increase in interstitium in the hypertrophying right ventricle (point-counting method of stereology).

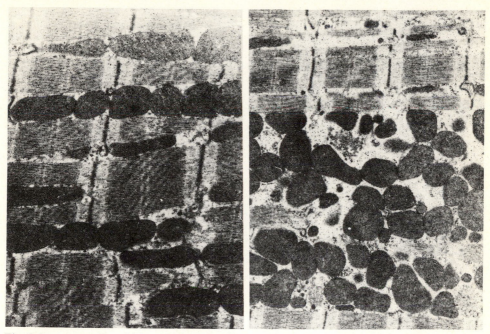

Fig. 5. Rat myocardium (right ventricle, electron microsocpe, Mag.: × 8,000). Left: untreated control animal with regularly distributed mitochondria of nearly the same size and shape. Right: animal from the 4th week of hypobaric conditions: focally increased mitochondria of varying shapes in areas with focal loss of myofibrils.

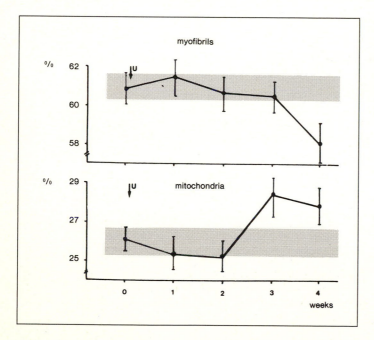

Fig. 6. Variations in the amount of myofibrils and mitochondria in hypertrophying right ventricular muscle cells (point-counting method of stereology).

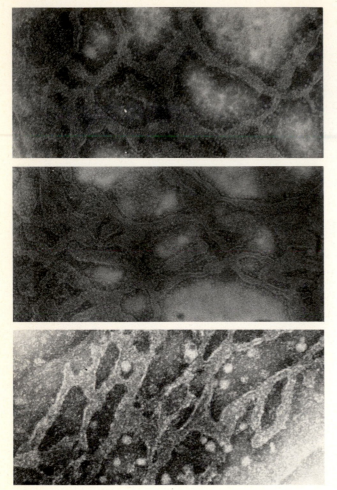

Fig. 7. Demonstration of mitochondrial F1 ATPase by negative staining (electron microscope, Mag.: × 100,000). Top: untreated control animal. The small buds of the ATPase complexes are of normal size (about 9 mm) and distributed symmetrically. Middle: animal from the 2nd week of hypobaric conditions. The mitochondrial cristae seem to be more twisted, the ATPase buds are smaller and seem to be increased. Below: animal from the 4th week of hypobaric conditions. The ATPase complexes are dissolved by the cristae. They accumulate focally, forming large balls.

and DNA content. The protein content decreased slightly, and the DNA content remained nearly unchanged. Also, the amount of interstitium did not decrease under normobaric conditions (Fig. 8).

Reactions of the left ventricle

As shown in Table 1, the left ventricle also exhibited an increase of about 30% in wet weight.

This was due to a hypertrophy of myocardial cells. The DNA content (about 10 mg) remained unchanged. By autoradiographic methods, only a minimal proliferation of interstitial cells could be observed, as manifest by a slight increase in labeled nuclei (from 8 to 12%). After cessation of hypobaric conditions no changes in the weight of the left ventricle could be observed (Table 2).

Table 2. Main data of regression of myocardial hypertrophy after cessation of hypobaric conditions. Abbreviation: n.b. = period of normobaric conditions.

	Lung Small pulmonary arteries wallthickness (µm)	Right ventricle				Left ventricle			
		wet weight (mg)	dry weight (mg)	protein content (mg)	DNA content (mg)	wet weight (mg)	dry weight (mg)	protein content (mg)	DNA content (mg)
Last week in the hypobaric chamber	3.9±0.5	350±28	72±6.0	49±3.6	4.9±3.6	602±51	145±12	84±7.3	10.2±1.0
1st week (n.b.)	3.0±1.2	310±32	70±6.2	42±4.0	4.7±0.4	620±61	155±14	95±8.9	10.1±0.9
2nd week (n.b.)	2.8±0.4	304±31	64±6.1	40±3.8	4.6±0.5	710±68	156±17	102±9.7	10.3±0.8
3rd week (n.b.)	2.5±0.3	302±35	61±6.8	38±3.9	4.2±0.4	650±62	152±15	110±10.2	10.0±1.1
4th week (n.b.)	2.7±0.3	297±29	58±6.1	35±3.9	4.4±0.3	630±63	151±14	101±10.4	9.9±1.1
8th week (n.b.)	2.4±0.2	283±31	56±6.0	33±3.2	4.3±0.3	635±63	157±17	98±9.3	10.2±0.9

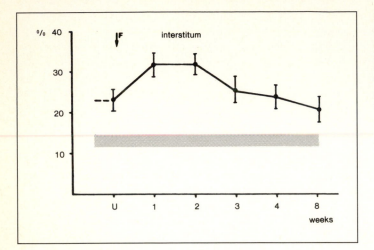

Fig. 8. Interstitial changes in the right ventricle after cessation of hypobaric conditions: no complete resolution takes place (point-counting method of stereology).

But, according to the increasing body weight of the animals under normobaric conditions, the total ventricular mass also increased. Detailed examination of this difficult problem of a corresponding increase in ventricular mass is not yet completed. The results are in preparation and will be published soon.

Discussion

In the model of right heart hypertrophy used in this study, the results clearly demonstrate that the animals develop cor pulmonale comparable to that occurring in humans (2, 6, 14, 21, 58). The findings suggest that this form of myocardial hypertrophy exhibits, not a steady development, but rather a series of distinctive events, which can be classified into three stages (Table 3). These results confirm those of Meerson (38, 39). Comparable ideas and speculations have been published recently by other authors, too (18, 20, 60, 63). From this point of view, different forms of myocardial hypertrophy may exist.

Table 3. Stages of right heart hypertrophy (hypobaric conditions).

2. (1st—2nd week):
   Pure hypertrophy with extensive stimulation of protein synthesis.
2. (2nd—3rd):
   Steady state of biochemical cell composition.
   No myocardial cell alteration.
   Increase of mitochondrial ATPase.
   Proliferation of interstitium.
   (Hyperplasia of cardiomyocytes?)
3. (4th week):
   Decrease in myofibril content of cardiomyocytes.
   Severe alterations in mitochondria.
   (Monitoring signs of myocardial insufficiency?).

Earlier concepts, implying that pressure stress to myocardium is more favourable in functional tolerance than volume overload seem questionable, from this point of view. Perhaps only the rate of development of heart hypertrophy is different under these conditions (33, 51, 52). Thus, a differentiation of physiologic and pathologic hypertrophy seems reasonable (5, 32, 43).

Phase 1 of myocardial hypertrophy is characterized by mere protein synthesis and, dependent on this, an increase in heart muscle cell mass (9, 34, 37). No other developments take place in this phase. Indeed, myocardial hypertrophy is completely reversible at this stage of development. This form of hypertrophy is comparable to training hypertrophy in humans and animals (22, 23).

The beginning of imminent problems in myocardial hypertrophy results from the second stage, in which the ventricular mass increases and expansion of the interstitium takes place, perhpas together with hyperplasia of cardiomyocytes (5, 15, 28). The increases in DNA content and in the amount of interstitial tissue seem not to be reversible, as shown by the present study and by other authors (12, 21, 37, 53). This stage of myocardial hypertrophy may be classified as the compensated stage and constitutes the most often published phenomenon of myocardial hypertrophy. During this period, functional compensating processes are starting, especially by increasing mitochondrial ATPase activity. Observations of stage 3 of myocardial hypertrophy are rarely published. Indeed, in our model, the animals died if the hypobaric conditions were maintained over a period of 6 to 8 weeks. The phenomenon of sudden and unexpected death in patients with myocardial hypertrophy is well known (55, 57). Perhaps the demonstrated loss of myofibrils and the decreasing activity of mitochondrial ATPase may be an appropriate explanation for this (19, 27, 50, 60, 61). Myocardial hypertrophy at this stage of development is not completely reversible if the inducing stress is completely eliminated. But there is a catch to the results: in our experimental study the pulmonary hypertension also failed to resolve completely (Table 2).

The surprising result that the left heart ventricle also increased in volume mass cannot be explained definitely. Comparable investigations are extremely rare. The observations of pathologists that during the growth of a heart ventricle the corresponding one is also involved to a minor degree, has been confirmed in a few studies (4, 17, 26, 29, 41, 54). Perhaps there is an interior mechanism of regulation of ventricular weights which aims to balance the normal ratio of right to left ventricle at 1 to 3. More studies will be needed to elucidate this curious phenomenon.

Summary: Male Wistar rats were exposed, in a hypobaric chamber, to a simulated altitude of 6000 m for up to four weeks. The animals quickly developed pulmonary hypertension with an important media hypertrophy of the pulmonary arteries, followed by severe right heart hypertrophy (cor pulmonale). Right heart hypertrophy is evident in three morphologically and biochemically definable stages.

In stage 1 (1st—2nd week) a manifest thickening of heart muscle cells develops due to increased protein synthesis. In stage 2 (2nd—3rd week) one can find, in the regular biochemical composition of heart muscle, an activation of mitochondrial ATPase, a multiplication of mitochondria, a proliferation of interstitial cells and an increase in interstitial volume. In stage 3 (3rd—4th week) the hypertrophied myocardium exhibits signs of biochemical and morphological decompensation.

Besides a loss of myofibrils and a reduction in mitochondrial ATPase, DNA and protein concentrations sink to subnormal values. Only myocardium from stage 1 of hypertrophy shows complete reversibility after cessation of hypobaric conditions, but not so in stage 3.

Parallel with the developing cor pulmonale, the animals also react with a small hypertrophy of the left heart ventricle. This concomitant growth persists under normobaric conditions, too. These investigations document that growth of myocardium under extreme conditions shows a phasic development. Severe forms of myocardial hypertrophy do not always seem to be reversible.

References

1. Aherne WA, Dunhill MS (1982) Morphometry. Edward Arnold, London
2. Alexander AF, Will DN, Grove RF, Reeves JT (1960) Pulmonary hypertension and right ventricular hypertrophy in cattle at high altitude. Am J Vet Res 21: 199—208
3. Alpert NR (1983) Myocardial hypertrophy and failure. Raven Press, New York
4. Anversa P, Beghi C, McDonald SL, Levicky V, Kikkawa Y, Olivetti G (1984) Morphometry of the right ventricular hypertrophy induced by myocardial infarction in the rat. Am J Pathol 116: 504—513
5. Badeer HS (1972) Development of cardiomegaly. A unifying hypothesis explaining the growth of muscle fibers, blood vessels and collagen of heart. Cardiology 57: 247—261
6. Bardsley P, Evely R, Howard P (1986) Hypoxic cor pulmonale: A review. Herz 11: 155—168
7. Beyersdorf F (1983) Ultrastrukturelle Veränderungen der Myocardzellen während Herzhypertrophie, -degeneration und -ischämie. Thieme, Stuttgart, New York
8. Bishop SP (1984) Cardiac hypertrophy with congenital heart disease and cardiomyopathy. In: Zak R (ed) Growth of the heart in health and disease. Raven Press, New York, pp 241—274
9. Bozner A, Meessen H (1969) Die Feinstruktur des Herzmuskels der Ratte nach einmaligem und nach wiederholtem Schwimmtraining. Virchow Arch (B Cell Path) 3: 248—269
10. Burton K (1956) A study of the conditions and mechanisms of the diphenylamine reaction for the colorimetric estimation of DNA. Biochem J 62: 315—323
11. Caroll JD, Gaasch WH (1981) Left ventricular volume, mass and function following surgical correction of chronic aortic regurgitation. Herz 6: 131—137
12. Cutiletta AF, Dowell RT, Rudnick M, Arcillar A, Zak R (1975) Regression of myocardial hypertrophy. I. Experimental modell changes in heart weight, nucleic acids and collagen. J Mol Cell Cardiol 7: 767—781
13. Dische Z (1930) Über einige neue charakteristische Farbreaktionen der Thymonucleinsäure und eine Mikromethode zur Bestimmung derselben in tierischen Organen mit Hilfe dieser Reaktion. Mikrochemie 8: 4—32
14. Duke HN (1957) Observations on the effects of hypoxia on the pulmonary vascular bed. J Physiol 135: 45—51
15. Ebert L, Pfitzer P (1977) Nuclear DNA of myocardial cells in the peripher of infarction and scars. Virchow Arch (B Cell Path) 24: 209—217
16. Fishman AP (1976) Hypoxia and its effects on the pulmonary circulation. How and where it acts. Circ Res 38: 221—231
17. Fluck DL, Chandrasekar RG, Gardner FV (1966) Left ventricular hypertrophy in chronic bronchitis. Br Heart J 29: 92—97
18. Grimm AF, Kubota RBS, Whitehorn WV (1966) Ventricular nucleic acid and protein levels with myocardial growth and hypertrophy. Circ Res 19: 552—558
19. Gudbjarnason S, Telerman M, Bing RJ (1964) Protein metabolism in cardiac hypertrophy and heart failure. Am J Physiol 206: 294—298

20. Hatt PY, Jouannot P, Moravec J, Swynghedauw B (1974) Current trends in heart hypertrophy. Basic Res Cardiol 69: 479—483
21. Heath D, Edwards C, Winson M, Smith P (1973) Effects on the right ventricle, pulmonary vasculature and carotid bodies of rat of exposure to, and recovery from simulated high altitude. Thorax 28: 24—28
22. Hort W (1951) Morphologische und physiologische Untersuchungen an Ratten während eines Lauftrainings and nach Training. Virchow Arch 320: 197—237
23. Hort W, Frenzel H, Höltermann W, Schnürch HG, Novi A (1983) Myocardial hypertrophy. Development and regression. In: Just H, Schuster HP (eds) Myocarditis — Cardiomyopathy. Springer, Berlin, Heidelberg, New York, Tokyo, pp 135—142
24. Jacob R, Gülch RW, Kissling G (1983) Cardiac Adaptation to hemodynamic overload, training and stress. Dr. Dietrich Steinkopff, Darmstadt
25. Kaltenbach M, Epstein SE (1982) Hypertrophic cardiomyopathy. Springer, Berlin, Heidelberg, New York
26. Khaja F, Parker JO (1971) Right and left ventricular performance in chronic obstructive lung disease. Am Heart J 81: 319—327
27. Kisch B (1960) A new concept of cardiac failure. Am J Cardiol 5: 383—389
28. Klinge O (1967) DNS-Synthese and Kernteilung im normalen und im infarcierten Rattenherzen. Verh Dtsch Ges Path 51: 157—161
29. Knierim HJ (1972) Morphologische Grundlagen der Herzhypertrophie. Verh Dtsch Ges Kreisl 38: 1—21
30. Köhler E, Völz G, Haerten K, Hartkotte D, Körfer R, Loogen F (1981) Echokardiographische Verlaufsbeobachtungen der linksventrikulären Größe und Funktion bei Patienten vor und nach prothetischem Aortenklappenersatz. Z Kardiol 70: 660—669
31. Konno S, Sakakibara S (1963) Endo-Myocardial biopsy. Dis Chest 44: 345—350
32. Kuhn H (1982) The definition of ventricular hypertrophy. Eur Heart J 3 (Suppl A): 5—8
33. Kunkel B, Schneider M, Kober G, Bussmann WD, Hopf R, Kaltenbach M (1982) Die Morphologie der Myocardbiopsie und ihre klinische Bedeutung. Z Kardiol 71: 787—794
34. Loud AV, Beghi C, Olivetti G, Anversa P (1984) Morphometry of right and left ventricular myocardium after strenous exercise in preconditioned rats. Lab Invest 51: 104—111
35. Lowry DH, Rosebrough NJ, Farr AL, Randall RJ (1951) Protein measurement with the Folin Phenol reagent. J Biol Chem 193: 265—275
36. Mall G, Otto HF (1985) Herzhypertrophie, Springer, Berlin, Heidelberg, New York, Tokyo
37. Medugorac I, Jacob R (1983) Myocardial mass and collagen content in Crotalaria spectabilis-induced pulmonary hypertension of young and adult rats. In: Jacob R, Gülch RW, Kissling G (eds) Cardiac adaptation to hemodynamic overload, training and stress. Dr Dietrich Steinkopff, Darmstadt, pp 341—348
38. Meerson FZ (1969) The myocardium in hyperfunction, hypertrophy and heart failure. Circ Res (Suppl II) 25: 1—163
39. Meerson FZ (1983) The failing heart, Raven Press, New York
40. Mellerowics H (1972) Trainingswirkungen auf Herz und Kreislauf. In: Baitsch H, Bock HE, Bolte M, Bokler W, Grupe O, Heidland HW, Lotz F (eds) Sport im Blickpunkt der Wissenschaften. Springer, Berlin, Heidelberg, New York, pp 236—248
41. Oberpriller JO, Ferrans VJ, Carroll RF (1984) DNA-Synthesis in rat atrial myocytes as a response to left ventricular infarction. An autoradiographic study of enzymatically dissociated myocytes. J Mol Cell Cardiol 16: 1119—1126
42. Parsons DF (1963) Negative staining of thinly spread cells and associated virus. J Cell Biol 16: 620—626
43. Rapaport E (1982) Pathophysiological basis of ventricular hypertrophy. Eur Heart J 3 (Suppl A): 29—33
44. Reindell H, Dickhut HH, Keul J (1983) Anpassungsvorgänge des Herzens an Dauerbelastungen unter Berücksichtigung von Herzvolumen und echokardiographischen Befunden. In: Kaltenbach M, Klepzig H (eds) Röntgenologische Herzvolumenbestimmung, Springer, Berlin, Heidelberg, New York, pp 26—35

45. Ressl J, Urbanová D, Widimsky J, Ostadal B, Pelouch V, Prochazka J (1974) Reversibility of pulmonary hypertension and right ventricular hypertrophy induced by intermittent high altitude hypoxia in rats. Respiration 31: 38—46

46. Riede UN, Reith A (1980) Morphometry in Pathology. Gustav Fischer, New York

47. Ross W (1967) Karyometrische Untersuchungen normaler und durch Lauftraining hypertrophierter Herzmuskel von Ratten. Beitr Path Anat 135: 183—212

48. Schwarz F, Flameng W, Schaper J, Herrlein F (1978) Correlation between myocardial structure and diastolic properties of the heart in chronic aortic valve disease. Effects of corrective surgery. Am J Cardiol 42: 895—903

49. Sill V (1971) Einfluß von Arbeits- und Druckbelastung auf den rechten Ventrikel. Verh Dtsch Ges Kreislforsch 37: 196—200

50. Singal PK, Dhillon KS, Dhalla NS (1983) Cardiac muscle function during the development of hypertrophy in pigs due to pressure overload. In: Jacob R, Gülch RW, Kissling G (eds) Cardiac adaptation to hemodynamic overload, training and stress. Dr Dietrich Steinkopff, Darmstadt, pp 189—196

51. Spann JF (1984) Functional changes in pathologic hypertrophy. In: Zak R (ed) Growth of the heart in health and disease. Raven Press, New York, pp 421—466

52. Staiger J, Stolze H, Adler CP (1975) Nuclear deoxyribonucleic acid content in congenital cardiac malformations. In: Fleckenstein A, Rona G (eds) Recent advances in studies on cardiac structure and metabolism, Vol 6. University Park Press, Baltimore, pp 357—363

53. Taylor RR, Papadimitriou JM, Hopkins BE (1972) Structure and function in myocardial hypertropy. Adv Cardiol 12: 246—253

54. Turek Z, Grandtner M, Kreuzer F (1972) Cardiac hypertrophy, capillary and muscle fiber density, muscle fiber diameter, capillary radius and diffusion distance in the myocardium of growing rats, adapted to a simulated altitude of 3,500 m. Pflügers Arch 335: 19—28

55. Wagner BM (1986) Left ventricular hypertrophy and sudden death. (Editorial) Hum Pathol 17: 1

56. Weibel ER, Gomez DM (1962) A principle for counting tissue structures on random sections. J Appl Physiol 17: 343—348

57. Weitzenblum E, Mamosser M, Ehrhart M (1986) Evolution and prognosis of pulmonary hypertension in chronic obstructive pulmonary disease. Herz 11: 147—154

58. Widimsky J (1981) Pulmonale Hypertonie. Thieme, Stuttgart, New York

59. Widimsky J, Urbanová D, Ressl J (1975) Chronic pulmonary hypertension induced by intermittent high altitude exposure. Prog Resp Res 9: 121—125

60. Wikman-Coffelt J, Parmley WW, Mason DT (1979) The cardiac hypertrophy process. Circ Res 45: 697—707

61. Wollenberger A, Schulze WJ (1961) Mitochondrial alterations in the myocardium of dogs with aortic stenosis. J Biophys Biochem Cytol 10: 285—288

62. World Health Organization (1963) Chronic cor pulmonale. Report of an expert committee. Circulation 27: 594—615

63. Zak R (1984) Growth of the heart in health and disease. Raven Press, New York

Authors' address
Markward Schneider, Zentrum der Pathologie, Universitätsklinik, Theodor-Stern-Kai 7, D-6000 Frankfurt/M, FRG

Myocardial structure and left ventricular function in hypertrophic and dilative cardiomyopathy and aortic valve disease

B. Kunkel, M. Schneider

Medizinische Poliklinik der Universität Erlangen und Zentrum der Pathologie des Klinikums der Universität Frankfurt, F.R.G.

Introduction

Left ventricular biopsies from patients with latent cardiomyopathy, dilative cardio-myopathy and hypertrophic cardiomyopathy and aortic valve disease were analyzed in order to evaluate possible correlations between myocardial structure and left ventricular function.

Patients and Methods

Left ventricular biopsies from three patient groups with different myocardial diseases were investigated. Group 1 included 126 patients with mild (EF 50—60%, n = 21) and advanced (EF < 50%, n = 45) dilative cardiomyopathy and 66 patients with "latent" cardiomyopathy. The latter was defined as having normal ejection fraction under resting conditions and elevated left ventricular filling pressure at rest and/or under exercise according to the definition of Kuhn (4). Group 2 consisted of 18 patients with aortic valve disease. 13 had normal ejection fraction while in five patients left ventricular function was reduced (EF < 50%). Group 3 included 22 patients with hypertrophic cardiomyopathy.

During the diagnostic procedure, right and left heart catheterization, including selective coronary angiography and biplane ventriculography, and in aortic valve disease an additional aortography were performed. Two left ventricular biopsies were excised from the left ventricular posterior free wall. One was fixed in formalin and embedded in paraplast for light microscopy. The sections were routinely stained with hematoxylin-eosin and Goldner stains for microscopic analysis. The second specimen was fixed in 2.5% glutaraldehyde and embedded in Vestopal. Ultrathin sections were examined by electron microscope (Siemens Elmiscope 101).

The following parameters were measured by light microscopy:
1. Mean muscle cell diameter: 100 myocytes were measured at the site of the nucleus. The degree of hypertrophy was graded according to the mean cell diameter: Below 16 μm was considered normal, 16—20 μm as mild, 21—25 μm as moderate and over 25 μm as severe hypertrophy.

2. The volume density of the nuclei of the muscle cells (nuclear volume) and the interstitial fibrous tissue content were calculated according to the principles of Weibel (10). The sections were divided into adjacent areas, upon which a square grid, consisting of 121 points, was superimposed. For the calculation of the nuclear volume of the myocytes, usually 17 test areas per biopsy with a total number of 2057 points were analyzed. In a few cases the number of areas analyzed could be increased or had to be reduced according to the size of the specimen. For calculation of the interstitial fibrous tissue, ten test areas were analyzed.

On the electron microscopic level, the volume fractions of myofibrils, mitochondria and sarcoplasma were measured. Ten randomly sampled pictures were analyzed from each specimen at a magnification of 10 000. The pictures did not include parts of the nucleus or interstitium. The total number of test points analyzed in each specimen was 1210.

The volume fraction of a particular structure (connective tissue or nucleus or myofibrils or mitochondria) was calculated by the formula $Ps \times 100 : Pt$ = volume density of a given structure in percent. Ps = number of points falling on a particular structure. Pt = total number of test points. For analysis of the nuclear volume, Pt represented all points falling on myocytes. The results therefore indicate the percentage of nuclei per myocardial cells. For the calculation of the interstitial fibrous tissue, Pt represented all test points.

The morphological results were plotted against the ejection fraction derived from biplane left ventricular angiograms.

Results

The correlation between myocardial cell diameter and left ventricular function in latent and dilative cardiomyopathy is demonstrated in Fig. 1a. With deterioration of the left ventricular function, an increase in muscle cell diameter was observed. Although there was a considerable overlap, the result is statistically significant due to the large number of patients. As in dilative and latent cardiomyopathy, identical patterns were found in aortic valve disease (Fig. 1b). In cases with reduced left ventricular function, myocardial hypertrophy was more pronounced than in patients presenting with normal ejection fraction. Patients with hypertrophic cardiomyopathy present cell diameters similar to those of the patients with latent cardiomyopathy (Fig. 1c). In conclusion, myocardial hypertrophy is more pronounced in aortic valve disease and in advanced dilative cardiomyopathy than in hypertrophic or latent cardiomyopathy.

Figures 2a—c demonstrate the correlation between nuclear volume of the cardiocytes and ventricular function in the different groups. In group 1, the nuclear volume of the patients with normal ejection fraction (latent cardiomyopathy) ranged between 0.5% and 0.9% of the myocytes. The nuclear size increased significantly with reduction of the ventricular function. In patients with markedly depressed ejection fraction (dilative cardiomyopathy), the nuclear volume exceeded 1% of the total volume of the myocytes, up to 2% in a few cases (Fig. 2a). The result is statistically highly significant. Similar observations were made in patients with aortic valve disease. The nuclear volume increased significantly with reduction of the left ventricular ejection fraction. In aortic valve dis-

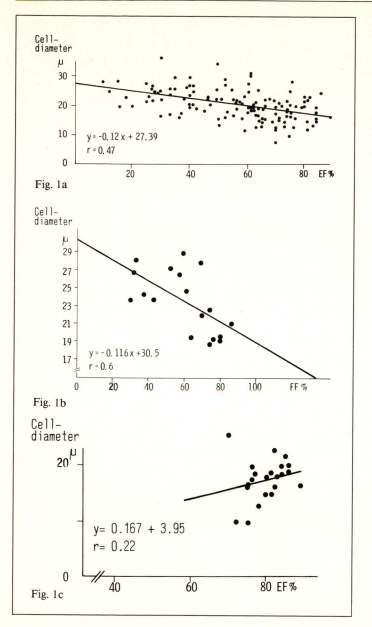

Fig. 1a—c: Correlation between the fiber diameter and ejection fraction in patients with (a) latent and dilative cardiomyopathy (b) aortic valve disease (c) hypertrophic cardiomyopathy. In (a) and (b) muscle cell diameter increases with decreasing ejection fraction.

Fig. 1a

Fig. 1b

Fig. 1c

ease, nuclear volumes were found to be higher in patients with both normal and impaired ventricular function (Fig. 2b).

Patients with HCM had normal ejection fractions. Normal nuclear volumes ($< 1\%$ of the myocytes volume) were found in nine patients, whereas 16 showed nuclear enlargement (Fig. 2c). This observation again demonstrates that there were several patients

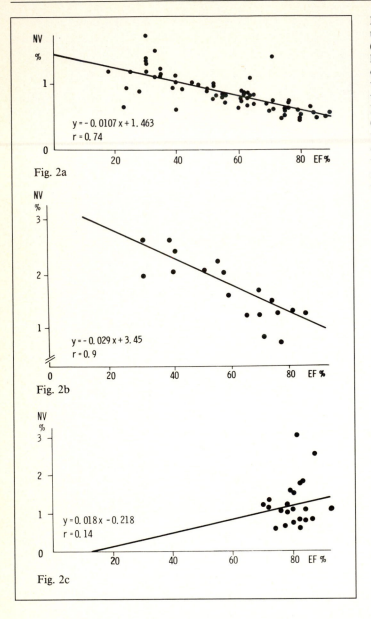

Fig. 2a

Fig. 2b

Fig. 2c

Fig. 2a—c: Nuclear volume of the myocytes (NV) in patients with (a) latent and dilative cardiomyopathy (b) aortic valve disease (c) hypertrophic cardiomyopathy. In (a) the nuclear volume (in % of the muscle volume) increases with depression of the ventricular function. In (c) normal enlarged nuclear volumes were observed.

without bioptical evidence of myocardial hypertrophy in the group with HCM, while others presented with severe forms of hypertrophy.

The mean mitochondrial density was 23% in the normal and hypertrophied myocardium, independent of the underlying disease (Table 1). In group I patients, the mitochondrial volume remained constant in normal and depressed left ventricular function.

Table 1. The volume density of the mitochondria, which remains nearly constant in cases with normal and depressed ventricular function independent from the underlying disease.

Mitochondrial Volume	EF > 65%	EF 50—64%	EF > 50%
Latent and dilative cardiomyopathies	23.3 ± 3.7	23.2 ± 6.4	23.3 ± 6.5
Aortic valve disease	19.7 ± 7.6	24.0 ± 2.9	23.6 ± 2.4
Hypertrophic cardiomyopathy	24.5 ± 5.5	—	—

In aortic valve disease, the mitochondrial volume was found to be nonsignificantly increased in patients with mild reduction of ventricular function and returned to normal volume with further impairment of the ventricle. Patients with hypertrophic cardiomyopathy presented with similar volume fractions of mitochondria as in the other diseases. The observation of nearly constant volume fractions of mitochondria in different stages of hypertrophy and ventricular function indicates an augmentation of mitochondrial mass during the course of hypertrophy. Duplication of myocardial mass leads to a duplication of the mitochondrial mass. While the volume density of mitochondria remained constant during the various stages of hypertrophy, abnormally small and irregularly shaped mitochondria were constantly found in patients with reduced left ventricular function.

The volume density of myofibrils of the normal myocardium was 54% in our study. The volume density of the myofibrils continuously decreased with worsening of left ventricular function. Patients with latent cardiomyopathy showed a normal or slightly decreased content of myofibrils (Fig. 3a). In patients with dilative cardiomyopathy and markedly reduced ejection fraction, low volume densities of myofibrils were observed. Extreme loss of myofibrils (20—30%) was found in individual cases. Similar values were obtained from patients with aortic valve disease (Fig. 3b).

Again the myofibrillar volume decreased from 50% in conditions with normal ejection fraction, to less than 40% in cases with reduced left ventricular function. In HCM patients, normal myofibrillar volumes were observed in one third of the patients, while others presented with mild to moderate reduction of the myofibrils (Fig. 3c). A significant reduction of the contractile elements, as usually seen in dilative cardiomyopathy or aortic valve disease with impaired left ventricular function, was not observed in HCM. The reduction of the myofibrillar volume is compensated by an increase in the portion of the sarcoplasm and certain structures such as t-system, sarcoplasmic reticulum and glycogen, which were not separately quantified in this study. The sarcoplasm increased from 30% in normal ventricular function to 40—50% in patients with severely reduced ejection fraction.

Discussion

Our results demonstrate that worsening of left ventricular function is associated with increasing myocardial hypertrophy. This could be shown by various independent parameters such as cell width and nuclear volume. Increasing cell diameters associated with

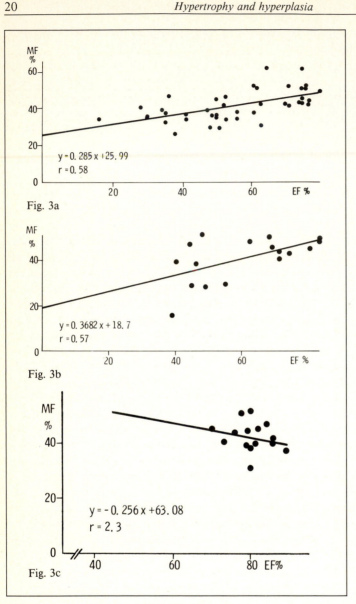

Fig. 3a

Fig. 3b

Fig. 3c

Fig. 3a—c: Volume density of the myofibrils in (a) latent and dilative cardiomyopathy and (b) aortic valve disease and (c) hypertrophic cardiomyopathy. In (a) and (b) the volume of myofibrils decreased with worsening of the left ventricular function. In (c) normal or moderately decreased myofibrillar volumes were found.

depressed left ventricular function have also been reported in dilative cardiomyopathies, in left ventricular biopsies by Schwarz (7), and by Frenzel (3) in right ventricular biopsies. Unverferth (9) has shown an increasing nuclear area associated with increasing hypertrophy in biopsies from various heart diseases.

On the ultrastructural level, increasing hypertrophy and worsening of the left ventricular function was associated with a decreasing volume density of myofibrils. This has also been observed for dilative cardiomyopathies, including latent cardiomyopathy, by

Schwarz (7) and in our own laboratories (5). Schwarz and Schaper (8) reported identical patterns in aortic valve disease. As can be expected from these findings, it has also been demonstrated that the extent of loss of myofibrils has prognostic implications in DCM (2).

The mitochondrial density remained constant during all stages of myocardial hypertrophy. This was also seen in various degrees of hypertrophy in aortic valve disease (8). On the other hand, small and abnormally shaped mitochondrial populations in the myocardium from hypertrophied hearts were constantly observed. The functional capacity of these "abnormal" mitochondria has not been investigated so far. Considering that many biochemical reactions are related to surface membranes, the changes of the mitochondrial size and shape may be regarded as a compensatory mechanism rather than as sign of degeneration.

From a qualitative point of view, no difference could be found between dilative cardiomyopathy and aortic valve disease; HCM cannot reliably be diagnosed from the small biopsy samples. Different pathogenetic myocardial injuries (mechanical overload, idiopathic, toxic, viral and others) seem to induce an unique response of the myocardium leading to myocardial hypertrophy and interstitial fibrosis of various degrees. The various structural changes of the myocardium are not confined to a peculiar disease. The stage of hypertrophy is obviously correlated with ventricular function. Similar results were obtained by Unverferth (9) who also could not find principle difference in biopsies from patients with valvular, idiopathic and alcohol-induced myocardial failure. In doxorubicin-induced cardiomyopathies, however, little or no hypertrophy was observed, while the amount of fibrosis was markedly increased. Doxorubicin intercalates DNA and interferes with protein production. Thus hypertrophy-responsive myocardial injury is prevented.

In our series, 24% of the patients with hypertrophic cardiomyopathy had surprisingly no evidence of myocardial hypertrophy in biopsy specimens. The fiber diameters in HCM were comparable to those in the patients with latent cardiomyopathy, while myocardial hypertrophy was found more pronounced in DCM and aortic valve disease. This might be due to the fact that hypertrophy is irregularly distributed in the heart of patients with hypertrophic cardiomyopathy. In most cases, the basal intraventricular septum is more thickened than the free posterior wall, but the anterolateral and inferior wall and the apical septal region and other areas can also be involved. From echocardiography four different types of distribution of myocardial hypertrophy have been elaborated by Maron (6). It is unknown, however, whether these differences in wall thickness are associated with different fiber diameters in these areas. In post mortem studies and analysis of operatively-excised specimens from the ventricular septum, no excessive hypertrophy have been observed in these regions (see chapter by Frenzel, this volume, pp 14—19). Within a definite area, no major variability of the mean cell diameters occur, according to our own experience. On the other hand, similar heart weights, which means similar degrees of hypertrophy, have been found in patients with hypertrophic cardiomyopathy and dilative cardiomyopathy. Thus it may be speculated that hyperplasia might play an important role in the hypertrophic cardiomyopathies.

In most patients with dilative cardiomyopathy and aortic valve disease with reduced ventricular function, burnt-out late stage hypertrophy of the myocardium can easily be recognized from the biopsy. In HCM, however, normal myofibrillar volumes or mild reduction of the contractile elements is observed comparable to the findings in latent cardiomyopathy. The bioptical findings in HCM in this respect are compatible with the compensated stage of hypertrophy, according to Meerson's hypothesis.

Summary: Left ventricular biopsies from 126 patients with advanced (EF < 50%, n = 45) and mild (EF 50—60%, n = 21) and latent cardiomyopathy (EF > 60%, n = 60) and 18 additional patients with aortic valve disease and 22 cases with hypertrophic cardiomyopathy were analyzed to define possible correlations between myocardial structure and function.

Deterioration of ventricular function was combined with increasing muscle cell diameters (r = 0.47) and increasing nuclear size of the myocytes (r = 0.74) in latent and dilative cardiomyopathies and in patients with aortic valve disease (cell diameter, r = 0.6; nuclear size, r = 0.9). Patients with HCM showed a wide range of cell diameter and nuclear size. 24% of the latter patients had no bioptic evidence of myocardial hypertrophy.

The mitochondrial volume of the myocytes was 23% in the normal and hypertrophied myocardium independent of the kind of disease and ventricular function.

The volume fraction of the myofibrils continuously decreased with worsening of the left ventricular function in patients with latent and dilative cardiomyopathy (from 45 ± 6.9 to 37.6 ± 6.3%) and aortic valve disease (from 46.2 ± 3.4 to 27.9 ± 9.3%). Patients with hypertrophic cardiomyopathy presented with normal or slightly decreased values of myofibrils consistent with normal ventricular function (42.5 ± 5.0). The data demonstrate that the degree of myocardial hypertrophy and certain ultrastructural findings are inversely correlated with left ventricular function.

References

1. Ferrans VJ, Massumi RA, Shugoll GJ, Ali N, Roberts WD (1973) Ultrastructural studies of myocardial biopsies in 45 patients with obstructive or congestive cardiomyopathy 231—272. In: Bajusz E, Rona S, Brink AJ (eds) Recent advances in cardiac structure and metabolism. Cardiomyopathies. University Press, Baltimore
2. Figulla HR, Rahlf F, Nieger M, Luig H, Kreuzer H (1985) Spontaneous hemodynamic improvement or stabilization and associated biopsy findings in patients with congestive cardiomyopathy. Circulation 71: 1095—1104
3. Frenzel H, Kasper M, Kuhn H, Lösse B, Reifschneider G, Hort W (1985) Licht und elektronenmikroskopische Befunde in Früh- und Spätstadien der Herzinsuffizienz. Untersuchungen an Endomyokardbiopsien von Patienten mit latenter (LCM) und dilatativer (DCM) Kardiomyopathie. Z Kardiol 74: 135—143
4. Kuhn H, Knieriem HJ, Lösse B, Breithard G, Köhler E, Seipel L, Loogen F (1978) Prognosis and possible presymptomatic manifestations of congestive cardiomyopathy. Postgrad Med J 54: 451—459
5. Kunkel B, Schneider M, Kober G, Bußmann WD, Hopf R, Kaltenbach M (1982) Die Morphologie der Myokardbiopsie und die klinische Bedeutung. Z Kardiol 71: 787—794
6. Maron B, Gottdiener JS, Epstein E (1982) Echocardiographic identification of patterns of left ventricular hypertrophy in hypertrophic cardiomyopathy. In: Kaltenbach M, Eptein SE (eds) Hypertrophic Cardiomyopathy — the therapeutic role of calcium antagonists. Springer Verlag, Berlin—Heidelberg—New York, pp 18—37

7. Schwarz F, Mall G, Zebe H, Blickle J, Derks H, Manthey J, Kübler W, Quantitative, morphologic findings of the myocardium in idiopathic dilated cardiomyopathy. Am J Cardiol 51: 501
8. Schwarz F, Schaper J, Kitstein D, Flameng W, Walter P, Schaper W (1981) Reduced volume fraction of myofibrils in myocardium of patients with decompensated pressure overload. Circulation 63: 1299—1304
9. Unverferth EV, Fetters JK, Unverferth BJ, Leier CV, Magorien RD, Arn AR, Baker PB (1983) Human myocardial histologic characteristics in congestive heart failure. Circulation 68: 1194—1200
10. Weibel E, Kistler GS, Scherle WF (1966) Practical stereological methods for morphometric cytology. J Cell Biol 30: 23—38

Authors' address:

Prof. B. Kunkel, Medizinische Poliklinik der Universität Erlangen, Östliche Stadtmauerstraße 29, 8520 Erlangen, F.R.G.

Evidence for muscle fiber hyperplasia in the septum of patients with hypertrophic obstructive cardiomyopathy (HOCM). Quantitative examination of endomyocardial biopsies (EMCB) and myectomy specimens.

H. Frenzel[1], B. Schwartzkopff[2], P. Reinecke[1], K. Kamino[1], and B. Lösse[2]

[1] Institute of Pathology and [2]Medical Hospital (Department of Cardiology, Pneumology and Angiology) University of Düsseldorf, F.R.G.

Introduction

In hypertrophic cardiomyopathy, muscle mass is increased for no apparent reason (6). A familial occurrence in 20% of the cases indicates a genetic disposition. The most important feature of HOCM is a thickening of the septum disproportionate to the hypertrophied free left ventricular wall, whereas the cavity remains normal or is narrowed (14, 18). The catenoid-shaped septum bulges into the outflow tract of the left ventricle and results in its systolic obstruction (8). This obstruction is mainly located in the subaortic region, rarely in the middle or apical parts of the left ventricle (9). The disorganization of muscle fibers is the second hallmark of HOCM. Fiber disarray can be observed in various heart diseases as well as in normal hearts (1, 2, 17, 20), but when its distribution is diffuse (4) and quantitatively substantial (11, 12) it is quite specific to hypertrophic cardiomyopathy.

To a great extent, the structural basis of the asymmetric thickening of the septum is not yet known. It has been shown that the extent of fiber disarray does not correlate with the thickness of the septum (11). A massive local hypertrophy of the fiber or a local hyperplasia of muscle cells are under discussion as a possible morphologic substrate. Investigation of the hearts of deceased patients with HOCM has indicated an increase in muscle fiber layers in the asymmetrically thickened septum (5).

In the present study, quantitative evaluation of endomyocardial biopsies (EMCB) from the right side of the septum and myectomy specimens from the left side ascertained a combination of hypertrophy and hyperplasia of myocytes in the thickened septum of hearts with HOCM.

Materials and Methods

Endomyocardial biopsies and myectomy specimens from three groups of patients were evaluated quantitatively. The data of these patients are listed in Table 1.

1st group: seven patients with a heart of normal shape and normal size (N). Hemodynamic parameters at rest were within normal limits. Coronary arteriograms showed

Table 1. Mean values and standard deviation of clinical data relating to patients with hearts of normal shape (N), HOCM patients with EMCBs from the right side of the septum (HOCM 1), and HOCM patients with EMCBs from the right side of the septum and myectomy specimens from the left side (HOCM 2).

Patients	N	HOCM 1	HOCM 2
Number of patients	7	7	7
Male / female	1/6	6/1	4/3
Age (years)	39.8±12.1	45.1± 7	44.1±13.3
Left ventricular gradient at rest (mm Hg)	–	15.7± 6.1	38.8±36
Blood pressure (mm Hg) systolic	118 ± 7.5	132.8±31	112.5±19
diastolic	73 ±10	84.2±10.9	70 ±11.4
septal thickness (mm)	9.7± 1.2	18.7± 2.9	24.3± 6.3

Brackets indicate that the difference between the two values is significant ($p \leq 0.05$)

normal findings in all patients. On account of atypical angina pectoris, endomyocardial biopsies were performed to exclude myocarditis, small vessel disease or storage disease.

2nd group: seven consecutively examined patients with HOCM (HOCM 1).

3rd group: seven patients with HOCM, of whom EMCBs from the right side of the septum (HOCM 2-B) as well as myectomy specimens from the left side of the septum (HOCM 2-M) were available.

At least four biopsy samples from different parts of the right side of the septum were obtained from each patient, using an Olympus bioptome. The thickness of the septum in each patient was determined by echocardiography. In addition, the pressure gradient at rest between the left ventricular apex and the subaortic region was determined by catheterization of the left heart. Hyperplasia of the muscle fibers, as a possible cause of septal thickening, was studied by comparing group N with HOCM 1, HOCM 2-B and HOCM 2-M. The correlation between the thickness of the muscle fibers and that of the septum in HOCM patients was determined for HOCM 1 and HOCM 2-B.

Preparation of the tissue

The EMCB samples were immediately fixed in 2.5% cacodylate-buffered glutaraldehyde (360—380 mosmol/l), dehydrated and embedded in paraffin. The myectomy specimens were fixed in 4% formalin, dehydrated and embedded in paraffin. Hematoxylin-eosin and elastica van Gieson staining were performed on 5 μm-thick paraffin sections of EMCB and myectomy specimens.

Morphometry

At a magnification of × 1250, 100 longitudinally cut muscle fibers were measured to determine their width in the area of the nucleus. At the same magnification, the volume density of the interstitium and fibrous tissue was measured in paraffin sections with elastica van Gieson staining, using the point-counting method with a 100-point lattice. The interstitium was defined as the entire space between the myocytes. Fibrous tissue was defined as all structures stained reddish by the elastica van Gieson staining. At a magnification of × 1250, the total number of muscle fiber nuclei and the percentage of muscle fibers with two nuclei within the 100-point lattice were ascertained in respect of 5 μm-thick paraffin sections stained with hematoxylin-eosin. At ten points evenly distributed over the whole length of the sectioned endocardium, the thickness of the endocardium was measured at a magnification of × 160 (10).

Statistics

The mean and standard deviation for each parameter were calculated from the repeated measurements performed on the biopsy or myectomy specimens from each patient. The mean values for each different group were calculated from the mean values of each patient within the group concerned. To test the statistical significance of the differences in values relating to EMCBs in the three different groups of patients, an analysis of variance was carried out using Link and Wallace's test at $p \leq 0.05$. With regard to those patients from whom both EMCB and myectomy specimens were available, a paired t-test at $p \leq 0.05$ was carried out to investigate the statistical significance of differences in values between the right side of the septum and the left side.

Results

The results relating to the three groups of patients are given in Table 2. In comparison with hearts of normal shape (group N), the thickness of the septum in HOCM 1 had doubled and that in HOCM 2 had increased 2.5 times. The differences between the three groups are statistically significant.

The thickness of the muscle fibers in the EMCBs from hearts of normal shape (N) does not differ significantly from that in the hearts of HOCM 1 patients. However, the muscle fibers in the EMCBs of HOCM 2-B patients are significantly thicker than in the other two groups of patients. A significant difference exists in HOCM 2 patients with regard to the thickness of the muscle fibers in the EMCBs from the right side of the septum in comparison with that found in myectomy specimens from the left side of the septum. The thickness of the septum correlates significantly with the thickness of the muscle fibers measured in the EMCBs of HOCM 1 and HOCM 2 patients ($r = 0.78$) (Fig. 1).

Two nuclei were found in 7% of the muscle cells in the EMCBs obtained from hearts of normal shape (N). The percentage of muscle cells with two nuclei continuously increases in line with the growth in the thickness of the muscle fibers in hearts with HOCM. The differences between the groups are significant, except between HOCM 1 and hearts of normal shape (N).

In HOCM 1 the volume fraction of the interstitium increases by about 29% and in HOCM 2-B by about 40% in comparison with hearts of normal shape (N). The difference between the volume density of the interstitium in HOCM 1 and that in HOCM 2-B is not significant; however, there is a significant difference between the volume density measured in EMCBs and that in myectomy specimens from HOCM 2 patients. This

Table 2. Summary of morphometric data (mean values and standard deviation) relating to hearts of normal shape (N), HOCM hearts with EMCBs from the right side of the septum (HOCM 1), and HOCM hearts with EMCBs from the right side of the septum (HOCM 2-B) and myectomy specimens from the left side (HOCM 2-M).

	N	HOCM 1	HOCM 2 Biopsy (B)	Myectomy (M)
Number of patients	7	7	7	7
Septal thickness (mm)	9.7 ± 1.2	18.7 ± 2.9	24.3 ± 6.3	
Endocardial thickness (μm)	27.45±22.90	23.70± 16.67	10.75± 4.20	405.8±498
Muscle fiber thickness (μm)	11.41± 0.63	11.98± 1.80	16.56± 1.91	19.55± 1.80
Volume density interstitium (%)	16.14± 2.50	20.77± 0.78	22.60± 2.80	37.80± 7.90
Volume density fibrous tissue (%)	1.97± 0.55	2.60± 0.53	2.60± 1.25	20.20± 7.90
Myocytes with two nuclei (%)	7.08± 3.58	11.52± 4.93	17.82± 2.59	21.40± 5.73
Estimated number of septal muscle fiber layers	715 ±93	1242 ±149	1119 ±177	810 ±232

Brackets indicate that the difference between two values is significant ($p \leq 0.05$)

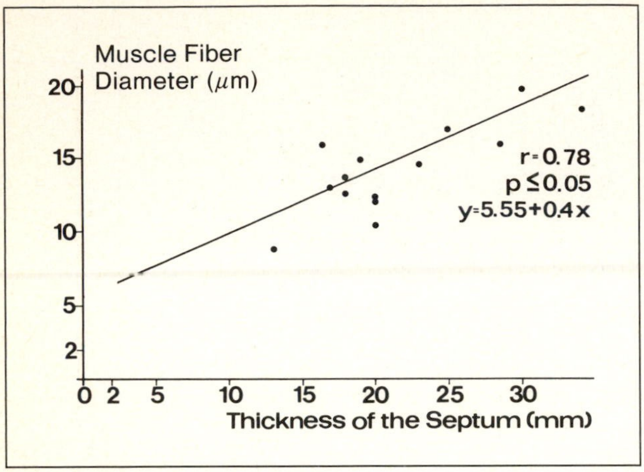

Fig. 1. Correlation between the echocardiographically determined thickness of the septum and the thickness of the muscle fibers measured in EMCBs from the right side of the septum of HOCM patients. (Significance at $p \leq 0.05$).

striking disparity between the volume density of the interstitium on the right side of the septum and that on the left side is caused by a significantly increased quantity of fibrous tissue in the myectomy specimens. The width of the endocardium varies greatly; the difference between this value in the EMCBs (HOCM 2-B) and that in the myectomy specimens (HOCM 2-M) is significant.

The number of septal muscle fibers can be calculated if the tickness of the septum and the endocardium, the volume density of the interstitium and the thickness of the muscle fibers are known, and if the muscle fibers of the septum do not run in a transverse direction:

Number of septal muscle fiber layers:

$$\frac{\text{Thickness of septum} - \text{Thickness of endocardium} - \text{Volume density of interstitium}}{\text{Thickness of muscle fibers}}$$

If the values of the EMCBs (HOCM 1 and HOCM 2-B) from the right side of the septum are assumed for the whole septum, the number of septal muscle fiber layers appears to increase by about 74% in HOCM 1 and by about 57% in HOCM 2. However, calculation on the basis of the values of the myectomy specimens from HOCM 2 patients (HOCM 2-M) indicates a lower number of muscle fiber layers in comparison with HOCM 2-B (Fig. 2).

Discussion

The thickness of the septum is dependent upon the thickness of the muscle fibers, the number of muscle fiber layers, the width of the interstitium and the thickness of the endocardium. The object of this study was to estimate, on the basis of EMCBs and myectomy specimens, the significance of these variables with regard to the asymmetric thickening of the septum in the hearts of patients with HOCM.

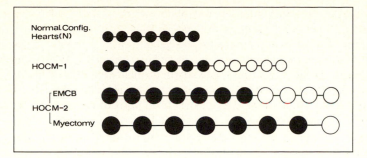

Fig. 2. Schematic diagram of the septum in seven patients with hearts of normal shape (N), in seven HOCM patients with EMCBs from the right side of the septum (HOCM 1), and in seven HOCM patients with EMCBs from the right side of the septum and myectomy specimens from the left side (HOCM 2). The continuous line indicates the thickness of the septum, excluding the endocardium. The septum is significantly thicker in HOCM hearts than in hearts of normal shape. One black or white circle corresponds to 100 muscle fibers; the distance between the circles illustrates the volume density of the interstitium. (●) indicates that portion of the septum for which calculations were made on the basis of the observed muscle fiber thickness, the volume density of the interstitium in HOCM, and the estimated number of transseptal muscle fiber layers in hearts of normal shape. (○) indicates the numerical increase in muscle fibers (hyperplasia) which is required to fill the echocardiographically determined thickness of the septum. For HOCM patients with EMCBs and myectomy specimens (HOCM 2) the calculated results shown relate to measurements on EMCBs (above) and myectomy specimens (below).

In the hearts of HOCM patients, the echocardiographically determined thickness of the septum was twice (respectively, 2.5 times) as great as that found in hearts of normal shape. Because the increased volume density of the interstitial space is not an adequate explanation for the significantly greater width of the septum in HOCM patients, a significant role in the asymmetric thickening of the septum in HOCM can be attributed to an increase in the thickness or number of the myocytes. In the septum of normally configurated hearts, no regional difference of muscle fiber thickness could be found (19).

In EMCBs from the right septum of patients with hearts of normal shape (N) and in those from consecutively investigated patients with HOCM upon whom no myectomy was performed (HOCM 1), we found muscle fibers of approximately equal thickness in spite of a doubling of the septal thickness in the patients with HOCM. In principle, this finding allows two interpretations: firstly, the region of the ventricular septum surveyed in the biopsy may be excluded from the process of an etiologically unclarified hypertrophy, whilst a substantial thickening of the muscle fibers in the middle and left portion of the septum would have to be postulated, as these were not surveyed in the biopsy. Likewise an unsynchronous thickening of the fibers may be of significance, with a disease-specific hypertrophy initially in the middle and left portions of the septum, and with a thickening of the muscle fibers of the right septum possibly occurring only at a later phase of the disease. As could be shown by calculations made on the data of the myectomy specimens, the degree of hypertrophy of the left and middle part of the septum is not sufficient to explain the increased septal thickness.

The second, more probable explanation, could be an increment of the fibers in the septa of HOCM hearts as an etiologically unclarified but disease-specific change.

If the morphometric data of the EMCBs from the right septum were valid for the entire breadth of the septum, then an increase in fibers by 74% for the group of patients with HOCM 1 and 57% for the group of patients with HOCM 2, in comparison with the non-

HOCM patients (N), would be necessary in order to explain the increases of 100% and 150%, respectively in the thickness of the septum in these HOCM patients. If one takes the data from the myectomy specimens as the basis for the calculation of the muscle fiber layers, then an increase of 15% in the muscle cells would suffice, especially on account of the greater volume density of the interstitium, to explain a thickening of the septum by 150% in comparison with that in hearts of normal shape. This calculation makes it clear that here, too, hypertrophy alone cannot be the structural basis of the asymmetric thickening of the septum in hearts with HOCM. As the EMCBs cover a subendocardial area of about 1 mm in size and the myectomy data relate to a portion of the septum of up to 1.5 cm wide, the degree of hyperplasia in our HOCM patients can be estimated as being about 30—40%. The calculations concerned with the asymmetrical septal thickening in HOCM are made on the precondition of a harmonious growth of the myocytes in their length and thickness. A disproportionately large increase in myocytic length could induce a rearrangement of myocytes in the septum which would explain a septal thickening even without an increment in myocytes.

It is remarkable that the calculated degree of hyperplasia in all HOCM patients is of an approximately equal order of magnitude. Measurements on the hearts of autopsied patients with HOCM revealed an increase of barely 30% in the number of muscle fibers in the septum, compared with that in normal hearts (5).

The factors that induce hyperplasia of myocytes in the septa of HOCM hearts are not yet known. In the context of normal cardiac development in humans, the capability of mitosis is restricted to the intrauterine phase and a brief postnatal period. But various findings indicate that the final number of muscle cells may be increased by physiological and pathological stimuli which affect the heart, not only during this period, but also during adulthood (16). According to a hypothesis put forward by Ferrans and Rodriguez (3), hyperplasia of myocytes in the asymmetrically thickened septa might be determined by a hypercontractile state during the developmental phase before birth.

Our investigation revealed significant differences concerning the quantitative myocardial structure in the right and left side of the septum in HOCM hearts. In the septum of normally shaped hearts, without pathological changes, no regional differences, or only those of a small degree, have been described (7, 19). However, comparison of the EMCBs and myectomy specimens from our group of HOCM 2 patients revealed that on the left side of the septum, the muscle fibers were 17% thicker, the proportion of binucleate muscle cells was higher, and the volume density of the interstitium was about 70% greater. These regional differences may be secondary changes which develop only in the course of a HOCM and therefore do not rank among the characteristic, but etiologically unclarified symptoms of HOCM. The significant thickening of the septum is accompanied by a disproportionately large increase in collagenous fibers. This focally accentuated fibrosis possibly originates as a replacement fibrosis after a loss of muscle cells. A disseminated loss of muscle cells during the advanced stage of a HOCM could be, on the one hand, the consequence of degeneration under severe hypertrophy or, on the other hand, the result of a local disturbance of the circulation. Qualitatively, in the myectomy specimens we have not infrequently observed small arteries with a stenosing fibro-elastosis of the intima, which have been described and quantified in HOCM hearts by Maron et al. (14). A disseminated loss of myocytes would, in turn, cause a compensatory hypertrophy of the remaining muscle fibers.

Our investigations furthermore revealed a clear correlation between the thickness of the muscle fibers measured in the EMCBs and the thickness of the septum in hearts with HOCM. It thus follows that individual differences in the thickness of the septum in HOCM patients are most probably an expression of a diverse degree of hypertrophy of the muscle fibers, which may intensify over the course of the disease. It was shown by echocardiographic follow-up that a notable thickening of a formerly normal septum can develop in young persons and adults (13). Early or less severely pronounced forms of HOCM may therefore be characterized predominantly by hyperplasia in the septum with or without slight hypertrophy (HOCM 1 patients), with severe and advanced forms of the disease being characterized by hyperplasia and a more severe degree of hypertrophy (HOCM 2 patients).

In conclusion, our study has shown a combination of hyperplasia and hypertrophy of myocytes as the structural basis for the asymmetric thickening of the septum in the hearts of patients with HOCM. Differences in the septal thickness of HOCM hearts are mainly attributable to different degrees of hypertrophy. The increase in the volume density of the interstitium in the left part of the septum, in conjunction with a disproportionately large increment of collagenous fibers, points to a regional loss of myocytes with consequent replacement fibrosis.

Summary: Asymmetric thickening of the septum is one of the hallmarks of hypertrophic obstructive cardiomyopathy (HOCM). Endomyocardial biopsies (EMCB) from the right side of the septum and myectomy specimens from its left part were morphometrically investigated to determine the size of septal myocytes, as well as the volume density of the interstitium and fibrous tissue, and to estimate the number of transseptal muscle fiber layers.

EMCBs of seven patients with normally shaped hearts, taken as controls (N), EMCBs of seven consecutively examined patients with HOCM (HOCM 1), and of seven HOCM patients with additionally available myectomy specimens (HOCM 2) were evaluated. In myectomy specimens muscle fiber thickness and volume density of the interstitium and fibrous tissue were significantly increased, as compared with the findings in the EMCBs. The echocardiographically determined septal thickness was increased by 93% in HOCM 1 and by 150% in HOCM 2 compared with controls; however, the increase in muscle fiber thickness and volume density of the interstitium did not give a sufficient explanation for the increased septal thickness in both groups of HOCM. Based on EMCB data, the estimated number of septal muscle fiber layers was 715 ± 93 in group N, 1242 ± 149 in HOCM 1, and 1119 ± 177 in HOCM 2, while 810 ± 232 layers were estimated according to the findings from myectomy specimens. Taking into account that EMCB represent only 1 mm of septal thickness, and myectomy specimens up to 15 mm, an increase in the septal muscle cell layers of about 30% can be estimated in HOCM hearts. The significant correlation between muscle fiber thickness, derived from EMCB, and septal thickness, indicates that the extent of muscle cell hypertrophy is the main cause of variant septal thickness in patients with HOCM. It is concluded that a combination of hyperplasia and hypertrophy of muscle fibers is the morphologic basis of asymmetric septal thickening in HOCM hearts.

References

1. Becker AE, Caruso G (1982) Myocardial disarray: A critical review. Br Heart J 47: 527—538
2. Bulkley BH, Weisfeldt M, Hutchins GM (1977) Asymmetric septal hypertrophy and myocardial fiber disarray: features of normal developing and malformed hearts. Circulation 56: 296—298
3. Ferrans VJ, Rodriguez ER (1983) Specifity of light and electron microscopic feature of hypertrophic obstructive and nonobstructive cardiomyopathy. Qualitative, quantitative and etiologic aspects Eur Heart J 4, Suppl 7: 2—22
4. Fujiwara H, Hoshino T, Fujiwara T, Kawai C, Hamashima Y (1982) Classification and distribution of myocardial fascicle and fiber disarray in 14 hearts with hypertrophic cardiomyopathy in 25 μ thick sections. Jpn Circ J 46: 225—234
5. Fujiwara H, Hoshino T, Yamana K, Fujiwara T, Furuta M, Hamashima Y, Kawai C (1983) Number and size of myocytes and amount of interstitial space in the ventricular septum and in the left ventricular free wall in hypertrophic cardiomyopathy. Am J Cardiol 52: 818—823
6. Goodwin JF (1970) Congestive and hypertrophic cardiomyopathies. A decade of study. Lancet i: 731—739
7. Hoshino T, Fujiwara H, Kawai C, Hamashima Y (1983) Myocardial fiber diameter and regional distribution in the ventricular wall of normal adult hearts, hypertensive hearts and hearts with hypertrophic cardiomyopathy. Circulation 67: 1109—1116
8. Hutchins GM, Bulkley BH (1978) Catenoid shape of the intervenricular septum: possible cause of idiopathic hypertrophic subaortic stenosis. Circulation 58: 392—397
9. Kuhn H, Mercier J, Köhler E, Frenzel H, Hort W, Loogen F (1983) Differential diagnosis of hypertrophic cardiomyopathies: typical (subaortic) hypertrophic obstructive cardiomyopathy, atypical (mid-ventricular) hypertrophic obstructive cardiomyopathy and hypertrophic non-obstructive cardiomyopathy. Eur Heart J 4, Suppl F: 93—104
10. Loud AV, Anversa P (1984) Biology of disease. Morphometric analysis of biologic process. Lab Invest 50: 250—261
11. Maron BJ, Roberts WC (1979) Quantitative analysis of cardiac muscle cell disorganization in the ventricular septum of patients with hypertrophic cardiomyopathy. Circulation 59: 689—706
12. Maron BJ, Epstein SE (1980) Hypertrophic cardiomyopathy: Recent observations regarding the specifity of three hallmarks of the disease: asymmetric septal hypertrophy, septal disorganization and systolic anterior motion of the anterior mitral leaflet. Am J Cardiol 45: 141—154
13. Maron BJ, Spirito P, Wesley Y, Arce J (1986) Development and progression of left ventricular hypertrophy in children with hypertrophic cardiomyopathy. N Engl J Med 315: 610—614
14. Maron BJ, Wolfson JK, Epstein SE, Roberts WC (1986) Intramural ("small vessel") coronary artery disease in hypertrophic cardiomyopathy. J Am Coll Cardiol 8: 545—547
15. Olsen EGJ (1980) The pathology of idiopathic hypertrophic subaortic stenosis (hypertrophic cardiomyopathy). A critical review. Am Heart J 100: 553—562
16. Rakusan K (1984) Cardiac growth, maturation, and aging. In: Zak R (ed) Growth of the Heart in Health and Disease, Raven Press, New York, pp 131—164
17. Roberts WC, Ferrans VJ (1975) The pathologic anatomy of the cardiomyopathies (idiopathic dilated and hypertrophic types, infiltrative types and endomyocardial disease with and without eosinophilia). Human Pathol 6: 287—342
18. Teare D (1958) Asymmetrical hypertrophy of the heart in young adults. Br Heart J 20: 1—8
19. Unverferth DV, Baker PB, Swift SE, Chaffee R, Fetters IK, Uretsky BF, Thompson ME, Leier CV (1986) Extent of myocardial fibrosis and cellular hypertrophy in dilated cardiomyopathy. Am J Cardiol 57: 816—820
20. Van der Bel-Kahn J (1977) Muscle fiber disarray in common heart disease. Am J Cardiol 40: 355—364

Authors' address:
Prof. Dr. Hartmut Frenzel, Institute of Pathology, University of Düsseldorf, Moorenstr. 5, 4000 Düsseldorf, F.R.G.

Evidence of myocyte hyperplasia in hypertrophic cardiomyopathy and other disorders with myocardial hypertrophy?

V. J. Ferrans, and E. R. Rodríguez

Ultrastructure Section, Pathology Branch, National Heart, Lung and Blood Institute, National Institutes of Health, Bethesda, Maryland, U.S.A.

The mechanisms that mediate the increase in cardiac mass which occurs in patients with hypertrophic cardiomyopathy remain uncertain. The disease is characterized microscopically by an increase in the size of the myocytes, which often show a bizarre type of cellular and intracellular disarray, and by an increase in the amount of interstitial fibrous connective tissue (35). It is considered that the greatest contribution to the increased cardiac mass is made by the myocytes. Nevertheless, it is not clear at the present time whether this is mediated not only by an increase in the size of the cells (hypertrophy) but also by an increase in the number of cells (hyperplasia) or by a combination of these two factors. This question is particularly relevant to the process of asymmetric hypertrophy that affects the ventricular septum in hypertrophic cardiomyopathy. Before considering this question in detail, it is convenient to review our knowledge of the mechanisms involved in hypertrophy and hyperplasia of cardiac myocytes.

The increase in cardiac mass that occurs during embryonic development is due to hyperplasia and is mediated by mitotic division of the cardiac myocytes. Under normal circumstances, this mitotic activity ceases 2 to 3 weeks after birth, after which time hypertrophy becomes the mechanism by which further increases in cardiac mass are attained (5, 7, 8, 17, 34, 42). Nevertheless, evidence has been presented to show that under certain conditions DNA synthesis and cellular division can occur in adult myocytes. This evidence is reviewed in detail below. The reasons for the cessation of mitotic activity in cardiac myocytes of newborn humans and animals are not clear. It has been suggested that this change in growth pattern may be brought about by an increase in the functional demands placed on the developing heart. The activity of adenylate cyclase and the concentration of cyclic AMP increase progressively during cardiac development, and it has been demonstrated that agents that increase the intracellular concentrations of cyclic AMP accelerate the normal events that occur as the cardiac myocytes undergo terminal differentiation (8, 9). These events are temporally correlated with the anatomical and physiological development of the adrenergic nerves of the heart. Thus, it has been hypothesized that the physiological signal for the heart to change its growth pattern from hyperplasia to hypertrophy is functional adrenergic innervation, with norepinephrine and cyclic AMP serving as chemical mediators (8, 9).

The control of the cell cycle and cell division is thought to reside in the factors that control initiation and regulate the rate of DNA synthesis. The adrenergic nervous system may influence DNA synthesis and, hence, cell proliferation, by a programmed and selective repression in the genes coding for the enzymes and proteins needed for DNA replication (8, 9). The activities of two of these enzymes, DNA polymerase α and thymidine kinase, disappear from cardiac myocytes as these cells lose their ability to replicate DNA (9). In addition, thyroid hormone may affect the development and differentiation of cardiac muscle cells by influencing the maturation of sympathetic neurotransmission in the heart (9). The increased functional demands placed on the heart after birth would cause a response of differentiation characterized by increased production of contractile elements and by a cessation of cell division. The presence of contractile elements may serve as a barrier to prevent complete cell division. This concept is in accord with observations showing that mitosis in cardiac myocytes is associated with marked disruption of the contractile elements (particularly of the Z bands), which become reconstituted after completion of cell division (37, 42).

DNA synthesis can occur in cardiac myocytes after birth. Such a synthesis goes well beyond that needed for DNA repair and it can result in polyploidy, binucleation or multinucleation, or complete cell division. Polyploidy occurs normally, as a function of age, in the hearts of humans and primates, in which species it develops to a greater extent than in the hearts of rodents (1, 37). According to Adler (1), polyploidy in human hearts develops normally during late childhood. Polyploidy may involve the selective amplification of certain parts of the genome rather than complete multiplication of all genetic material. Nevertheless, polyploidy may also result from complete synthesis of DNA which is not followed by nuclear division. The extent to which polyploidy occurs in human hearts is increased considerably in cardiac hypertrohy, including the hypertrophy related to hypertrophic cardiomyopathy (1, 2, 13, 17, 25).

Binucleation or multinucleation of cardiac myocytes results from nuclear division (karyokinesis) that is not followed by cytoplasmic division (cytokinesis); however, it also can result from cell fusion and from amitotic division of polyploid nuclei. Binucleated nuclei are very common in human and rodent hearts, as demonstrated by counts of mononucleated and binucleated cardiac myocytes at different ages (4—7, 20, 21, 24, 26, 42). Myocytes of newborn rats are predominantly uninucleated, but by 12—14 days of age, 80 % of the myocytes are binucleated (23, 26, 42). Binucleated cardiac myocytes have also been observed in other species, including dogs and rabbits [see (23) for review]; most myocytes of pigs and miniature swine are multinucleated (16).

In vivo studies of lower vertebrates, including frog ventricle and newt ventricle, have demonstrated the potential of adult cardiac myocytes to undergo division in response to injury [see (31, 32, 36, 37) for review]. More importantly, Rumyantsev (36, 37) and Oberpriller (31, 32) have shown that atrial myocardium is a suitable model system for studying the DNA synthesis that occurs in association with the hypertrophy that develops in response to the overload stress produced by left ventricular infarction created by left coronary artery ligation. Using a series of tritiated thymidine injections, Rumyantsev (36, 37) demonstrated that 51 % of the myocytes in left atrium and 35 % of the myocytes in right atrium respond by undergoing DNA synthesis after ventricular infarction. In contrast to the large atrial response, a much smaller response (9 %) was found in the left ventricle in the surviving myocytes of the subepicardium in the perinecrotic area of the infarct. Oberpriller et al. (31) studied myocytes from the atria of young male Sprague-Dawley rats, at 11 days after left coronary artery ligation and showed that binucleation is a major response of atrial myocytes to ventricular infarction. In sham-operated animals, 23 % of left and 15.5 % of right atrial myocytes were binucleated, compared to 77.8 % of left and 40.5 % of right atrial myocytes in infarcted animals. Microfluorimetric studies have demonstrated that the degree of ploidy increased considerably in the atrial myocytes of rats undergoing coronary ligation (31). In a subsequent study, Oberpriller et al. (32) found that in infarcted animals, 37.1 % of left atrial myocytes were binucleated and were labeled by tritiated thymidine, and 6.5 % were labeled and mononucleated; 13 % of right atrial myocytes were labeled and binucleated, and 12.7 were labeled and mononucleated. For both the left and the right atria, the incidence of tritiated thymidine label in myocytes of the sham-operated group was similar to that of the unoperated controls, indicating that the surgical procedure itself did not stimulate DNA synthesis in atrial myocytes. A low level of labeling occurred in myocytes and non-myocytes in unoperated animals, indicating that a small amount of DNA synthesis was occurring in atrial tissue in the young growing rats used in this study (32). These studies were carried out using enzymatically dissociated myocytes in order to avoid the problems related to the evaluation of binucleation in tissue sections, in which one of the nuclei could be out of the section plane, and in which it is often difficult to be certain whether or not a given nucleus belongs to a myocyte or to a connective tissue cell. These studies have established in a definitive way that DNA synthesis and nuclear division can be induced in adult rat atrial myocardium; however, they have not determined to what extent these events are followed by cytokinesis under the conditions of the experiment. This would require the direct demonstration of an increase in the total number of myocytes in the atria.

Linzbach (27) has suggested that myocyte proliferation occurs in human cardiac hypertrophy after the heart has reached a "critical weight" of 500 g. This concept was based on (1) calculations of the total numbers of myocytes in variously hypertrophied hearts, based on data of cell counts and measurements of cell diameters and lengths, and (2) the finding that up to 500 g of heart weight there is a linear correlation between myocyte size and cardiac weight, from which it may be concluded that the increase in cardiac mass, up to the critical weight, can be accounted for on the basis of increased cellular size. After this critical heart weight has been reached, further increments in cardiac mass are not accompanied by a corresponding increase in myocyte dimensions, and for this reason Linzbach postulated that these increments are mediated by the formation of new myocytes. Linzbach also postulated that a process of "amitotic" division or splitting leads to the formation of new myocytes; however, such a process has not been observed. More recently, Astorri et al. (3) carried out studies similar to those of Linzbach (27) and reported similar conclusions with respect to the relationships between cardiac weight and myocyte size. The hypothesis of the critical heart weight has not been tested in experimental animal models, as in most of these models the resulting degree of hypertrophy does not show the massive increases in cardiac weight found in human cardiac hypertrophy. The studies of Linzbach and Astorri et al. do not exclude the possibility that mitotic division of cardiac myocytes occurs at a very slow rate during the development of increases in cardiac mass, but, because of its low frequency, it is not detected by visual observation of mitotic figures. Such a phenomenon could be demonstrated only by multiple injections of tritiated thymidine, as was done by Rumyantsev (36, 37) and Oberpriller et al. (31, 32).

If the critical heart weight hypothesis is correct, it would follow that some degree of hyperplasia would occur in many patients with hypertrophic cardiomyopathy, simply because of the pronounced increase in cardiac mass that such patients have. Nevertheless, some uncertainties remain about this hypothesis. The calculations involved in the estimation of the total numbers of myocytes in hypertrophied hearts are complex and subject to a number of sources of potential errors, especially with respect to the calculations of myocyte volumes using data derived from tissue sections. Perhaps because of these problems, estimates by different investigators of the total numbers of myocytes in rat hearts have varied widely (15). Such problems would appear to be considerably reduced by using enzymatically dissociated myocytes to obtain the myocyte volume data needed for the total and regional cell counts.

Of direct relevance to the problem of the morphogenesis of hypertrophic cardiomyopathy, is the pathologic increase in cardiac weight that can be experimentally induced during neonatal life. Several studies have concluded that hyperplasia of myocytes can be induced by anemia (30), hypoxia (21), and aortic banding (10) in very young rats. These studies suggest, as does a study of aortic banding in young dogs (5), that the time of cessation of mitosis in cardiac myocytes can be extended when the heart is overloaded during the neonatal period. Nevertheless, this generalization cannot be extended to all models of hypertrophy, because Gerdes et al. (14) showed that the administration of thyroxine to newborn rats causes true hypertrophy (primarily by increasing cell length) and inhibits rather than accelerates hyperplastic growth.

In many patients, hypertrophic cardiomyopathy is a genetically transmitted disorder, and it seems very likely that the stimulus to increase cardiac mass in this disorder is present from a very early age, so that it eventually gives rise to clinical manifestations of hypertrophy. In some patients, the transition from the preclinical to the clinical phase of the disease occurs during childhood. These observations suggest the possibility that the increase in cardiac mass occuring in hypertrophic cardiomyopathy is mediated in part by hyperplasia. Ferrans and Rodríguez (11) have previously presented this hypothesis, which is summarized in Table 1. The central elements of it are: (1) the basic defect in hypertrophic cardiomyopathy is an inappropriate or exaggerated response of the cardiac myocytes to contractile stimuli [see review by Perloff (33)]; (2) this response is already present during the fetal period; (3) this response causes an abnormal exaggeration of the extent to which myocyte hyperplasia occurs during the prenatal period; (4) the increased hyperplasia may have a focal distribution (both in the ventricular septum and in the ventricular free walls), perhaps reflecting local differences in the mechanical forces exerted by myocyte contraction; (5) the asymmetric cardiac hypertrophy that occurs in hypertrophic cardiomyopathy (which in most patients involves the ventricular septum, but in some patients is localized to unusual regions of the left ventricle [29]) may be a consequence of the focal distribution of this hyperplasia, and (6) the ventricular septal asymmetry that normally occurs during fetal life would fail to regress, as it normally, should, because of the increased numbers of myocytes present in the ventricular septum. Thus, the genetic defect in hypertrophic cardiomyopathy would lead first to increased

Table 1. Hypertrophic cardiomyopathy: Hypothetic stages of development.

Stage of life	Normal	Hypertrophic Cardiomyopathy
Fetal period	1. Normal contractility 2. Hyperplasia is the main mechanism of cardiac growth 3. Some septal asymmetry develops	1. Hypercontractility 2. Hyperplasia is exaggerated in certain areas, particularly in the ventricular septum, because of mechanical forces produced by hypercontractile cells 3. Degree of septal asymmetry is exaggerated as numbers of myocytes in septum are increased over normal
Newborn	1. Mitosis stops in myocytes and increase in cell size becomes the mechanism of further cardiac growth 2. Septal asymmetry regresses as growth of free walls exceeds that of septum	1. Mitosis stops in myocytes (delayed cessation?) and increase in cell size becomes the mechanism of further cardiac growth 2. Septal asymmetry is maintained; either it regresses less than normal of fails to regress because of increased number of myocytes in septum
Childhood and young adulthood	1. Cardiac growth is completed 2. Result of this growth is normal gross anatomic cardiac structure 3. Regulation of growth prevents development of hypertrophy in the absence of increased workload	1. Excessive cell growth develops in association with hypercontractility. This process is influenced by other factors. 2. The resulting hypertrophy is asymmetric with respect to ventricular septal growth 3. Progression of hypertrophy leads to clinically overt disease

hyperplasia of myocytes during the fetal period, thus creating certain permanently disturbed patterns of cardiac gross anatomy, and subsequently to progressive hypertrophy after the switch from hypertplastic to hypertrophic growth. One can only speculate as to whether or not the time of this switch is accelerated or delayed in hypertrophic cardiomyopathy.

The concept that myocyte hyperplasia is involved in the morphogenesis of hypertrophic cardiomyopathy provides an explanation for the asymmetric septal hypertrophy that occurs in hypertrophic cardiomyopathy. A recent study has concluded that the anatomic reason for this asymmetric septal hypertrophy is that the ventricular septum in this condition contains an abnormally large number of layers of myocytes (rather than abnormally large myocytes or an abnormally large component of fibrous tissue) (12). The number of layers of myocytes in ventricular septum (630 ± 80) was found to be increased in comparison to that present in normal patients (490 ± 70) and in patients with hypertensive heart disease (510 ± 80), and a good correlation was found between the numbers of layers of myocytes and the degree of asymmetric septal thickening. In contrast to these findings, the diameters of the myocytes did not differ significantly in ventricular septum (19 ± 3 μ) and posterior left ventricular free wall (21 ± 2 μ) of patients with hypertrophic cardiomyopathy. Thus, these data indicate that the number of cells in the ventricular septum of patients with hypertrophic cardiomyopathy is larger than normal, and the increase in septal mass corresponds to the increased number of layers of myocytes, rather than to a degree of hypertrophy greater than that oberved in the left ventricular free wall (12, 22). It remains to be determined whether this is due to: (1) abnormal amounts of cell division (hyperplasia) during development and/or later in life; (2) abnormal patterns of myocyte migration during development; (3) failure of regression of the fetal pattern of disproportionate septal thickening that is seen normally (28) during fetal life (and which seems to have a delayed regression in the infants of diabetic mothers [18, 19, 41]), or (4) a combination of two or more of these factors. The effects of adrenergic influences on these phenomena are poorly understood, but are of particular interest because of the many findings that suggest a link between hypertrophic cardiomyopathy and abnormal or exaggerated effects of catecholamines (33). As mentioned previously, the development of adrenergic innervation may play an important role in the switch from hyperplastic to hypertrophic growth. Of interest in this regard are recent studies showing that norepinephrine stimulates the development of hypertrophy in primary myocyte cultures of neonatal rat ventricle, and this stimulation seems to be an alpha$_1$ adrenergic effect, since it is not blocked by propranolol or by the alpha$_2$ adrenergic antagonist yohimbine, but is blocked by the nonselective alpha adrenergic antagonist phentolamine and by the alpha$_1$ adrenergic antagonists prazosin and terazosin (38—40).

In conclusion, the evidence reviewed in this communication shows that hyperplasia normally occurs during the prenatal phase of cardiac development and stops soon after birth, at which time hypertrophy becomes the main mechanism by which cardiac mass increases. Under certain circumstances, the ability of cardiac myocytes to synthesize DNA and undergo mitotic division can be restored; however, it is uncertain to what extent this results in complete cell division or only in either polyploidy or bi- or multinucleation. It is proposed that in hypertrophic cardiomyopathy, increased hyperplasia of cardiac myocytes occurs early in life and leads to permanently disturbed patterns of cardiac gross anatomy; then it is followed by a phase of progressive hypertrophy, after the switch from hyperplastic to hypertrophic growth. It is also possible that hyperplasia continues to occur after the usual time of this switch. It is also proposed that the increased number of myocyte layers in the ventricular septum of patients with hypertrophic cardiomyopathy is a consequence of exaggerated hyperplasia during development.

Summary: A review is presented of the mechanisms that mediate the increase in cardiac mass that occurs in patients with hypertrophic cardiomyopathy. This increase in mass is mediated by an increase in the total mass of the myocytes and the total mass of interstitial fibrous connective tissue. The increase in myocyte mass is the most important of these two components. However, it is not clear at the present time whether this increase is mediated not only by an increase in the size of the cells (hypertrophy), but also by an increase in the numbers of myocytes (hyperplasia) or by a combination of these two factors.

Hyperplasia normally occurs during the prenatal phase of cardiac development and stops soon after birth, at which time hypertrophy becomes the main mechanism by which cardiac mass increases. Under certain circumstances, the ability of cardiac myocytes to synthesize DNA and undergo mitotic division can be restored; however, it is uncertain to what extent this results in complete cell division or only in either polyploidy or bi- or multinucleation. It is proposed that in hypertrophic cardiomyopathy, increased hyperplasia of cardiac myocytes occurs early in life and leads to permanently disturbed patterns of cardiac gross anatomy; it is then followed by a phase of progressive hypertrophy after the switch from hyperplastic to hypertrophic growth. It is possible that hyperplasia continues to occur after the usual time of this switch. It is also proposed that the increased number of layers of myocytes in the ventricular septum of patients with hypertrophic cardiomyopathy is a consequence of exaggerated hyperplasia during development.

References

1. Adler CP (1976) DNS in Kinderherzen. Biochemische und Zytophotometrische Untersuchungen. Beitr Pathol 158: 173—202
2. Adler CP, Sandritter W (1980) Alterations of substances (DNA, myoglobin, myosin, protein) in experimentally induced cardiac hypertrophy and under the influence of drugs (isoproterenol, cytostatics, strophanthin). Basic Res Cardiol 75: 126—138
3. Astorri E, Bolognesi E, Colla B, Chizzola A, Visioli O (1977) Left ventricular hypertrophy: A cytometric study on 42 human hearts. J Mol Cell Cardiol 9: 763—775
4. Baroldi G, Falzi G, Lampertico P (1967) The nuclear patterns of the cardiac muscle fiber. Cardiologia 51: 109—123
5. Bishop SP (1973) Effect of aortic stenosis on myocardial cell growth, hyperplasia, and ultrastructure in neonatal dogs. Recent Adv Stud Card Struct Metab 3: 637—656
6. Bishop SP (1983) Ultrastructure of the myocardium in physiologic and pathologic hypertrophy in experimental animals. Perspect Cardiol Res 7: 127—147
7. Bugaisky L, Zak R (1979) Cellular growth of cardiac muscle after birth. Tex Rep Biol Med 39: 123—138
8. Claycomb WC (1983) Cardiac muscle cell proliferation and cell differentiation in vivo and in vitro. Adv Exp Med Biol 161: 249-2659.
9. Claycomb WC, Bradshaw HD, Jr (1983) Acquisition of multiple nuclei and the activity of DNA polymerase α and reinitiation of DNA replication in terminally differentiated adult cardiac muscle cells in culture. Dev Biol 99: 331—337
10. Dowell RT, McManus RE III (1978) Pressure induced cardiac enlargement in neonatal and adult rats: left ventricular functional characteristics and evidence of cardiac muscle cell proliferation in the neonate. Circ Res 42: 303—310
11. Ferrans VJ, Rodríguez ER (1983) Specificity of light and electron microscopic features of hypertrophic obstructive and nonobstructive cardiomyopathy. Qualitative, quantitative and etiologic aspects. Eur Heart J 4 (Suppl F): 9—22
12. Fujiwara H, Hoshino T, Yamana K, Fujiwara T, Furuta M, Hamashima Y, Kawai C (1983) Number and size of myocytes and amount of interstitial space in the ventricular septum and in the left ventricular free wall in hypertrophic cardiomyopathy. Am J Cardiol 52: 818—823
13. Fukuda M, Nakanishi K, Takamatsu T (1983) DNA of hypertrophied heart muscle. Byouri to Rinsho 1: 717—726
14. Gerdes AM, Kriseman J, Bishop SP (1983) Changes in myocardial cell size and number during the development and reversal of hyperthyroidism in neonatal rats. Lab Invest 48: 598—602
15. Gerdes AM, Moore JA, Hines JM, Kirkland PA, Bishop SP (1986) Regional differences in myocyte size in normal rat heart. Anat Rec 215: 420—426
16. Grabner W, Pfitzer P (1974) Number of nuclei in isolated myocardial cells of pigs. Virchows Arch B: Zellpathol 15: 279—294

17. Grove DK, Nair G, Zak R (1969) Biochemical correlates of cardiac hypertrophy. III. Changes in DNA content. The relative contributions of polyploidy and mitotic activity. Circ Res 25: 463—471
18. Gutgesell HP, Mullins CE, Gillette PC, Speer M, Rudolph AJ, McNamara DG (1976) Transient hypertrophic subaortic stenosis in infants of diabetic mothers. J Pediatr 89: 120—125
19. Gutgesell HP, Speer M, Rosenberg HS (1980) Characterization of the cardiomyopathy in infants of diabetic mothers. Circulation 61: 441—450
20. Henschel E (1952) Über Muskelfasermessungen und Kernveränderungen bei numerischer Hyperplasie des Myokards. Virchows Arch A: Pathol Anat 321: 283—294
21. Hollenberg M, Honbo N, Samorodin AJ (1976) Effects of hypoxia on cardiac growth in neonatal rat. Am J Physiol 231: 1445—1450
22. Hoshino T, Fujiwara H, Kawai C, Hamashima Y (1983) Myocardial fiber diameter and regional distribution in the ventricular wall of normal adult hearts, hypertensive hearts and hearts with hypertrophic cardiomyopathy. Circulation 67: 1109—1116
23. Katzberg AA, Farmer BB, Harris RA (1977) The predominance of binucleation in isolated rat heart myocytes. Am J Anat 149: 489—500
24. Klinge O (1970) Karyokinese und Kernmuster im Herzmuskel wachsender Ratten. Virchows Arch Zellpathol 6: 208—219
25. Kompmann M, Paddags I, Sandritter W (1966) Feulgen cytophotometric DNA determination on human hearts. Arch Pathol 82: 303—308
26. Korecky B, Sweet S, Rakusan K (1979) Number of nuclei in mammalian cardiac myocytes. Can J Physiol Pharmacol 57: 1122—1129
27. Linzbach AJ (1960) Heart failure from the point of view of quantitative anatomy. Am J Cardiol 5: 370—382
28. Maron BJ, Verter J, Kapur S (1978) Disproportionate ventricular septal thickening in the developing normal human heart. Circulation 57: 520—526
29. Maron BJ, Gottdiener JS, Bonow RO, Epstein SE (1981) Hypertrophic cardiomyopathy with unusual locations of left ventricular hypertrophy undetectable by M-mode echocardiography. Identification by wide-angle two-dimensional echocardiography. Circulation 63: 409—418
30. Neffgen JF, Korecky B (1972) Cellular hyperplasia and hypertrophy in cardiomegalies induced by anemia in young and adult rats. Circ Res 30: 104—113
31. Oberpriller JO, Ferrans VJ, Carroll RJ (1983) Changes in DNA content, number of nuclei and cellular dimensions of young rat atrial myocytes in response to left coronary artery ligation. J Mol Cell Cardiol 15: 31—42
32. Oberpriller JO, Ferrans VJ, Carroll RJ (1984) DNA synthesis in rat atrial myocytes as a response to left ventricular infarction. An autoradiographic study of enzymatically dissociated myocytes. J Mol Cell Cardiol 16: 1119—1126
33. Perloff JK (1981) Pathogenesis of hypertrophic cardiomyopathy: hypotheses and speculations. Am Heart J 101: 219—226
34. Rakusan K, Korecky B, Mezl V (1983) Cardiac hypertrophy and/or hyperplasia? Perspect Cardiol Res 7: 103—109
35. Roberts WC, Ferrans VJ (1975) Pathologic anatomy of the cardiomyopathies. Idiopathic dilated and hypertrophic types, infiltrative types, and endomyocardial disease with and without eosinophilia. Hum Pathol 6: 287—342
36. Rumyantsev PP (1974) Ultrastructural reorganization, DNA synthesis and mitotic division of myocytes in atria of rats with left ventricular infarction. Virchows Arch (Cell Pathol) 20: 29—342
37. Rumyantsev PP (1977) Interrelations of the proliferation and differentiation processes during cardiac myogenesis and regeneration. Internat Rev Cytol 51: 187—273
38. Simpson P (1983) Norepinephrine-stimulated hypertrophy of cultured rat myocardial cells is an alpha$_1$ adrenergic response. J Clin Invest 72: 732—738
39. Simpson P, Savion S (1982) Differentiation of rat myocytes in single cell cultures with and without proliferating nonmyocardial cells. Circ Res 50: 101—116
40. Simpson P, McGrath A, Savion S (1982) Myocyte hypertrophy in neonatal rat heart cultures and its regulation by serum and by catecholamines. Circ Res 51: 787—801

41. Way GL, Ruttenberg HD, Eshaghpour E, Nora JJ, Wolfe RR (1976) Hypertrophic obstructive cardiomyopathy in infants of diabetic mothers. Circulation 53-54 Suppl II: II-105
42. Zak R (1974) Development and proliferative capacity of cardiac muscle cells. Circ Res 34—35 Suppl II: 17—26

Authors' address:
Victor J. Ferrans, M.D., National Institutes of Health, Bethesda, Maryland 20892, U.S.A.

Variability and reproducibility of morphologic findings in endomyocardial biopsies of patients with hypertrophic obstructive cardiomyopathy

B. Schwartzkopff[1], B. Ühre[2], B. Ehle[3], B. Lösse[1], H. Frenzel[2]

Medical Hospital, Department of Cardiology, Pneumology and Angiology[1], Institute of Pathology[2] and Institute of Medical Statistics 3, University of Düsseldorf, F.R.G.

Introduction

Since its introduction in 1962, endomyocardial catheter biopsy has become an established method of investigation in cardiomyopathies, permitting the study of fresh tissue samples from the heart (16). Morphometric methods of investigation of biopsy samples make it possible to estimate the size and arrangement of myocytes, as well as to quantify the thickness of the endocardium, and the amount of interstitium and fibrous tissue.

Hypertrophic obstructive cardiomyopathy (HOCM) is a myocardial disease of unknown etiology. It is macroscopically defined as an asymmetrical thickening of the septum, that might be evident at birth or may develop later in life (14). Septal thickness is mainly determined by the number and size of muscle fibers, the total amount of interstitium and the thickness of endocardium. Besides a progressive hypertrophy of the individual myocyte, hyperplasia is discussed as an additional cause of septal thickening (4).

Before applying endomyocardial biopsy as a promising tool for the evaluation of the morphologic-functional relationship and the follow-up of the morphologic course of cardiac disease in the individual patient with HOCM, it is mandatory to determine the variation of morphologic findings in different biopsy specimens from a well defined part of the heart, chosen as a representative locus of the disease. It is to be expected that the right ventricular septum, technically quite easily to reach, is involved in the pathogenetic process of septal hypertrophy. In view of the small amount of information available about the variability and reproducibility of findings in endomyocardial biopsies from the right ventricular septum, we studied multiple biopsies of 25 patients with HOCM, to reveal the variability of morphologic findings between patients, between multiple biopsies from one heart and between measurements in one biopsy. From these data we propose a protocol for the sampling and evaluation of right ventricular biopsies in patients with HOCM.

Materials and Methods

Patients

In 25 consecutively investigated patients (six females and 19 males, of mean age, 38.3 ± 15.2 years) hypertrophic obstructive cardiomyopathy was diagnosed by left ventricular heart catheterization and angiogram.

Mean systolic blood pressure was 126.8 ± 21.1 mm Hg and mean diastolic blood pressure was 75.2 ± 19.5 mm Hg. Two patients suffered from essential high blood pressure (systolic, 180 and 170 mm Hg, respectively; diastolic, 100 mm Hg in both patients). Echocardiography could be evaluated in 22 patients showing mean asymmetrical septal thickness of 22 ± 6.7 mm. In three patients, quantitative echocardiographic analysis was not technically possible. In 18 patients, cardiac catheterization revealed a gradient from 5 to 75 mm Hg at rest between the apex and the subaortal region of the left ventricle. Seven patients had no gradient at rest. In one patient an additional valvular aortic stenosis with a gradient of 5 mm Hg was disclosed; in another, moderate stenosis of the left anterior descending coronary artery. Under provocation by Valsalva maneuver and/or orciprenalin, a mean maximal left ventricular outflow tract gradient of 99.2 ± 56.6 mm Hg was observed in 24 patients. In one patient no provocation was performed. Eight patients had a right ventricular gradient at rest (mean 18.62 ± 12.1 mm Hg). Right ventricular endomyocardial biopsies were gained before angiography and during catheterization, by transvenous technique using a King's bioptome. Four or more biopsies were planned per patient from the right ventricular septum for morphometric evaluation.

Before catheterization and right ventricular myocardial biopsy, the patients were informed and gave their written consent to the investigation.

Tissue preparation

Specimens were immediately fixed in 2.5% cacodylate buffered glutaraldehyde. Each biopsy sample was divided into two. One half was embedded in paraffin, 5 µm thick sections were stained with hematoxylin-eosin (HE) and with elastic van Gieson (EvG). The other half was dehydrated in a graded ethanol series and embedded in epon. Semi-thin sections of 1 µm thickness were stained with methylene blue.

Morphometric methods

Biopsy size was determined by the point counting method using a grid with 100 points (Zeiss Integration Okular II) at a magnification of ×160 (5—7, 11).

Muscle fiber diameters were determined by measuring 50 myocytes per biopsy at a magnification of ×1600 on methylene stained semi-thin sections. Longitudinally or obliquely cut muscle fibers were chosen, the sarcomeres of which were clearly visible and not hypercontracted (2). Measurements were performed across the nucleus at the shortest distance between the cell membranes. At the left upper corner of the specimen, the measurements were started and meanderingly continued, until 50 suitable myocytes per biopsy had been evaluated. If fewer measurements were done, the biopsy was not accepted.

In EvG stained sections, the volume density of the reddish-stained fibrous tissue and the total non-myocytic tissue, the interstitium, were determined by the point counting method with a 100 points grid at a magnification of ×1250 (Zeiss Integration Okular II). 15 units (total area 0.126 mm²), were evaluated of the EvG stained specimens (5). Large artificial spaces and hemorrhages were avoided. Samples were not accepted if less than 15 fields were found per biopsy.

Endocardium was measured in HE stained specimens at a magnification of ×160 at ten points at a regular distance.

Muscle fiber disarray was quantified in HE stained sections projected on a board of 30 cm² underlined with a grid of 100 test points. At a magnification of ×920, the crossing of vertically running myocytes, abnormal branching or whorls of myocytes were quantified as muscle fiber disarray by counting cross points, expressed as a percentage of the total specimen. This examination was done by two observers.

Statistics

To describe the variability of morphologic findings in patients with HOCM, we considered three different sources of variability of the mean for muscle fiber diameter, volume density of interstitium and fibrous tissue and thickness of endocardium: (a) patients, (b) multiple biopsies from one heart (sampling variability), (c) multiple measurements in one biopsy. Variability of muscle fiber disarray could only be given for (a) and (b).

The mean (M) and the standard deviation (SD) were calculated for each variable at each of the defined levels, for all available biopsies.

To describe the variability of the mean at each level, according to our protocol, we used the coefficient of variation (CV), which is defined by $CV = SD/M \times 100\%$. The coefficient of error (CE) defined by $CE = CV/\sqrt{n}$ (n = number of measurements) was used to describe the precision of the estimates (5, 6, 15).

The measurements were assumed to follow a hierarchical variance component model. To estimate the main source of variance at the different levels, hierarchical analysis of variance was carried out in 13 patients, each of whom had four suitable biopsies to determine myocardial diameter, volume density of interstitium and fibrous tissue. Eight patients had three biopsies of good quality for the quantification of endocardial thickness; eight patients had four biopsies for the characterization of muscle fiber disarray. From the variance between multiple biopsies from one heart, we estimated the increase or decrease in one parameter, necessary to promise statistical significance at $p \leq 0.05$ with 90% probability ($\beta = 0.9$), in dependence on the number of biopsies and measurements:

$$\sqrt{\frac{\text{Variance of biopsies}}{n \text{ biopsies}} + \frac{\text{Variance of measurements}}{n \text{ measurements}}} \times (1.96 + 1.28) \times \sqrt{2}$$

From the observed SD of multiple biopsies from one heart, we roughly estimated the number of biopsies necessary for each variable to reach a coeficient of error (CE) of 5%, regarded as an acceptable degree of precision for the estimation of biological parameters (15).

Reproducibility

To define the variability of repeated studies of biopsies, we used the standard deviation of the differences between the initial and repeat studies. For this purpose, 16 randomly chosen biopsies were evaluated, twice by one observer and once by another. Likewise, the standard deviations of the difference between the two studies of one observer and between the first studies of two observers were used to define same observer and inter-observer reproducibility. To disclose significant differences between mean values of different studies for each variable, analysis of variance and an appropriate test were performed. The reproducibility of the measurements was expressed as the CV of the mean of two studies.

By analysis of variance and F-test we looked for significant differences between multiple biopsies from the same heart for each variable at $p \leq 0.05$.

Results

Size of biopsy samples and technical suitability

There were no clinical complications in any of the 25 patients and no interruption of the biopsy procedure was necessary. Between two and seven biopsies could be obtained per patient. A total of 112 biopsies were gained for morphometric investigation. Mean biopsy size was 0.755 ± 0.567 mm². 32 biopsies (28.6%) could not be used for morphometric studies, reducing the mean available number of biopsies per patient from 4.48 ± 1.15 to 3.2 ± 1.05.

14 of the non-suitable biopsies (12.5%) were too small to fulfil the predetermined criteria, having a mean size of 0.28 mm² (range: 0.038—0.39), 14 (12.5%) completely consisted of fibrous tissue, three (2.7%) contained extensive hemorrhage and one (0.9%) was extremely distorted. In several biopsies pinch artifacts were observed, which did not seriously hamper morphometric investigations.

Means and variability at different levels for muscle fiber diameter, thickness of endocardium, volume density of interstitium, fibrous tissue and muscle fiber disarray

Mean muscle fiber diameter was 16.42 µm deduced from findings from 25 patients. The variability of measurements of a single biopsy was 22.2%; sampling variability reached only a CV of 5.1% (Table 1). The total mean volume density of interstitium, including fibrous tissue, was 19%; the mean volume density of fibrous tissue alone reached 4%. The variability of measurements for volume density of interstitium was 28.4%, of fibrous tissue 60.7%, deduced from 80 biopsies of 25 patients. The sampling variability reached 8.8% for volume density of interstitium, 17.2% for fibrous tissue (Table 1). 56 biopsies contained parts of endocardium, mean endocardial thickness was 10.95 µm, CV was 79.3% for biopsies of one heart, with a CV of 44.9% for the measurements in a biopsy. The mean amount of muscle fiber disarray in a biopsy was 6.32%. In all but one patient muscle fiber disarray was observed (96%). Sampling variability reached a CV of 99.8%.

Components of variance

Analysis of variance revealed that the variance of measurements is the main component influencing the estimation of muscle fiber size, volume density of interstitium and

Table 1. Means, standard deviations and variability of morphologic findings in HOCM.

	Mean	Patients ($n = 25$)		Biopsies ($n > 2$)		Measurements		CE %
		SD	CV %	SD	CV %	SD	CV %	
Muscle fiber diameter	16.42	± 1.68	10.2	± 0.84	5.1	± 3.65	22.2	3
Interstitium (VV %)	19.0	± 4.13	21.7	± 1.68	8.8	± 5.41	28.4	7
Fibrous tissue (VV %)	4.0	± 2.36	59.0	± 0.69	17.2	± 2.43	60.7	16
Endocard. thickness (µm)	10.95	± 5.38	49.1	± 8.69	79.3	± 4.92	44.9	14
Muscle fiber disarray (VV %)	6.32	± 5.53	87.5	± 6.31	99.8	–	–	–

SD = standard deviation, CV = coefficient of variation, CE = coefficient of error.

Table 2. Analysis of variance in patients with HOCM.

Source	SS	DF	MS	C.o.V	CV%
Muscle fiber diameter					
Patient	7 266	12	605.52	2.83	10.18
Biopsy	1 535	39	39.37	0.504	4.3
Measurement	36 068	2548	14.15	14.15	22.7
$m = 16.5$ µm; SD = ± 1.74, $n = 13$ patients, 4 biopsies/patient					
Volume density of interstitium					
Patient	11 405	12	950	15.27	20.51
Biopsy	1 321	39	33.87	0.178	2.21
Measurement	22 709	728	31.19	31.19	29.31
$m = 19.05$ VV %, SD = ± 3.98, $n = 13$, 4 biopsies/patient					
Volume density of fibrous tissue					
Patient	2 938	12	244.83	3.93	50.83
Biopsy	333	39	8.53	0.2	11.46
Measurement	4 066	728	5.58	5.58	60.56
$m = 3.9$ VV %, SD = ± 2.017, $n = 13$, 4 biopsies/patient					
Thickness of endocardium					
Patient	12 041	7	1720.2	2.95	15.06
Biopsy	26 107	16	1631.7	158.08	110.28
Measurement	10 982	216	50.84	50.84	62.54
$m = 11.4$ µm, SD = ± 7.57, $n = 8$ patients, 3 biopsies/patient					
Muscle fiber disarray					
Patient	461	7	65.9	3.57	35.92
Biopsy	1 325	24	55.18	55.2	141.24
$m = 5.26$ VV %, SD = ± 4.16, $n = 8$ patients, 4 biopsies/patient					

SS = sum of squares, DF = degrees of freedom, MS = mean squares, m = mean values, SD = standard deviation, n = number of patients, C.o.V. = component of variance, CV = coefficient of variation.

fibrous tissue for the individual patient, whereas multiple biopsies of the same heart contribute only a small part. In contrast to this, variation of endocardium and muscle fiber disarray are mainly determined by sampling variability (Table 2). CV deduced from the components of variance (Table 2) reached comparable values at the different levels for each variable as shown in Table 1. Components of variance of biopsies were significant at $p < 0.05$ for muscle fiber diameter, fibrous tissue and thickness of endocardium.

Reproducibility of repeated studies

Results of repeated studies are given in Table 3. The means of the three studies did not differ significantly for any variable, indicating that there was no systematic mistake. The CV of 5% for intra- and 8% for interobserver variation of muscle fiber diameter were less than those observed for volume density of interstitium and fibrous tissue. Reproducibility, expressed as CV, similarly, was nearly as high as sampling variability for these variables (Tables 1, 3). For endocardial thickness and muscle fiber disarray, the CV of repeated studies of a biopsy were remarkable but less than the sampling variability.

In respect of these data there were only significant differences between multiple biopsies of the same heart for endocardial thickness at $p < 0.05$. Muscle fiber disarray was not tested, because one measurement per biopsy does not permit a meaningful test.

Increasing precision by the number of measurements

As shown in Table 1, the estimates of the variables were of different precision for one biopsy. For muscle fiber size, an error coefficient of 5% would be achieved with 20 measurements, whereas volume density of interstitium and fibrous tissue would demand 33 and 148 measurements, respectively. These high numbers may explain why reproducibility with only 15 measurements per biopsy was so hampered for these variables. More measurements are hard to derive from one biospsy. With regard to the fact that the precision of an estimate is mainly described by the coefficient of error (CE) of units, as in our study, by the CE of the means of multiple biopsies from the same heart (15), and considering the described reproducibility, an estimate of the increasing degree of precision by increasing numbers of biopsies is given in Fig. 1, according to our protocol.

To detect smaller changes in hypertrophy, more biopsies are needed, as shown in Table 4. For instance, to disclose an increase in muscle fiber diameter of 12%, four biopsies (a total of 200 measurements) are desirable, whereas from one bopsy (50 measurements) only a change of 25% or more can be detected.

Discussion

Various studies of post-mortem hearts of patients with hypertrophic obstructive cardiomyopathy have disclosed typical morphologic findings in the septum, such as muscle fiber hypertrophy, fibrosis and muscle fiber disarray, which help to support the diagnosis (3, 4). Morphometric investigations of endomyocardial biopsies from the right ventricular septum might be a promising approach to determine the morphologic status and course of the disease in the individual patient. To describe a useful sampling of endomyocardial biopsies from the right ventricular septum, we investigated 112 biopsies from

Table 3. Reproducibility of repeated studies in 16 biopsies.

	1st Observer		2nd Observer
	1. Study	2. Study	1. Study
Muscle fiber diameter (µm)			
Mean	15.47	15.23	15.38
SD	± 1.3	± 1.33	± 0.98
Difference	$a =$ 0.24		$b =$ 0.09
SD	±0.8		±1.22
CV %	5		8
Interstitium (VV %)			
Mean	18.47	17.9	19.56
SD	± 2.5	± 2.04	± 2.59
Difference	$a =$ 0.57		$b = -1.09$
SD	±1.54		±2.36
CV %	9		12
Fibrous Tissue (VV %)			
Mean	3.28	3.38	2.92
SD	±1.78	±2.09	±1.4
Difference	$a = -0.10$		$b =$ 0.36
SD	±0.69		±2.2
CV %	21		71
Endocardium (µm)			
Mean	15.97	15.54	15.28
SD	±13.25	±11.04	± 9.4
Difference	$a = -0.43$		$b =$ 0.69
SD	±3.76		±3.93
CV %	24		25
Muscle fiber disarray			
Mean	7.93	8.65	
SD	±9.01	±9.72	
Difference	$a = - 0.72$		
SD	±4.9		
CV %	59		

SD = standard deviation, a) = difference between measurements of the first and second study of the 1st observer; b) = difference between the first study of the 1st observer and the study of the 2nd observer. CV = coefficient of variation for the differences.

myocardial biopsies from the right ventricular septum, we investigated 112 biopsies from 25 consecutively investigated patients with HOCM.

Biopsy size and quality

The size of the average biopsy, 0.755 mm² in our study, was comparable to those reported by other authors also using a King's bioptome (1, 2, 12). As in our study, Baan-

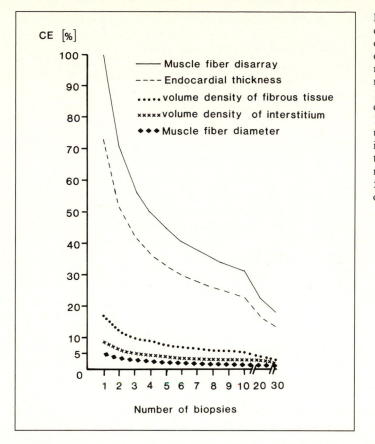

Fig. 1. Estimate of the decrease of the coefficient of error (CE) by increasing numbers of right septal biopsies, muscle fiber disarray = 1 categorization/biopsy, endocardial thickness = 10 measurements, volume density (VV %) of interstitium and fibrous tissue = 15 units/biopsy, muscle fiber diameter = 50 measurements/biopsy.

Table 4. Change in myocardial diameter, volume density of interstitium and fibrous tissue and thickness of endocardium, to reach significance ($p < 0.05$) with 90% probability in dependance on the number of available biopsies.

		Number of biopsies/patient			
		4	3	2	1
Muscle fiber	μm	±2.03	2.35	2.86	4.07
size	%	12	14	17	25
Volume density	VV %	± 3.42	3.95	4.83	6.83
of interstitium	%	18	21	25	36
Volume density of	VV %	± 1.71	1.97	2.42	3.42
fibrous tissue	%	44	51	62	88
Thickness of	μm	±29.00	34.00	41.00	58.00
endocardium	%	154	198	259	409

% = change as percentage of the mean, from our findings. Muscle fiber size = 50 measurements per biopsy, volume density of fibrous tissue and interstitium = 15 unit measurements, thickness of endocardium = 10 measurements.

drup et al. (1) bisected many samples to provide material for both light and electron microscopic investigation. In our study the number of non-suitable biopsies was remarkably high, at 28.6%, which can be explained by the number of measurements demanded to be performed in one biopsy. By accepting 20 or more muscle fibers and 10 or more random units for the estimation of volume fraction of interstitium and fibrous tissue, Baandrup et al (1) had only 16.9% biopsies of a poor quality that did not permit morphologic categorization. We demanded 50 muscle fibers, 15 units for volume density of interstitium and fibrous tissue per biopsy, which can be regarded as the upper number of measurements in most of the biopsies.

Muscle fiber diameter

We observed a mean muscle fiber diameter of 16.42 µm, indicating a mild to moderate hypertrophy of myocytes in the right ventricular septum. Data reported by other authors ranged from 11.2 to 16.2 µm (1, 4, 9, 18) in normally configurated hearts, evaluated from post-mortem or bioptic specimens from the right ventricular septum. In patients with HOCM, mean myocytic diameter ranged from 14 to 20.7 µm (1, 4, 9) always found to be thicker than control values. Besides a different severity of the disease in several studies, variations in fixation and embedding of specimens, use of post-mortem or bioptic specimens or different study protocols may be reasons for the differing results (17). The structure of the septum itself shows regional differences, with up to 10% thicker muscle fibers on the left side of the septum (9, 18) in normally shaped hearts. In HOCM, Hoshino et al. (9) found an altered structure of the septum with muscle fiber size of 14.1 µm for the right, 16 µm for the mid protion and 13 µm for the left ventricular side of the septum, indicating that right septal biopsies may give good information about septal hypertrophy.

Sampling variability of muscle fiber diameter was only 5.1% in terms of the coefficient of variation (CV), showing that one biopsy is highly representative of the right ventricular septum. Mall et al. (12) reported a CV of 6% for muscle fiber diameter derived from two left ventricular endomyocardial biopsies in each of 26 patients with dilatative cardiomyopathy. Baandrup et al. (2), not distinguishing between right or left ventricular biopsy pairs, found a CV of 18.6% in 79 patients with different forms of heart disease.

From our data, it becomes obvious that the small differences between right septal biopsies of one heart are also overlapped by the reproducibility of measurements, having a CV of 5% for the intra-observer and 8% for the interobserver variation. The limited reproducibility of morphologic studies can be explained by the fact that in every new study not all previously observed fibers or units are exactly found again nor are measured by the same angle nor the same side. Each new analysis of the same specimen also yields some new information, depending on its size and the number of measurements performed. From one biopsy, 20 measurements give only a rough estimate of muscle fiber size, whereas 200 measurements (affording approximately four biopsies) would enable the observer to give quite a precise statement about hypertrophy, disclosing significant changes of ca. 12% in the pathological course of the disease in the individual patient.

Interstitium

We found a mean volume density of interstitium of 19% in our patients with HOCM. Baandrup et al. (1) reported 17.2%, in right septal biopsies of patients with normal ventricles and 18.5% in patients with HOCM. Fujiwara et al. (4) described a relatively high amount of interstitium, at 44% for controls and 45% in ten post-mortem investigated hearts of patients with HOCM. Sampling variability in our study was 8.8%, less than reported by Baandrup et al (2), who described 28.9% in 55 patients with different forms of heart disease. We did not find significant differences between multiple biopsies from one heart, making three biopsies desirable for adequate precision with an error coefficient of 5%. Also, for the volume density of interstitium, intraobserver reproducibility was better than interobserver's, proposing that use of the same observer for the evaluation of a series of biopsies will advise a higher degree of precision.

Fibrous tissue

The volume density of fibrous tissue was 4% in our patients. Unverferth et al. (18) reported 3% for the right and 4% for the left septal side of normal hearts. Baandrup et al. (1) found 0.8% for the right and 1.1% for the left ventricle in controls; in patients with HOCM, the content of fibrous tissue rose to 2.7% for the whole septum. Variability from one biopsy to the next was quite high, with a CV of 17.2% in our study. Mall et al. (11) reported a CV for the volume density of fibrous tissue of 43% in 26 patients with dilative cardiomyopathy, the mean content of fibrosis reached 10.4% in the left ventricular biopsies. Baandrup et al. (2) observed a sampling error of 80.5% for two biopsies in each of 49 patients with various cardiomyopathies; the mean volume density of fibrosis reached only 2.1%. Repeated studies of our biopsies disclosed hampered reproducibility which reduced the differences between biopsies from one heart. To increase the precision of the estimate to an error coefficient of 5% (15) 148 measurements (or approximately 9 biopsies) are necessary. Four biopsies, which seems a reasonable number, can push the coefficient of error at least to under 10%.

Endocardial thickness

Mean endocardial thickness was 10.5 μm. Baandrup et al. (1) found 21.6 μm for the right and 21.2 μm for the left unsuspiciously shaped ventricle, but 27.3 μm for the righ ventricular endocardium in 12 patients with HOCM. We performed measurements at several points at regular distances across the endocardium, whereas Baandrup et al. (1) measured the thickest point of endocardium. Sampling variability was remarkable, with a CV of 79.3%. High variations of endomyocardial thickness may be induced by regional alterations of cusp motions and the blood stream, but also shrinkage artifacts and the direction of cutting can be the cause of high sampling variability. Even large numbers of biopsy samples do not yield very precise data, making it an uncertain variable in morphometric evaluation.

Muscle fiber disarray

Maron et al. (13) found an extent of fiber disarray of 35% of the septal area in 52 patients with hypertrophic cardiomyopathy, but only 2% in patients with other congenital or acquired heart disease. Particularly marked free wall and septal disorganization was present in 14 patients younger than 25 years, in whom sudden death was the initial manifestation of cardiac disease, reinforcing the suspicion that this pattern is an important determinant of clinical outcome in certain patients. Fujiwara et al. (3) found an extent of muscle fiber disarray of 30% in patients with hypertrophic cardiomyopathy and only 10% in controls. The main disarray was noted mostly in the middle three fifths of the septum. The mean volume density of muscle fiber disarray was 6.32% in biopsies from our 25 patients with HOCM. Hoshino et al. (8) found 9% of disarray in 11 post-mortem hearts from patients with hypertrophic cardiomyopathy, and 4% in the subendocardial region in controls. The frequency of occurrence of disarray in this part was 38% in HCM and 20% in controls. We observed muscle fiber disarray in 96% of our patients. Hoshino et al. (8) reported that significant differences between HCM and controls are to be expected only for the upper part of the right ventricular septum, not for the lower half. Also, in left septectomy specimens, the density of disarray reached only 7%, compared with 20% for the whole septal area in 18 patients who died after operation (10).

The high variability in the amount of disarray from one biopsy to the next, reaching a CV of nearly 100% in our study, might also be explained by regional differences, as in cut-induced artifacts. Besides this, repeated studies of a specimen are necessary because of hampered reproducibility. It should be considered that bioptical specimens are quite small. Abnormal large fascicles may be falsely regarded as the true direction. From the reported data it becomes obvious that the total amount of septal disarray is not estimable even by numerous endomyocardial biopsies. It is open to speculation whether the highest amount of disarray derived from one out of a few biopsies, gives more important information than the mean. Hoshino et al. (8) pointed out that a degree of disarray of more than 76% in a biopsy specimen was specific for HOCM.

Conclusion

In view of the literature and our data, five right septal biopsies are desirable, considering the fact that 25—30% are of limited quality. With four useful biopsies, good estimates of muscle fiber diameter and volume density of interstitium and limited, but acceptable ones for fibrous tissue can be evaluated. Maximum values of muscle fiber disarray and endocardial thickness, derived from these biopsies, might be of more diagnostic importance than mean values, which are quite inaccurate because of high sampling variability.

Summary: Morphometric investigations of endomyocardial catheter biopsies (EMCB) promise to give more insight in the morphologic-functional relationship in patients with hypertrophic obstructive cardiomyopathy (HOCM), and may disclose the morphologic course of the disease. Variability and reproducibility of morphologic findings in EMCB of patients with HOCM are still undefined.

We investigated 112 right ventricular biopsies of 25 patients with HOCM of a mean age of 38.3 ± 15.2 years (six women, 19 men). Mean EMCB size was 0.755 ± 0.567 mm^2. 28.6% of EMCB were not suitable for morphometric investigation. Variability of morphologic findings was investigated by analysis of variance and described by the coefficient of variation (CV).

Sampling variabilities of muscle fiber diameter (CV = 5%), volume density of interstitium (CV = 9%) and fibrous tissue (CV = 17%) differed. Reproducibility in terms of intra- and interobserver variations for these variables reached a comparable level, diminishing observed differences between biopsies from the same heart, which became non-significant. Sampling variability of endocardial thickness (CV = 79%) and muscle fiber disarray (CV = 100%) were higher than intra- and interobserver variations.

For an estimate of muscle fiber size, one EMCB specimen is sufficient, three for volume density of interstitium and nine for fibrous tissue. High sampling variability of endocardial thickness and muscle fiber disarray demand numerous biopsies; here the greatest measured value from a few biopsies may be of more clinical relevance.

From our data, five EMCB are desirable, and give the most information at an acceptable strain.

References

1. Baandrup U, Olsen EGJ (1981) Critical analysis of endomyocardial biopsies from patients suspected of having cardiomyopathy. Br Heart J 45: 475—486
2. Baandrup U, Florio RA, Olsen EGJ (1982) Do endomyocardial biopsies represent the morphology of the rest of the myocardium? Europ Heart J 3: 171—178
3. Fujiwara H, Hoshino T, Fujiwara T, Kawai C, Hamashima Y (1982) Classification and distribution of myocardial fascicle and fiber disarray in 14 hearts with hypertrophic Cardiomyopathy in 25 μ thick sections. J Circ J 46: 225—234
4. Fujiwara H, Hoshino T, Yamana K, Fujiwara T, Furuta M, Hamashima Y, Kawai C (1983) Number and size of myocytes and amount of interstitial space in the ventricular septum and in the left ventricular free wall in hypertrophic cardiomyopathy. Am J Cardiol 52: 818—823
5. Gundersen HJG (1977) Notes on the estimation of the numerical density of arbitrary profiles: the edge effect. J Microscopy 111: 219—223
6. Gunderson HJG, Osterby R (1981) Optimizing sampling efficiency of stereological studies in biology: or "Do more less well!". J Microscopy 121: 65—73
7. Gupta M, Mayhew T M, Bedi K S, Sharma A K, White FH (1983) Inter-animal variation and its influence on the overall precision of morphometric estimates based on nested sampling designs. J Microscopy 131: 147—154
8. Hoshino T, Fujiwara H, Kawai C, Hamashima Y (1982) Diagnostic value of disarray in endomyocardial biopsy specimens in hypertrophic cardiomyopathy. J Circ J 46: 1281—1291
9. Hoshino T, Fujiwara H, Kawai C, Hamashima Y (1983) Myocardial fiber diameter and regional distribution in the ventricular wall of normal adult hearts, hypertensive hearts and hearts with hypertrophic cardiomyopathy. Circulation 67: 1109—1116
10. Isner GM, Maron BJ, Roberts WC (1980) Comparison of amount of myocardial cell disorganization in operatively excised septectomy specimen with amount observed at necropsy in 18 patients with hypertrophic cardiomyopathy. Am J Cardiol 46: 42—47
11. Loud AV, Anversa P (1984) Biology of disease. Morphometric analysis of biologic process. Lab Invest 50: 250—261
12. Mall G, Schwarz F, Derks H (1982) Clinicopathologic correlations in congestive cardiomyopathy. Virchows Archiv (Pathol Anat) 397: 67—82
13. Maron BJ, Anan TJ, Roberts WC (1981) Quantitative analysis of the distribution of cardiac muscle cell disorganization in the left ventricular wall of patients with hypertrophic cardiomyopathy. Circulation 63: 882—894
14. Maron BJ, Spiriti P, Wesley Y, Arce J (1986) Development and progression of left ventricular hypertrophy in children with hypertrophic cardiomyopathy. Engl J Med 315: 610—614
15. Mathieu O, Cruz-Orive L M, Hoppeler H, Weibel E R (1980) Measuring error and sampling variation in stereology: Comparison of the efficacy of various methods for planar image analysis. J Microscopy 121: 75—88

16. Sakakibara S, Konno S (1962) Endomyocardial biopsy. Jpn Heart J 3: 537—543
17. Schwartzkopff B, Heusch A, Frenzel H (1984) Makroskopisch, lichtmikroskopisch und elektro-nenmikroskopisch-morphometrische Befunde bei der Autolyse des Herzmuskels. Verh Dtsch Ges Path 68: 510
18. Unverferth D V, Baker P B, Swift S E, Chaffee R, Fetters J K, Uretsky B F, Thompson M E, Leier CL (1986) Extent of myocardial fibrosis and cellular hypertrophy in dilated cardiomy-opathy. Am J Cardiol 57: 816—820

Authors' address:
Dr. Bodo Schwartzkopff, Department of Cardiology, Moorenstr. 5, D-4000 Düsseldorf 1, F.R.G.

Myocardial biopsy in patients with hypertrophic cardiomyopathy: Correlations between morphologic and clinical parameters and development of myocardial hypertrophy under medical therapy

B. Kunkel, M. Schneider, A. Eisenmenger, B. Bergmann, R. Hopf, M. Kaltenbach

Medizinische Poliklinik der Universität Erlangen und Zentrum der Inneren Medizin und Zentrum der Pathologie des Klinikums der Universität Frankfurt, F.R.G.

Introduction

Except for a few patients with myocarditis or other specific heart muscle diseases, such as amyloidosis, sarcoidosis and others, the diagnotic value of myocardial biopsy is limited. It has been shown, however, that there are certain correlations between structure and function of the myocardium. This has been demonstrated in patients with dilative cardiomyopathy and in aortic valve disease. An analysis of structure and function of the myocardium in hypertrophic cardiomyopathy has not been performed so far.

Medical treatment with calcium blockers has been shown to improve cardiac symptoms in a majority of patients with hypertrophic cardiomyopathy. The question of whether the underlying hypertrophic process can be influenced by this treatment is, however, a matter of discussion. This study was designed, therefore, to evaluate possible correlations between morphology and clinical parameters and the development of myocardial hypertrophy under medical treatment.

Patients and Methods

Left ventricular biopsies from 38 patients with hypertrophic cardiomyopathy were analyzed in the study. The diagnosis was established by echocardiography and right and left heart catheterization including coronary angiography and biplane ventriculography. There were 31 male and seven female patients. The mean age was 40.5 ± 11.7 years. 28 patients presented with an intraventricular pressure gradient of more than 30 mmHg while ten had no gradient.

A second biopsy procedure was performed in 11 patients with hypertrophic cardiomyopathy after medical therapy of 33 ± 12.6 months. Among these 11 patients, nine were treated with verapamil and two with propranolol. In one of the latter, the betablocker therapy was replaced by verapamil because of clinical deterioration.

During the initial diagnostic catheterization and the control angiography under medical treatment, two biopsy specimens were excised from the left ventricular posterior free wall. One was fixed in 4% formalin for light microscopy. The sections were routinely stained with hematoxylin-eosin and Goldner for microscopic analysis. The second specimen was fixed in 2.5% glutaraldehyde for electron microscopy.

The following parameters were measured:

1. Mean cell diameter (100 cells measured).
2. Size of the nuclei of the myofibers (volume density of the nuclei).
3. Interstitial fibrous tissue.
4. Volume density of the myofibrils (in patients with repeated biopsies).
5. Volume density of the mitochondria (in patients with repeated biopsies). (For details of the procedure see chapter „Myocardial structure and left ventricular function . . .").

The microscopic findings from patients with hypertrophic cardiomyopathy were compared with those obtained from 60 patients with advanced dilative cardiomyopathy. The morphological data were compared with various clinical data, such as intraventricular gradient, filling pressure, the radiologically measured heart volume, Sokolow-Lion-Index and the clinical stage.

Results

Histology

The histologic findings of the biopsies are compiled in Table 1. Myocardial hypertrophy was present in all patients with dilative cardiomyopathy and HNCM, while 29% of the HOCM cases had no evidence of myocardial hypertrophy in the biopsies from the left ventricular posterior wall. Disarray of myofibers was observed in 25% and 30% of the patients with HOCM and HNCM, respectively, but it was also seen in a small number of patients with dilative cardiomyopathy (8%). Degenerative changes of the myocytes

Table 1. Histologic findings in patients with HOCM, HNCM and DCM.

	HNCM (N = 10)		HOCM (N = 28)		DCM (N = 60)	
	N	%	N	%	N	%
Myocardial hypertrophy	10	100	23	82	60	100
Degenerative alterations of the myocytes	2	20	5	18	28	47
Irregular arrangement of the myocytes	3	30	7	25	5	8
Interstitial fibrosis	5	50	9	32	46	77
Endocardial fibrosis	1	10	3	11	23	38
Increase in fibrocytes fibroblasts and histiocytes	—	—	6	21	9	15
Inflammatory infiltrations	—	—	—	—	1	1.6
Normal myocardium	—	—	5	18	—	—
M. Fabry	—	—	1	3.5	—	—

and interstitial fibrosis were both seen more often and were more severe in dilative cardiomyopathies than in the hypertrophic form. Areas showing an increase in fibroblasts and histiocytes could be observed in both groups. In one patient with HOCM (pressure gradient 39 mmHg at rest and 64 mmHg after provocation) light and electron microscopy revealed an M. Fabry. All other changes listed in the table were seen in both HCM and DCM.

Morphology and clinical parameters

To analyze possible relations between myocardial structure and function, the morphological parameters, cell diameter, nuclear volume and interstitial fibrous tissue content were correlated with various clinical data, such as intraventricular gradient, filling pressure, heart volume, Sokolow-Lion-Index (Table 2). An analysis of whether high intraventricular pressure gradients or high enddiastolic filling pressure correlate with more pronounced forms of myocardial hypertrophy is shown in Figs. 1 and 2. A similar degree of myocardial hypertrophy was observed in patients with high and low pressure gradients and in the non-obstructive form of the disease. The filling pressure reflecting left ven-

Table 2. Correlations between clinical and morphologic findings.

	Correlation coefficiente	Nuclear volume	Connective tissue
Heart volume	0.28	0.20	0.11
Sokolow-Index	0.08	0.52	0.12
Filling pressure	0.20	0.19	0.02
Gradient	0.12	0.10	0.03
Muscle mass	0.26	0.19	0.08

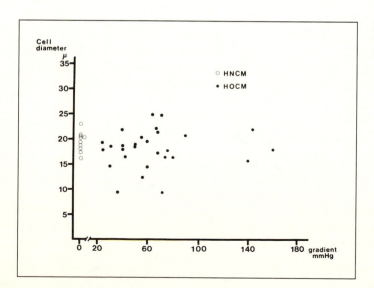

Fig. 1. Pressure gradient and myocardial hypertrophy.

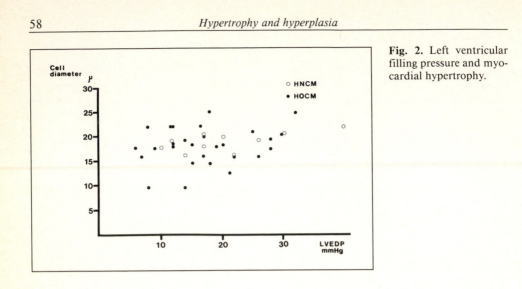

tricular compliance also showed no correlation with the severity of myocardial hypertrophy. Identical fiber diameters were found in patients with normal and elevated filling
pressures.

Neither the fiber diameter nor any other morphologic parameters tested, such as nuclear size, or connective tissue content of the biopsy specimen, showed any correlation
to various clinical parameters such as pressure gradient, filling pressure, Sokolow-Index
and the radiologic heart size (Table 2).

Morphologic changes under medical therapy

The development of myocardial hypertrophy could be analyzed in 11 patients after
2—5 years of medical treatment (Fig. 3). An increasing fiber diameter was observed in
the second biopsy in all 11 patients. In most of them, the increase in cell diameter was
mild, ranging between 1 and 4 μm. Three of the patients, however, showed a tremendous
growth of myocardial hypertrophy (increase in fiber size > 5 μm). The number of patients without and with mild forms of myocardial hypertrophy apparently decreases during the course of the disease, while more patients present with moderate and severe
hypertrophy. The histograms of all 11 patients revealed the typical signs of growing hypertrophy: Widening of the basis, shift of the mean diameter towards higher values and
flattening of the peak of the curve (Fig. 4).

The nuclear volume of the myocytes as another parameter of myocardial hypertrophy
increased in seven out of 11 patients, while in four cases, identical or slightly decreasing
values were noted (Fig. 5). Increasing nuclear volume represents an additional and independently measured parameter of growing hypertrophy in the course of the disease.
The mean fibrous tissue content increased from 6% to 12% (Fig. 6). The detailed analysis
revealed a slight decrease of interstitial fibrosis in two patients, another presented with
unchanged values while a significant increase in interstitial fibrous tissue was found in
eight patients.

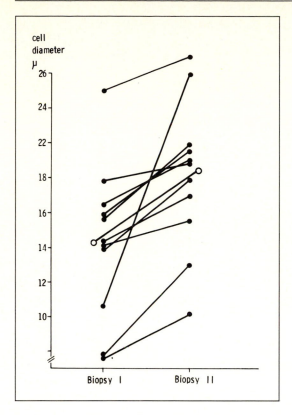

Fig. 3. Myocardial hypertrophy in HCM.

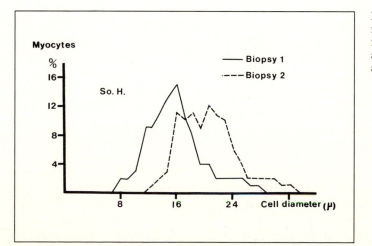
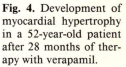

Fig. 4. Development of myocardial hypertrophy in a 52-year-old patient after 28 months of therapy with verapamil.

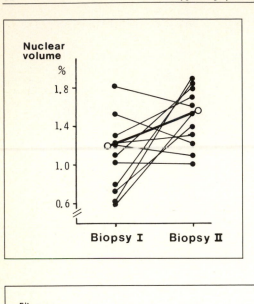

Fig. 5. Nuclear volume in HCM.

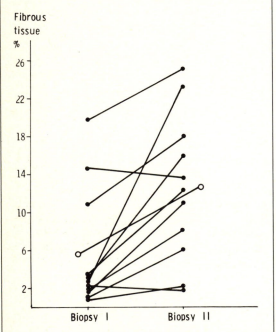

Fig. 6. Interstitial fibrous tissue in HCM.

The volume fraction of myofibrils, mitochondria and sarcoplasm were measured on the electron microscopic level in 11 patients.

In ten of them, a significant decrease in the volume fraction of myofibrils (48.8 ± 2.7% vs. 43.6 ± 5.3%) was observed during the observation period (Fig. 7). One patient pre-

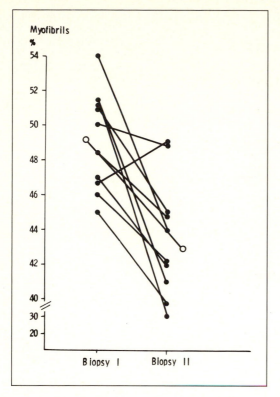

Fig. 7. Volume fraction of myofibrils in HCM.

sented with slightly increasing values. The mitochondrial volume remained unchanged (27.5 ± 3.9% vs. 28.3 ± 5.1%) while the volume fraction of the sarcoplasm increased (23.4 ± 3.5% vs. 27.7 ± 8.3%).

Morphologic changes and clinical course

After 33 ± 12.6 months of therapy, five patients were classified as unchanged from their clinical parameters (Fig. 8a). In all of them, an increase in cell diameter, nuclear volume and connective tissue was observed. Four patients were classified as clinically improved (Fig. 8b), and in all of them an increase in cell diameter was seen. The nuclear volume was increased in one patient and slightly reduced in another. The interstitial fibrous tissue showed an increase in three of these patients. Two patients deteriorated clinically (Fig. 8c). Both presented with severer forms of myocardial hypertrophy, as indicated by an increasing cell diameter and nuclear size. The connective tissue increased in one patient and decreased in the other.

Discussion

The characteristic histological appearance of hypertrophic cardiomyopathies consists of hypertrophied abnormally shaped, irregularly arranged muscle cells. Small foci of these

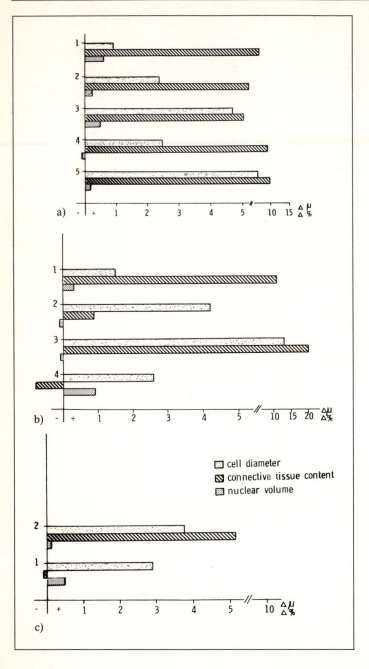

Fig. 8. Clinical course and morphology in patients classified as (a) unchanged ($N = 5$); (b) improved ($N = 4$); (c) deteriorated ($N = 2$).

cells can, however, be found under various other conditions: Ferrans (2) observed disarray of myofibers in 10% of patients with congestive cardiomyopathy and in 18% of patients with congenital heart disease associated with right ventricular hypertrophy and obstruction. Maron and coworkers (7) pointed out that it is not the presence of cell disorganization itself, but the number of cells involved that is characteristic of hypertrophic cardiomyopathy. The biopsy specimens, however, usually are too small to evaluate the true extent of fiber disarray of the total myocardium, even if a greater number of samples are taken into consideration. A positive diagnosis of hypertrophic cardiomyopathy in most cases cannot therefore be made from the myocardial biopsy (4).

While in most patients with dilative cardiomyopathy and aortic valve disease with reduced ventricular function, the burned out late stage hypertrophy of the myocardium can easily be recognized from the biopsy (5, 9), in HCM, normal or only mild reduction of the contractile elements was observed representing hypertrophy in the compensated stage. The various clinical abnormalities in hypertrophic cardiomyopathy seem to be caused by functional disorders or contractility and relaxation, more than by structural changes of the hypertrophied myocardium.

The hypertrophied myocardium forms the morphologic basis for the various clinical and hemodynamic signs of hypertrophic cardiomyopathies. Consequently, this study was designed to analyze whether the degree of myocardial hypertrophy shows correlations with various clinical parameters. Our results show, however, that no such correlations exist. Identical forms of hypertrophy were observed in patients with high and low intraventricular pressure gradient and in those without gradient. The left ventricular filling pressure also yielded no correlation with clinical and hemodynamic parameters. Also, the degree of interstitial fibrosis showed no correlation with various clinical parameters. Cellular disorganization yielded none, or only pure correlations with clinical symptoms: Maron (7) found no correlation between the extent of fiber disorganization and sex distribution, duration of symptoms, enddiastolic pressure, heart weight, septal thickness. He found the most marked disorganization in younger people without functional limitation and, in a number of patients, without outflow tract obstruction. In an echocardiography study, Spirito and coworkers (11) found the enddiastolic abnormalities to be more pronounced in patients with extensive wall thickening, compared to those with milder forms of hypertrophy. However, he pointed out that the diastolic abnormalities were also found in ventricular segments of normal thickness. Furthermore, from the clinical experience there is no clear correlation between the various functional expressions of the hypertrophic process, e.g. gradient, filling pressure, ECG and wall thickness and clinical symptoms. Although it is clear that the irregularly hypertrophied myocardium represents the basic condition of the hypertrophic cardiomyopathy, the pathophysiological mechanism of the various clinical and hemodynamic patterns and their relationship to the extent and severity of the hypertrophic process is not completely understood.

The clinical course in HOCM is slowly progressive in the majority of patients. However, absence of symptoms for life or constant clinical stages also occur (10). Progression of myocardial hypertrophy has been demonstrated by echocardiography and ECG in 13—20% of the patients (1, 6). Calcium antagonists have been shown to improve the clinical and hemodynamic symptoms in the majority of patients with HOCM (3). Reduction of the muscle mass and reduction of septal thickness have also been reported (3). This study represents the first bioptical analysis of the course of myocardial hypertrophy under medical treatment. It shows a progression of hypertrophy in all cases analyzed within a relatively short observation time. In addition, the increase in interstitial fibrous tissue content was found in most patients. This was observed regardless of the clinical outcome, which was improved in five and stable in four and worsened in two patients only. From our observations, it may be suggested that the clinical benefit of calcium channel blockers is achieved by functional pharmacologic effects on the contraction and relaxation of the myocardium, while the underlying hypertrophic process of unknown origin is not influenced. On the other hand, from the natural history of hypertrophic cardiomyopathy in larger studies it is unlikely that our observations can generally be transmitted to all patients with hypertrophic cardiomyopathy. This has to be analyzed in larger studies.

Summary: Left ventricular biopsies from 38 patients with hypertrophic cardiomyopathy (HOCM 28, HNCM 10) were investigated to evaluate possible correlations between morphological and clinical parameters.

No correlation was found between the degree of myocardial hypertrophy (muscle cell diameter), nuclear size of the myocytes, fibrous tissue content and various clinical data such as pressure gradient, left ventricular enddiastolic pressure, Sokolow index and heart volume. In 11 patients with HOCM, a second biopsy was performed after medical therapy (verapamil, n = 9; propranolol, n = 2) over 33 ± 12 months. Increasing myocardial hypertrophy (cell diameter $16.2 \pm 4.4\,\mu$ vs. $20.3 \pm 4.2\,\mu$) was observed in all 11 patients. The interstitial fibrous tissue content increased from 5.7 ± 6.3 to $12.7 \pm 6.8\%$. The volume fraction of myofibrils decreased (48.8 ± 2.7 vs. $43.6 \pm 5.3\%$). The morphological changes were observed regardless of the clinical outcome which was improved in four, unchanged in five and worsened in two cases. The underlying hypertrophic process in HCM seems to be slowly progressive in most patients and cannot be influenced by medical treatment.

References

1. Domenicucci S, Lazzeroni E, Roelandt J, Ten Cate FJ, Vletter WB, Arntzenius AC, Das SK (1985) Progression of hypertrophic cardiomyopathy. A cross sectional echocardiographic study. Br Heart J 53: 405—411
2. Ferrans VJ (1978) Myocardial ultrastructure in human cardiac hypertrophy. In: Kaltenbach M, Loogen F, Olsen EGJ (eds) Cardiomyopathy and myocardial biopsy. Springer Verlag, Berlin—Heidelberg—New York, pp 100—120
3. Kaltenbach M, Hopf R, Kober G, Bußmann WD, Keller M, Petersen Y (1979) Treatment of hypertrophic obstructive cardiomyopathy with Verapamil. Br Heart J 42: 35—42
4. Kunkel B, Schneider M, Hopf R, Kober G, Hübner K, Kaltenbach M (1982) Left ventricular biopsy in hypertrophic cardiomyopathy: Light and electron microscopic evaluation. In: Kaltenbach M, Epstein SE (eds). Hypertrophic cardiomyopathy. The therapeutic role of calcium antagonists. Springer Verlag, Berlin—Heidelberg—New York, pp 58—69
5. Kunkel B, Schneider M, Kober G, Bußmann WD, Hopf R, Kaltenbach M (1982) Die Morphologie der Myokardbiopsie und ihre klinische Bedeutung. Z Kardiol 71: 787—794
6. Deanfield J, Oakley CM, Goodwin JF (1982) The natural history of left ventricular hypertrophy in hypertrophic cardiomyopathy: an electrocardiographic study. Circulation 66: 1233—1240
7. Maron BJ, Roberts WC (1982) Distribution of cardiac muscle cell disorganization in the left ventricle of patients with hypertrophic cardiomyopathy: Evidence of a diffuse cardiomyopathic process. In: Kaltenbach M, Epstein SE (eds). Hypertrophic cardiomyopathy. The therapeutic role of calcium antagonists. Springer Verlag, Berlin—Heidelberg—New York, pp 38—57
8. Maron BJ, Roberts WC (1979) Quantitative analysis of cardiac muscle cell disorganization in the ventricular septum of patients with hypertrophic cardiomyopathy. Circulation 59: 689—706

9. Schwarz F, Schaper J, Kitstein D, Flameng W, Walter P, Schaper W (1981) Reduced volume fraction of myofibrils in myocardium of patients with decompensated pressure overload. Circulation 63: 1299—1304

10. Shah PM, Adelman AG, Wigle DD, Gobel FL, Burchell HB, Hardarson T, Curiel R, DelaCalzada C, Oakley CM, Goodwin JF (1973) The natural (and unnatural) course of hypertrophic obstructive cardiomyopathy. A multicenter study. Circ Res (Suppl II) 24; 25: 179—195

11. Spirito P, Maron BJ, Chiarella F, Belotti P, Tramarin R, Pozzoli M, Vecchio C (1985) Diastolic abnormalities in patients with hypertrophic cardiomyopathy: relation to magnitude of left ventricular hypertrophy. Circulation 72: 310—316

Authors' address:

Prof. Dr. B. Kunkel, Medizinische Poliklinik der Universität Erlangen,
Östliche Stadtmauerstraße 29, 8520 Erlangen, F.R.G.

Radionuclide ventriculography: acute and chronic response to verapamil in patients with hypertrophic cardiomyopathy[1]

F. D. Maul, R. Hopf, G. Hör, R. Standke, H. Richter, H. G. Olbrich, J. Happ

Division of General Nuclear Medicine and Cardiology,
J. W. Goethe University, Frankfurt, F.R.G.

Introduction

Procedures of nuclear cardiology are applied to the diagnosis and follow-up of hypertrophic cardiomyopathy in two aspects: (a) in the determination of myocardial thickening and (b) to document functional response to therapy. For morphological studies, Tl-201 myocardial scintigraphy was introduced by Bulkeley in 1975 (7). Using a gated SPECT technique for myocardial scintigraphy, the wall thickening in different myocardial regions could be recorded (25). Soon after their introduction, gated blood pool studies were utilized to image regional dimension and motion of the myocardial wall (17). Later, instead of gated blood pool studies, one and two dimensional echocardiography were employed (8, 16). Besides morphological parameters, regional functional data at rest are available which enable one to quantify regional disorders and responses to drugs (6, 9, 21, 24). Nuclear cardiological measurements of global left ventricular functions, based on analysis of the left ventricular volume curve (time activity curve), were introduced by Bonow (3) in patients with hypertrophic cardiomyopathy before and during verapamil treatment.

It was shown by echocardiography that left ventricular relaxation and filling characteristics could be impressively improved by verapamil, nifedipin, and even propanolol (6, 9, 15, 20, 21). Using radionuclide ventriculography at rest, parameters of global time and volume changes of the left ventricle were significantly improved, especially in the filling phase (3, 5, 12). The increase of peak filling rate correlated with the improvement in exercise capacity. The clinical response was more pronounced after 1—4 weeks as compared to results after 1—2 years (5).

By the use of radionuclide ventriculography, we (11) described a marked asynchronicity of left and right ventricular Fourier phases, in patients with hypertrophic cardiomyopathy, which synchronized under verapamil. Recently, Bonow et al (4) have presented data indicating functional improvements in patients with hypertrophic cardiomyo-

---

[1] Dedicated to Prof. Dr. H. Kriegel on the occasion of his 65th birthday.

pathy before and during treatment with verapamil, using global and regional parameters of radionuclide ventriculography.

Besides changes in global ventricular function, it may be assumed that hypertrophic cardiomyopathy also induces regional disorders both in the ejection and in the filling phase. This assumption is based on at least two findings: (a) patients have various degrees of regional hypertrophy and (b) in cases of outflow tract obstruction, regional functional disturbances in the ejection period must be expected and can be demonstrated (11).

The aim of this investigation was to study the therapeutic response of verapamil (a) on the left ventricle regionally, in combination with global parameters in systole and diastole and to quantify (b) the resynchronization of the left ventricular delay of Fourier phases.

Patients and Methods

Patients

We investigated 11 patients, eight males and three females (nine: seven males, two females) under short- or long-term verapamil treatment), with echocardiographically, angiographically, and hemodynamically confirmed hypertrophic cardiomyopathy. Their mean age was 43 (range 17 to 65 years). All patients underwent cardiac catheterization with measurement of left ventricular enddiastolic pressure and intraventricular systolic pressure gradient. Five patients had an obstruction of the outflow tract with a pressure gradient of 30 mmHg or more. Before the onset of verapamil therapy, three patients were free of complaints. Three patients were classified as stage II, two as stage III, and one as stage IV according to the New York Heart Association (Table 1).

Table 1. Patients.

Number of patients	11(9)*⁾
males	8(7)*⁾
females	3(2)*⁾
Age	
mean	43
range	17—65
Verapamil dosage	
mean	516 mg/day
range	320—640 mg/day
With obstruction (patients)	5
Clinical stage (NYHA (control period/during verapamil))	
stage I	3/5
stage II	3/3
stage III	2/1
stage IV	1/0
Number of controls (patients with coronary artery disease (with and without infarction))	17
number of radionuclide ventriculographies	2
time interval (min)	60

*⁾ ( ) under short- and long-term verapamil treatment.

Controls

17 patients with coronary heart disease served as untreated controls. These patients were investigated twice, at rest after withdrawal of medication, within an interval of 60 min between both studies.

Because the investigation of normal volunteers is not allowed in West Germany, all our standard values were derived from patients with single-vessel disease without myocardial infarction after successful transluminal angioplasty (23). Ventriculography and exercise ECG were entirely normalized and the patients were free of any clinical symptoms. The mean values of the sectors served as a standard profile.

Study design

The patients in the study group were investigated at rest during four different treatment phases:

First phase: initially nine out of 11 patients were under long-term verapamil treatment. The mean verapamil dose was 516 mg/day (range 320—640), and the mean duration of therapy was 57 months (range 14—84 months).

Second phase: control period 2 weeks after withdrawal of verapamil.

Third phase: immediately after phase 2, nine patients received 160 mg verapamil orally and were investigated 90 min later without a new application of radioactivity for the acute response. In two patients 50 mg gallopamil was given.

Fourth phase: the final radionuclide ventriculography was carried out 2 weeks after renewed verapamil treatment ($n = 9$).

Radionuclide ventriculography

We used a software package developed in our nuclear medicine division using a fully automated procedure of acquisition and processing which has been described earlier (22, 23). All investigations were carried out on patients at rest in an ECG-gated frame mode acquisition; a standardized acquisition time of 5 min was chosen. Time-activity curves were corrected for varying cycle length by scaling all frames to the same acquisition time and filtered by Fourier transformation. Left and right ventricular regions of interest (ROIs) were defined automatically. Ejection fraction (EF) and peak filling rate were calculated globally and in sectors. In addition, peak ejection rate, ejection time, rapid filling time were computed globally. The various cardiac cycle times were derived from the 1st and 2nd derivative of the time-activity curve.

For determining sectorial parameters, the left ventricular enddiastolic region of interest was divided in nine equiangular sectors around the center of gravity (Fig. 1). The profiles of ejection fraction were computed using the absolute sectorial values and the profiles of peak filling rate using the differences from the global peak filling rate. To reduce the amount of data, the sectorial results of basal sectors (1, 2, 7, 8, 9) and apical sectors (3—6) were combined and the mean deviation from the standard profile calculated.

Regional Fourier phase analysis was carried out using the method introduced by Adam and coworkers (1).

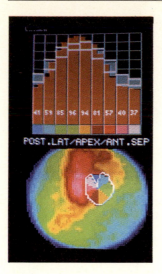

Fig. 1. Radionuclide ventriculography example of an untreated patient with HCM. Upper panel: supernormal ejection fraction in apical sectors. Rectangles indicate the normal range (22). Lower panel: enddiastolic image with the left ventricular region of interest subdivided in 9 equiangular sectors.

Data analysis

Mean values and standard deviations of all studies of each treatment phase were calculated. The parameters were compared with the paired value of each control phase. The number of pairs depends on the number of studies of the particular treatment phase. In the untreated control group, the first study was compared with the second. Wilcoxon nonparametric tests were used. The statistical significance of differences was assessed as significant at $p < 0.05$.

Results

Clinical findings

During long-term verapamil treatment, four out of nine patients presented with improvement of their clinical symptoms, four patients were unchanged and one patient worsened. No patient remained in stage IV or III according to the New York Heart Association classification (Table 1).

Heart rate

The heart rate increased significantly ($p < 0.01$) after acute oral administration (79.9 ± 14.8 l/min) compared with the control period (68.5 ± 10.2 l/min). Under short-term as well as under long-term verapamil therapy, the heart rate remained unchanged (70.0 ± 13.1, and 71.0 ± 14.5 l/min, respectively (Table 2)).

Enddiastolic volume

In the control period, EDV (166.1 ± 29.2) was within the normal range (124–226), and did not change significantly in any of the treatment phases (Table 2).

Table 2. Heart rate and enddiastolic volume (mean and standard deviation) in the control period (CP), after acute administration (AC), and during short-term (ST), and long-term (LT) verapamil treatment of patients with hypertrophic cardiomyopathy (HCM), as well as in a first and second radionuclide ventriculography at rest in patients with coronary artery disease (CAD), as a control.

	HCM				CAD	
	CP	AC	ST	LT	1st	2nd
n	11	11	9	8	17	17
Heart rate (l/min)	68.5	79.9	70.0	71.0	73.7	75.2
SD	10.2	14.8	13.1	14.4	16.9	16.9
compared with CP (1st)	—	p<0.01	n.s.	n.s.	—	n.s.
EDV (ml)	166.1	173.4	170.8	156.1	161.8	154.9
SD	29.2	35.5	35.4	48.0	45.0	39.0
compared with CP (1st)	—	n.s.	n.s.	n.s.	—	n.s.

Systolic parameters

Ejection time was significantly shortened after acute administration (from 309.5 ± 28.8 to 278.4 ± 50.1 ms ($p < 0.05$)) and also under short-term treatment (283.6 ± 29.1 ms ($p \leqslant 0.01$)). No change was observed under long-term therapy (312.1 ± 89.5 ms (Table 2)). The peak ejection rate did not change significantly under verapamil treatment at any time (Table 3).

Global EF during the control period (72.6 ± 11.1 %) was in the upper normal range (50—79) and decreased nonsignificantly under long-term treatment to 68.6 ± 12.1 % (Table 2). Global EF normalized in three of five patients with a supernormal (> 79 %) value in the control period.

Mean sectorial EF of apical and basal sectors were higher then the corresponding standard mean sectorial EF. However, the sectorial EF of apical sectors presented a slight but significant relative reduction compared with basal sectors in the control phase (untreated HCM patients) as well as after acute application of verapamil. This intraventricular EF difference was normalized under short-and long-term treatment (Table 3). The normalization was due to a regional improvement in the apical sectors and decreasing EF values in the basal sectors (Fig. 2).

Diastolic parameters

Time-to-peak filling rate after the withdrawal of verapamil was 185.7 ± 25.3 ms and decreased insignificantly to 180.6 ± 35.3 ms after acute administration and to 172.4 ± 18.6 ms under short-term treatment (Table 4). Under long-term treatment, time-to-peak filling rate remained nearly unchanged, compared to the control period (188.8 ± 65.7 ms). Rapid filling time only showed a tendency to decrease from 345.4 ± 112.8 to 314.5 ± 65.9 ms (acute administration), 313.1 ± 73.4 ms (short-term; N.S.), and 309.8 ± 98.5 ms (long-term; N.S.). In the control period, global peak filling rate was found to be normal (283.5 ± 61.2 %/EDV/s), and increased significantly ($p < 0.01$) after acute administration (325.5 ± 63.5). Under short- and long-term administration, no

Table 3. Left ventricular systolic parameters (mean and standard deviation) in the control period (CP), after acute administration of verapamil (AC), and during short-term (ST), and long-term (LT) verapamil treatment of patients with hypertrophic cardiomyopathy (HCM), as well as in a first and second radionuclide ventriculography at rest in patients with coronary artery disease (CAD), as a control.

	HCM				CAD	
	CP	AC	ST	LT	1st	2nd
n	11	11	9	8	17	17
ejection time (ms)	309.5	278.4	283.6	312.1	281.0	278.2
SD	28.8	50.1	29.1	89.5	50.3	49.9
compared with CP (1st)	—	$p<0.05$	$p<0.01$	N.S.	—	N.S.
peak ejection rate (%/EDV/s)	362.7	398.0	351.2	343.4	275.1	294.1
SD	70.3	76.6	74.1	105.8	59.7	65.8
compared with CP (1st)	—	N.S.	N.S.	N.S.	—	N.S.
global EF (%)	72.5	72.8	68.6	68.6	53.0	54.4
SD	11.1	11.5	10.1	12.1	11.1	11.2
compared with CP (1st)	—	N.S.	N.S.	N.S.	—	N.S.
mean basal EF (%)	13.3	11.8	8.3	8.1	9.1	7.4
SD	10.4	10.9	10.3	11.3	8.9	12.2
mean apical EF (%)	9.9	7.7	5.4	6.5	9.2	7.4
SD	11.7	13.1	10.7	12.7	13.6	13.6
basal vs. apical	$p<0.05$	$p<0.05$	N.S.	N.S.	N.S.	N.S.

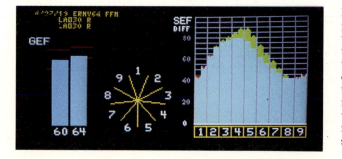

Fig. 2. Comparison of control phase with long-term verapamil treatment by means of differential profiles (right side) in a patient with hypertrophic cardiomyopathy. Left: global ejection fraction increased slightly from 60 % to 64 %. Right: under verapamil sectorial ejection fraction normalized in anteroseptal region (arrows).

significant increase could be seen (short-term, 289.6 ± 66.1; long-term 288.1 ± 94.8; Table 4).

Without verapamil, as well as under short-term treatment, sectorial peak filling rate was slightly but significantly reduced in apical compared to basal sectors and normalized after acute administration and under long-term treatment (Table 4, Fig. 3).

Left to right ventricular synchronicity

The shapes of left and right ventricular phase histograms were symmetric in patients with hypertrophic cardiomyopathy. However, in six out of 11 patients, the left ventricular

Table 4. Left ventricular diastolic parameters (mean and standard deviation) in the control period (CP), after acute administration of verapamil (AC), and during short-term (ST), and long-term (LT) verapamil treatment of patients with hypertrophic cardiomyopathy (HCM) as well as in a first and second radionuclide ventriculography at rest in patients with coronary artery disease (CAD), as a control.

	HCM				CAD	
	CP	AC	ST	LT	1st	2nd
n	11	11	9	8	17	17
rapid filling time (ms)	345.4	314.5	313.1	309.8	250.1	253.5
SD	112.8	65.9	73.7	98.5	39.8	33.3
compared with CP (1st)	—	N.S.	N.S.	N.S.	—	N.S.
time to peak filling (ms)	185.7	180.6	172.4	188.9	162.4	166.8
SD	25.3	35.3	18.6	65.7	27.8	20.6
compared with CP (1st)	—	N.S.	N.S.	N.S.	—	N.S.
global peak filling rate (%/EDV/s)	283.5	325.0	289.6	288.1	232.3	236.0
SD	61.2	63.5	66.2	94.8	63.8	65.8
compared with CP (1st)	—	$p<0.01$	N.S.	N.S.	—	N.S.
mean basal peak filling rate	14.1	0.4	13.0	2.3	5.3	6.1
SD	32.4	20.1	13.7	23.9	10.0	14.9
mean apical peak filling rate	−8.4	−8.2	−9.9	4.6	−12.6	−18.3
SD	44.9	21.1	19.5	45.6	8.3	8.1
basal vs. apical	$p<0.025$	N.S.	$p<0.05$	N.S.	$p<0.05$	$p<0.05$

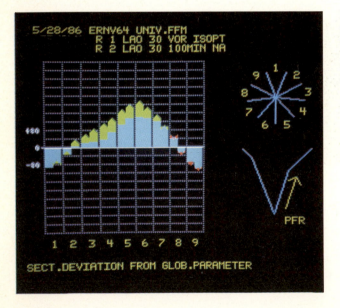

Fig. 3. Accentuated sectorial improvement of peak filling rate in apical sectors after acute verapamil administration in a patient with hypertrophic cardiomyopathy.

peak of Fourier phases presented a marked delay (Fig. 4a). As a measure of left ventricular phase delay, we calculated the difference of the mean phase of both ventricles. Untreated

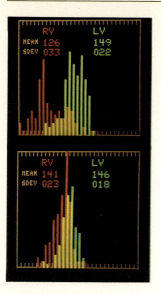

Fig. 4. Distribution of right and left ventricular Fourier phases: Control period (a), and long-term treatment with verapamil (b) in a patient with hypertrophic cardiomyopathy. The pathologic phase shift (a) between both ventricles was reduced markedly under long-term treatment (b).

patients had a mean phase delay of 11.7 ± 12.2 degrees. No significant change occurred after acute administration of verapamil, but during short-term therapy, the phases of both ventricles synchronized significantly ($p < 0.01$) and the mean phase difference was 1.4 ± 7.3 degrees. Under long-term therapy, the mean phase delay of the left ventricle remained decreased (Fig. 4b) at 4.1 ± 6.5 degrees (Table 5).

Controls

Globally, as well as sectorially, no significant differences could be observed between the first and second study of the untreated controls (patients suffering from coronary heart disease).

Table 5. Follow-up of left to right ventricular difference of Fourier phases (mean and standard deviation) in a control period (CP) (14 days after withdrawal of verapamil, after acute administration (AC), and during short-term (ST), and long-term (LT) treatment of verapamil in patients with hypertrophic cardiomyopathy (HCM) as well as in a first and second radionuclide ventriculography at rest in patients with coronary artery disease (CAD), as a control.

	HCM				CAD	
	CP	AC	ST	LT	1st	2nd
n	11	11	9	8	17	17
left/right phase delay	11.7	8.6	1.4	4.1	2.7	2.7
SD	12.2	9.8	9.8	6.5	5.3	5.2
compared with CP (1st)	—	N.S.	$p<0.01$	$p<0.05$	—	N.S.

Discussion

Diastolic function

Verapamil reduces the symptoms of patients with hypertrophic cardiomyopathy (10, 12—14, 18, 19). Recent publications support the hypothesis that in patients with hypertrophic cardiomyopathy, global left ventricular diastolic function primarily is improved by verapamil (3, 5, 9, 11, 12, 14). In our study, peak filling rate improved significantly only after acute oral administration but showed a nonsignificant increase under short and long term verapamil treatment. In concordance with these findings, no significant change of rapid filling time, and time-to-peak filling rate were observed. These results differ from those of other groups (2, 9, 15) especially those of Bonow (3, 5), in which a significant improvement of those diastolic parameters under verapamil and other Ca blocking agents could be seen. The most likely reason for these differences could be the acquisition in the gated frame mode, which is not sensitive enough to register smaller diastolic changes.

On the other hand, our data prove the hypothesis that the regional diastolic function of the left ventricle is improved by verapamil treatment. Calculating the mean deviation of sectorial peak filling rates of apical and basal sectors, verapamil normalized the relative decrease of the apical peak filling rate in patients with hypertrophic cardiomyopathy. Comparing sectorial with global results, our data — based on ECG gated frame mode acquisition — indicate that sectorial parameters of the left ventricular filling phase are more sensitive.

Systolic function

In patients with hypertrophic cardiomyopathy, systolic function as shown by ejection fraction, peak ejection rate, and ejection time do not indicate a negative inotropic response. Only the ejection fraction profile normalized by increasing fraction in the apical sectors, while basal sectors decrease relatively.

A slight negative response can only be assumed in patients with a supernormal global EF in the control phase which decreases to the normal range under verapamil in three out of five patients. No significant chronotropic response was found in our patients.

Left to right ventricular synchronicity

In contrast, during verapamil treatment, the contraction of left ventricle normalized in four out of nine patients as shown by adjusting the Fourier phases of the left ventricle to those of the right ventricle. According to the ECG, this response was interpreted as a reduction of an incomplete left ventricular bundle branch block (11). However, judging from the symmetrical shape of the left ventricular phase histogram, it is not the reduction of a left ventricular bundle branch block which is characterized by a posterolateral delay of sectorial phases but a homogeneous increase of the left ventricular contraction. Even if the underlying mechanism is unknown, delay and adjustment of Fourier phases can be assumed as a monitor of therapeutic response.

In conclusion: Our results indicate that verapamil causes a more pronounced improvement of regional diastolic function than global function. This is detectable as an acute response and is more pronounced as a long-term effect of verapamil. Regional improvement of diastolic function was not only more sensitive but also demonstrated a significant long-term response. No significant global negative verapamil effect could be seen. Regionally, the ejection fraction improved in the apical sectors. Under verapamil, a homogeneous delay of the left ventricular contraction which could be demonstrated in 40 % (4/9) of our patients was resynchronized in all phases of treatment.

Summary: Eleven patients with hypertrophic cardiomyopathy were investigated by repeated radionuclide ventriculography. Nine of them were studied for the first time while under long-term treatment for 14 to 84 months. In all eleven patients radionuclide ventriculography was performed after a withdraw of verapamil for at least 14 days or before the onset of therapy respectively (control period). A third investigation was carried out 60 to 90 min after acute administration of 90 mg oral verapamil. A last radionuclide ventriculography was perfomed following 2 weeks of therapy with 480 mg oral verapamil. After acute administration heart rate significantly increased from 69 ± 10 to $80 \pm 15/$ min. EDV was in the normal range. Left ventricular global ejection parameters showed no significant changes except for minimal decrease in ejection time from 309 ± 29 to 278 ± 50 ms after acute verapamil administration. The sectorial ejection fraction improved in apical sectors in relation to the basal one, while the global EF remained constant. The ventricular global peak filling rate increased significantly from 283 ± 61 to 325 ± 64 %/EDV/s after acute administration of verapamil and the sectorial peak filling rate increased in apical sectors compared to basal sectors following acute administration as well as long-term therapy. After withdrawal of verapamil, six out of 11 patients showed a homogeneous left ventricular delay of contraction by means of the Fourier phases which were normalized under short- and long-term verapamil treatment. In conclusion, verapamil caused a marked improvement of the left ventricular contraction delay without significant changes in global systolic function.

References

1. Adam WE, Tarkowaka A, Bitter F, Stauch M, Geffers H (1979) Equilibrium (gated) radionuclide ventriculography. Cardiovasc Radiol 2: 21—33
2. Betocchi S, Cannon III RO, Watson RM, Bonow RO, Ostrow HG, Epstein SE, Rosing DR (1985) Effects of sublingual nifedipine on hemodynamics and systolic and diastolic function in patients with hypertrophic cardiomyopathy. Circulation 72: 1001—1007
3. Bonow RO, Rosing DR, Bacharach SL, Green MV, Kent KM, Lipson LC, Maron BJ, Leon MB, Epstein SE (1981) Effects of verapamil on left ventricular systolic function and diastolic filling in patients with hypertrophic cardiomyopathy. Circulation 64: 787—796
4. Bonow RO, Vitale DF, Maron BJ, Bacharach SL, Frederick TM, Green MV (1987) Regional left ventricular asynchrony and impaired global left ventricular filling in hypertrophic cardiomyopathy: effect of verapamil. J Am Coll Cardiol 9: 1108—1116
5. Bonow RO, Dilsizian V, Rosing DR, Maron BJ, Bacharach ST, Green MV (1985) Verapamil-induced improvement in left ventricular diastolic filling and increased exercise tolerance in patients with hypertrophic cardomyopathy: short- and long term effects. Circulation 72: 853—864
6. Bourmayan C, Razavi A, Fournier C, Dussaule JC, Baragan J, Gerbaux A, Gay J (1985) Effect of propanolol on left ventricular relaxation in hypertrophic cardiomyopathy: an echographic study. Am Heart J 109: 1311
7. Bulkley BH, Rouleau J, Strauss HW, Pitt B (1975) Idiopathic hypertrophic subaortic stenosis: detection by Thallium 201 myocardial perfusion imaging. New Engl J Med 293: 1113—1116

8. Hanrath P, Mathey DG, Siegert R, Bleifeld W (1980) Left ventricular relaxation and filling pattern in different forms of left ventricular hypertrophy: an echocardiographic study. Am J Cardiol 45: 15—23
9. Hanrath P, Mathey DG, Kremer P, Sonntag F, Bleifeld W (1980) Effect of verapamil on left ventricular isovolumic relaxation time and regional left ventricular filling in hypertrophic cardiomyopathy. Am J Cardiol 45: 1258—1264
10. Hopf R, Keller M, Kaltenbach M (1976) Die Behandlung der hypertrophen obstruktiven Kardiomyopathie mit Verapamil. Verh dtsch Ges inn Med 82: 1054
11. Hopf R, Richter H, Kaltenbach M, Maul FD, Standke R, Hör G (1985) Radionuklidventrikulographie nach akuter und chronischer Verapamil-Medikation bei Patienten mit hypertropher Kardiomyopathie. In: Hör G, Kaltenbach M, Maul FD, Pabst HW (Hrsg.) Interventionelle Nuklearkardiologie, Kern & Birner Verlag, Frankfurt, pp 368—377
12. Hopf R, Rodrian S, Kaltenbach M (1986) Behandlung der hypertrophen Kardiomyopathie mit Kalziumantagonisten. Therapiewoche 36: 1433—1454
13. Kaltenbach M, Hopf R, Keller M (1976) Calcium-antagonistische Therapie bei hypertroph obstruktiver Kardiomyopathie. Dtsch Med Wochenschr. 101: 1284—1287
14. Kaltenbach M, Hopf R (1985) Treatment of hypertrophic cardiomyopathy: relation to pathological mechanisms. J Mol Cell Cardiol 17 (Suppl 2) 59—68
15. Lorell B, Paulus WJ, Grossman W, Wynne J, Cohn PF (1982) Modification of abnormal left ventricular diastolic properties by nifedipine in patients with hypertrophic cardiomyopathy. Circulation 65: 499—507
16. Maron BJ, Gottdiener JS, Epstein SE (1981) Patterns and significance of distribution of left ventricular hypertrophy in hypertrophic cardiomyopathy. A wide angle, two dimensional echocardiographic study of 125 patients. Am J Cardiol 48: 418—428
17. Pohost GM, Vignola PA, McKusick KE, Block PC, Myers GS, Walker HJ, Copen DL, Dinsmore RE (1977) Hypertrophic cardiomyopathy. Evaluation by gated cardiac blood pool scanning. Circulation 55: 92—99
18. Rosing DR, Kent KM, Borer JS, Seides SF, Maron BJ, Epstein SE (1979) Verapamil therapy: a new approach to the pharmacologic treatment of hypertrophic cardiomyopathy. I. Hemodynamic effects. Circulation 60: 1201—1207
19. Rosing DR, Kent KM, Maron BJ, Epstein SE (1979) Verapamil therapy: a new approach to the pharmacologic treatment of hypertrophic cardiomyopathy. II. Effects on exercise capacity and symptomatic status. Circulation 60: 1208—1213
20. Rosing DR, Condit JR, Maron BJ, Kent KM, Leon MB, Bonow RO, Lipson LC, Epstein SE (1981) Verapamil therapy: a new approach to the pharmacological treatment of hypertrophic cardiomyopathy: III. Effects of long-term administration. Am J Cardiol 48: 545—553
21. Senn M, Hess OM, Krayenbühl HP (1982) Nifedipin in der Behandlung der hypertrophen, nicht obstruktiven Kardiomyopathie. Schweiz med Wschr 112: 1312—1317
22. Standke R, Hör G, Maul FD (1983) Fully automated sectorial equilibrium radionuclide ventriculography. Proposal of a method for routine use: exercise and follow-up. Eur J Nucl Med 8: 77—83
23. Standke R, Hör G, Klepzig Jr H, Maul FD, Bussmann WD, Kaltenbach M (1985) Sectoranalysis of left ventricular function by fully automated equilibrium radionuclide ventriculography. Internat J Cardiac Imag 1: 87—97
24. Suwa M, Hirota Y, Kawamura K (1984) Improvement of left ventricular diastolic function during intravenous and oral diltiazem therapy in patients with hypertrophic cardiomyopathy: an echocardiographic study. Am J Cardiol 54: 1047—1053
25. Suzuki Y, Kadato K, Nohara R, Tamaki S, Kambara H, Yoshida A, Murakami T, Osakada G, Kawai C, Tamaki N, Mukai T, Torizuka K (1984) Recognition of regional hypertrophy in hypertrophic cardiomyopathy using Thallium-201 emission-computed tomography: comparison with two-dimensional echocardiography. Am J Cardiol 53: 1095—1102

Authors' address:
Dr. Frank-Dieter Maul, Abteilung für Allgemeine Nuklearmedizin, Klinikum der J. W. Goethe-Universität, Theodor-Stern-Kai 7, 6000 Frankfurt 70, F.R.G.

Effects of therapeutic interventions on minimal cardiac transit times and volume parameters in hypertrophic cardiomyopathy

B. Lösse and L. E. Feinendegen*

Dept. of Cardiology, Pneumology and Angiology, * Dept. of Nuclear Medicine, University of Düsseldorf, F.R.G.

Introduction

Hypertrophic cardiomyopathies are characterized by normal or small ventricular volumes, thickened ventricular walls and ventricular ejection fractions, usually in the upper normal range. Changes in cardiac volume ratios during exercise and/or after therapy are scarcely reported in hypertrophic cardiomyopathies and are then restricted to left ventricular volume parameters, due to the limitations of the methods employed, i.e. contrast angiography, radionuclide angiography or echocardiography (1, 6, 10, 26, 27). Measurements of the minimal transit times (MTTs) of a radioactive tracer through the heart allow, on the other hand, a separate estimation of the volume ratios of all cardiac compartments, i.e., both atria and both ventricles, and can be easily applied not only at rest but also during exercise. Using this method, it therefore seemed worthwhile to investigate the changes in atrial and ventricular volume ratios in a group of patients with hypertrophic obstructive and non-obstructive cardiomyopathy, before and after surgical therapy as well.

Patients and Methods

Patients

The study population consists of 45 patients with hypertrophic obstructive cardiomyopathy (HOCM) and 21 patients with hypertrophic non-obstructive cardiomyopathy (HNCM). The diagnosis was confirmed in all patients by means of angiocardiography and intracardiac pressure measurements. Age, hemodynamic findings at rest, exercise tolerance and distribution of patients according to the NYHA (New York Heart Association) functional classification, are summarized in Table 1. All patients had sinus rhythm at the time of measurement. Angiographic evidence of mitral regurgitation was present in 27 of the 45 HOCM and in four of the 21 HNCM patients. If present, the degree of regurgitation was usually minimal. Only six HOCM patients and one HNCM patient presented with moderate and one HOCM patient with substantial mitral regurgitation. Of the 45 HOCM patients, 12 underwent surgical therapy consisting of transaortal subvalvular myectomy (22). Pre- and postoperative (10.3 ± 1.8 months after sur-

Table 1. Age, resting hemodynamic findings and exercise tolerance (mean ± SEM) in 45 patients with hypertrophic obstructive cardiomyopathy (HOCM) and 21 patients with hypertrophic non-obstructive cardiomoyopathy (HNCM) grouped according to their functional limitation (NYHA classification).

		HOCM				HNCM		
		I (n = 6)	II (n = 12)	III (n = 25)	IV (n = 2)	I (n = 10)	II (n =7)	III (n = 4)
Age	(yrs)	34.0± 4.0	37.5± 3.5	39.1±1.7	40.5± 0.5	35.2±4.8	40.6±5.3	51.5± 2.5
LVEDP	(mm Hg)	16.7± 3.8	16.2± 2.5	17.4±1.5	29.3± 0.8	13.7±1.9	13.8±2.9	22.3± 5.6
LVΔP at rest	(mm Hg)	25.8±10.7	36.5± 8.9	59.3±8.5	107.5±57.6			
provoked	(mm Hg)	98.3±20.5	111.3±12.3	122.4±8.9	175 (n = 1)			
HR	(bpm)	77.7± 7.6	63.8± 2.9	79.3±4.0	76.0± 2.0	69.0±4.7	70.7±2.9	73.8± 8.9
SVI	(ml/m²)	50.3± 3.8	52.1± 2.9	42.2±2.5	28.5± 7.5	56.5±5.3	46.7±6.3	50.5± 5.7
CI	(l/min/m²)	3.9± 0.6	3.4± 0.2	3.2±0.2	2.0± 0.4	3.8±0.5	3.2±0.4	3.6± 0.3
PAP	(mm Hg)	16.7± 1.9	16.3± 1.2	18.4±0.9	27.0± 3.0	14.7±1.1	16.1±1.9	23.0± 5.8
max. exercise	(W)	95.8±15.0	82.5± 5.4	67.2±4.9	25.0± 0	101.4±9.4	78.6±6.5	50.0±10.2

Abbreviations: LVEDP = left ventricular enddiastolic pressure, LV ΔP = left ventricular outflow tract gradient, HR = heart rate, SVI = stroke volume index, CI = cardiac index, PAP = mean pulmonary artery pressure.

Table 2. Pre- and postoperative hemodynamic findings and exercise tolerance (mean ± SEM) in 12 patients with HOCM.

		preop.	postop.	*p* value
HR	rest	73.7±2.2	79.6±4.1	N.S.
(beats/min)	exercise	118.2±5.3	113.8±4.1	N.S.
SVI	rest	43.5±3.7	39.9±1.6	N.S.
(ml/m^2)	exercise	44.7±3.0	50.6±2.8	< 0.05
CI	rest	3.2±0.3	3.2±0.2	N.S.
(1/min/m^2)	exercise	5.3±0.4	5.7±0.4	N.S.
PAP	rest	19.7±1.5	15.9±1.0	< 0.05
(mm Hg)	exercise	45.9±3.8	33.2±1.8	< 0.025
max. exercise (W)		59.6±4.5	80.8±5.8	< 0.005

The hemodynamic values were measured in each individual at the highest common work load (57.7±7.3 W) reached in both the pre- and post-operative exercise test. Abbreviations: HR = heart rate, SVI = stroke volume index, CI = cardiac index, PAP = mean pulmonary artery pressure, SEM = standard error of the mean.

gery) hemodynamic findings at rest and during exercise, as well as changes in exercise tolerance, are summarized in Table 2.

Methods

The basic principles of cardiac minimal transit times (MTTs) of a radioactive tracer as an indicator of cardiac volume ratios have been described in detail elsewhere (7, 20, 21, 28, 29). In short, cardiac MTTs are defined as differences between the appearance times of the indicator in consecutive segments of the cardiopulmonary circulation. They are directly proportional to the quotient of the volume of interest (e.g. right atrium, right ventricle, lungs, left atrium, left ventricle, or total heart) to cardiac output (Fig. 1). Since cardiac output equals the product of heart rate and stroke volume, cardiac MTTs are, after correction for heart rate, inversely proportional to the ejection fraction of the volume compartment of interest. A formula has been derived (28) to calculate ejection fractions directly from segmental MTTs and has been experimentally validated in simultaneous biplane cineangiographic determinations of left ventricular ejection fractions (range: 17 % to 80 %) yielding a correlation coefficient of 0.92 (23) in evaluations by independent investigators.

All patients underwent bicycle ergometer exercise in the supine position, with a stepwise increase in work load. Pulmonary artery pressure was continuously measured using a Swan-Ganz catheter. Cardiac MTTs of an intravenously injected bolus of Indium 113m EDTA (0.8 mCi for the first measurement at rest, 3 mCi for the second measurement during exercise) were measured once at rest and once during exercise using a multicrystal gammaretina (7, 20). Appearance times of the indicator in the different compartments of the cardiopulmonary circulation were determined from time activity curves generated over the right atrium, right ventricle, pulmonary artery, left atrium, left ventricle and aortic root. Exact determination of the rapid upstroke of the time activity curve in the

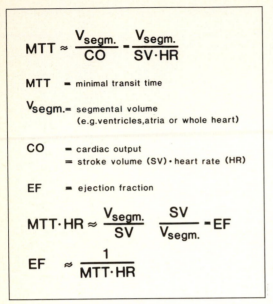

Fig. 1. Relationships between cardiac minimal transit times (MTT) and cardiac volume ratios.

$$MTT \approx \frac{V_{segm.}}{CO} - \frac{V_{segm.}}{SV \cdot HR}$$

MTT = minimal transit time

$V_{segm.}$ = segmental volume (e.g. ventricles, atria or whole heart)

CO = cardiac output
= stroke volume (SV) · heart rate (HR)

EF = ejection fraction

$$MTT \cdot HR \approx \frac{V_{segm.}}{SV} \quad \frac{SV}{V_{segm.}} = EF$$

$$EF \approx \frac{1}{MTT \cdot HR}$$

different compartments was facilitated by smoothing, according to the method of gliding averages. For better comparison, the measured MTTs were corrected for an arbitrary heart rate of 80 beats/min (21). To make deviations from the normal values (7) immediately obvious, an MTT index was calculated regarding the mean values for healthy control subjects as unity.

For statistical comparisons, Student's two-tailed *t*-test for paired data was used.

Results

Simultaneously measured mean pulmonary artery pressures and total cardiac MTTs (i.e. MTT from the right atrium to the aortic root, diminished by the MTT through the lungs), obtained in 45 HOCM patients at rest and on a mean exercise level of 31 W, are illustrated in Fig. 2. It can be seen that mean pulmonary artery pressure rose in all cases during exercise and exceeded the normal range in 70 % of them. Total cardiac MTTs, on the contrary, rose in less than half the patients and exceeded the upper border of the normal range in only 42 % of the cases. In the majority of cases they remained almost constant.

In the 21 HNCM patients, the behaviour of mean pulmonary artery pressures and total cardiac MTTs was similar (Fig. 3). Mean pulmonary artery pressure rose in all cases during exercise of an average 38 W and exceeded the upper normal range in 57 % of the patients. Total cardiac MTTs, on the other hand, remained constant in about one third of the cases and increased in the other two thirds, but exceeded the upper normal border in only 52 % of the patients.

The individual rate-corrected segmental MTTs through the cardiac compartments (right atrium, right ventricle, left atrium, left ventricle) and the lungs of all 45 HOCM patients are illustrated in Fig. 4. At rest, all left ventricular MTTs were within or below

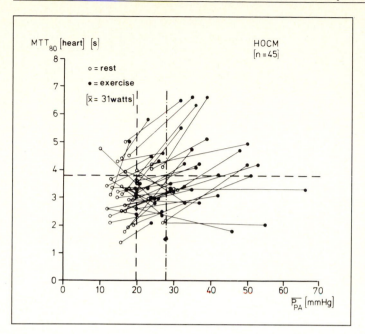

Fig. 2. Individual changes in rate-corrected (to a heart rate of 80 beats/min) total cardiac minimal transit times (MTT) and mean pulmonary artery pressure ($\overline{P}_{PA}$) during exercise in 45 patients with HOCM. Total cardiac MTT is the MTT of the tracer from the right atrium to the aortic root diminished by the MTT through the lungs. Broken lines indicate the upper borders of normal at rest (———) and during exercise (— · — · —), which are identical for MTTs.

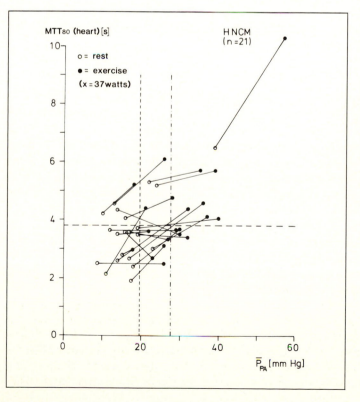

Fig. 3. Individual changes in rate-corrected (to a heart rate of 80 beats/min) total cardiac minimal transit times (MTT) and mean pulmonary artery pressure ($\overline{P}_{PA}$) during exercise in 21 patients with HNCM. Broken lines as in Fig. 1.

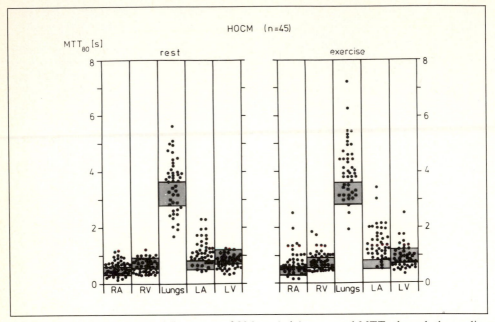

Fig. 4. Individual rate-corrected (heart rate of 80 beats/min) segmental MTTs through the cardiac compartments and the lungs in 45 patients with HOCM at rest and during exercise. The shadowed areas represent the normal range. RA = right atrium, RV = right ventricle, LA = left atrium, LV = left ventricle.

the normal range, corresponding to normal or increased ejection fractions. Nearly the same was true for the right ventricular MTTs. The majority of left atrial MTTs were, however, prolonged, as an expression of reduced atrial ejection fractions. Right atrial MTTs showed the same behavior, although to a lesser degree. MTTs through the lungs were grouped around the normal range, with a slight preponderance of prolonged values. Exercise caused prolongation of all segmental MTTs, most markedly in both atria. As a means of better comparison, MTT-indices were calculated, i.e., the relation between rate-corrected measuring values and normal values. The mean values of segmental MTT indices, illustrated in Fig. 5, show the marked increase in atrial MTTs during exercise, as compared to the slight increase in ventricular MTTs which remained within the normal range.

Figs. 6 and 7 illustrate the principally equal behaviour of rate-corrected segmental cardiac and pulmonary MTTs in 18 HNCM patients (in 3 of the 21 patients a correct subdivision into segmental MTTs was not possible). Again the marked prolongation of atrial MTTs with normal or near normal ventricular MTTs is clearly documented.

Surgical therapy in 12 HOCM patients caused impressive changes in segmental MTTs, especially during exercise (Fig. 8). At rest, only the increase in left ventricular MTTs to the upper normal range, which indicates a fall in left ventricular ejection fractions to the lower normal range, was significant ($p < 0.05$), whereas the other segmental MTTs

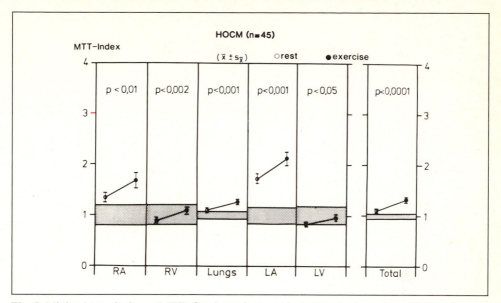

Fig. 5. Minimal transit times (MTT) for the entire heart including the lungs (= total) as well as for the individual cardiac chambers and the lungs at rest and during exercise in 45 patients with HOCM. The mean value for healthy control subjects is regarded as unity. Shadowed zones and abbreviations as in Fig. 4.

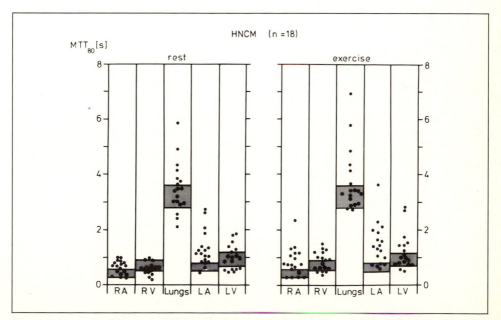

Fig. 6. Individual rate-corrected (heart rate of 80 beats/min) segmental MTTs through the cardiac compartments and the lungs in 18 patients with HNCM at rest and during exercise. Shadowed areas and abbreviations as in Fig. 4.

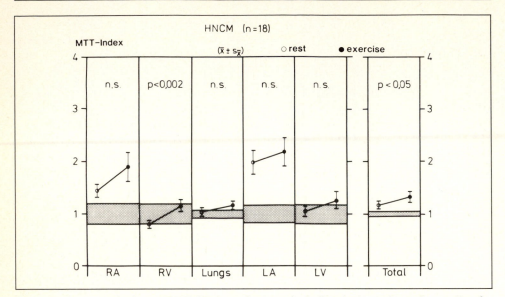

Fig. 7. Minimal transit times (MTT) for the entire heart including the lungs (= total) as well as for the individual cardiac chambers and the lungs at rest and during exercise in 18 patients with HNCM. The mean value for healthy control subjects is regarded as unity. Shadowed zones and abbreviations as in Fig. 4.

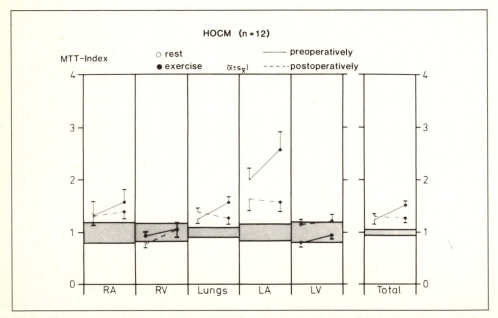

Fig. 8. Changes in minimal transit times (MTT) for the entire heart including the lungs (= total) as well as for the individual cardiac chambers and the lungs after surgical therapy in 12 patients with HOCM. As Fig. 7.

showed minor, insignificant changes. During exercise, however, a significant shortening of left atrial ($p < 0.01$) and pulmonary ($p < 0.05$) MTTs was also documented, as compared to the preoperative values, whereas the slight decrease in right atrial MTTs was not significant.

Discussion

Minimal cardiac transit times (MTTs) of a radioactive tracer reflect, after correction for heart rate, cardiac volume ratios (7, 20, 21, 29). They are proportional to the end-diastolic volume, inversely proportional to stroke volume, and thus related to ejection fraction (7, 23, 28, 29). Hence, prolongation of MTTs means a decrease in ejection fraction, whereas, in contrast, a rise in ejection fraction is reflected by a shortened MTT. Ejection fractions can be calculated from MTTs (23, 28). With concern to the left ventricle, ejection fractions derived from left ventricular MTTs have been shown to correlate strongly (correlation coefficient $r = 0.92$) to left ventricular ejection fractions derived from simultaneous contrast ventriculograms covering a range of 17 % to 80 % (23). Of special advantage, MTTs can be determined separately for the different cardiopulmonary compartments (right atrium, right ventricle, lungs, left atrium, left ventricle) and thereby enable a separate assessment of function of these compartments within one measurement. Due to the small radiation burden, repeat measurements at rest and during exercise can be performed. Simultaneous application of Swan-Ganz pulmonary artery catheterization renders a yet more comprehensive assessment of cardiac function since, in addition to cardiac volume ratios derived from MTTs, important pressure parameters are provided, e.g. right atrial and pulmonary artery pressures as well as left ventricular filling pressures (derived from pulmonary wedge pressures).

Our results of simultaneous measurements of cardiac MTTs and pulmonary artery pressures demonstrate no fundamental difference between obstructive and non-obstructive hypertrophic cardiomyopathy with regard to the relations between cardiac MTTs and pulmonary artery pressures at rest and during exercise. The characteristic features are: (1) normal left and right ventricular MTTs at rest and during exercise; (2) prolonged left and right atrial MTTs at rest with further prolongation during exercise; (3) increase in pulmonary artery pressure during exercise, in the majority of cases, above normal range.

Normal left ventricular and markedly prolonged left atrial MTTs are indicative of normal left ventricular and reduced left atrial ejection fractions. Since stroke volumes were normal (Table 1) — the detailed results have been published elsewhere (13, 14), — these findings can only be explained by increased left atrial volumes. Together with the increase in pulmonary artery pressures, the left atrial enlargement may be explained either by mitral regurgitation or by impaired blood inflow into the left ventricle. Since moderate or severe mitral regurgitation was present, however, only in 7 out of 45 HOCM patients and in one of 21 HNCM patients, impaired inflow into the left ventricle seems of predominant importance.

So far, these findings correlate well with the accepted pathophysiology of hypertrophic cardiomyopathies. Major determinants of pathophysiologic alterations are seen in the decrease in diastolic left ventricular relaxation and filling, common to both forms of hypertrophic cardiomyopathies, and in the left ventricular outflow obstruction present only in HOCM (1, 3—5, 8, 9, 12, 18, 24, 25, 30). Increased left ventricular filling pressures (as derived from pulmonary artery pressures) and impaired atrial emptying into the left ventricle, which showed no quantitative differences between HOCM and HNCM patients in our study, can be explained sufficiently by an impaired left ventricular diastolic function alone. An additional influence of left ventricular outflow obstruction in HOCM is, however, not ruled out.

Our data of slightly prolonged right atrial MTTs in connection with normal right ventricular MTTs suggest that this pathophysiological concept may be also applied, to a lesser degree, to the right ventricle. Our data further suggest that, according to the marked increase in atrial MTTs during exercise, inflow obstruction to both ventricles is aggravated during exercise. Furthermore, the slight prolongation of ventricular MTTs during exercise towards the upper border of the normal range indicates decreasing right and left ventricular ejection fractions. As far as left ventricular ejection fractions are concerned, corresponding findings have been presented in HOCM patients using radionuclide ventriculography: Borer et al. (6) described a slight decrease in the supernormal resting ejection fraction during exercise. Since stroke volume remained constant or rose during exercise in the majority of our patients, the MTT data suggest that both ventricles are capable of a certain enlargement of their enddiastolic volumes during exercise, in spite of the impaired distensibility caused by hypertrophy.

Surgical therapy of HOCM, which improves symptoms and hemodynamics more dramatically than medical therapy with propranolol or verapamil (2, 15, 16, 17, 19), causes significant changes in the cardiac volume ratios. The prolongation of left ventricular MTTs indicates a decrease in the preoperatively supernormal left ventricular ejection fractions towards the lower normal range, which is in agreement with recent radionuclide ventriculographic studies (6). Since postoperative stroke volumes do not decrease but, especially during exercise, increase, as compared to preoperative values (Table 2), these findings suggest an increase in left ventricular enddiastolic volume. Together with the impressive reduction in left ventricular enddiastolic pressure (11, 16, 17) and mean pulmonary artery pressure (Table 2), an improvement in left atrial ejection can be assumed, which explains the substantial shortening of left atrial and pulmonary MTTs. An additional role of the relief of outflow obstruction cannot, however, be ruled out.

Summary: 45 patients with hypertrophic obstructive cardiomyopathy (HOCM) and 18 patients with hypertrophic non-obstructive cardiomyopathy (HNCM) underwent simultaneous measurements of pulmonary artery pressure and minimal transit times (MTTs) of an intravenously injected bolus of indium-113m-EDTA through the heart at rest and during exercise in supine position. At rest, rate-corrected left and right ventricular MTTs were in the lower normal range, whereas left atrial and, to a lesser degree, right atrial MTTs were abnormally prolonged, indicative of high ventricular ejection fractions and impaired atrial ejection. During exercise, ventricular MTTs rose slightly but remained within the normal range, which corresponds to a slight fall in ventricular ejection fractions. Atrial MTTs exhibited, in contrast, a substantial further prolongation. Together with an abnormal increase in pulmonary artery pressure in the majority of patients, these findings suggest an aggravation of inflow impairment to both ventricles during exercise. There was no quantitative difference between HOCM and HNCM patients suggesting that impaired atrial ejection due to impaired diastolic function is of major pathophysiological importance irrespective of a possible additional role of left ventricular outflow obstruction in HOCM.

The influence of surgical therapy (transaortal septal myectomy) was studied in 12 patients with HOCM. A significant increase in left ventricular MTTs to the upper normal range, indicative of a depression of left ventricular ejection fractions to the lower normal range, and a significant shortening of left atrial and pulmonary MTTs were observed, whereas corresponding changes in the right heart were not significant. Together with the significant fall in pulmonary artery pressure and a rise in exercise stroke volume, these findings suggest a postoperative improvement in left ventricular diastolic function with an increase in left ventricular distensibility.

References

1. Anderson DM, Raff GL, Ports TA, Brundage BH, Parmley WW, Chatterjee K (1984) Hypertrophic obstructive cardiomyopathy: Effects of acute and chronic verapamil treatment on left ventricular systolic and diastolic function. Br Heart J 51: 523—529
2. Beahrs MM, Tajik AJ, Seward JB, Giuliani ER, McGoon DC (1983) Hypertrophic obstructive cardiomyopathy: Ten- to 21-year follow-up after partial septal myectomy. Am J Cardiol 51: 1160—1166
3. Betocchi S, Bonow RO, Bacharach SL, Rosing DR, Maron BJ, Green MV (1986) Isovolumic relaxation period in hypertrophic cardiomyopathy: Assessment by radionuclide angiography. J Am Coll Cardiol 7: 74—81
4. Bonow RO, Frederick TM, Bacharach SL, Green MV, Goose PW, Maron BJ, Rosing DR (1983) Atrial systole and left ventricular filling in patients with hypertrophic cardiomyopathy: Effect of verapamil. Am J Cardiol 51: 1386—1391
5. Bonow RO, Rosing DR, Bacharach SL, Green MV, Kent KM, Lipson LC, Maron BJ, Leon MB, Epstein SE (1981) Effects of verapamil on left ventricular systolic function and diastolic filling in patients with hypertrophic cardiomyopathy. Circulation 64: 787—796
6. Borer JS, Bacharach SL, Green MV, Kent KM, Rosing DR, Seides SF, Morrow AG, Epstein SE (1979) Effect of septal myotomy and myectomy on left ventricular systolic function at rest and during exercise in patients with IHSS. Circulation 60, Suppl I: 82—87
7. Feinendegen LE, Becker V, Vyska K, Schicha H, Freundlieb C, Bosiljanoff P, Lösse B, Gleichmann U (1980) Bestimmung globaler und regionaler Herzfunktion mit den minimalen Transitzeiten. Verh Dtsch Ges Herz- und Kreislaufforsch 46: 118—129
8. Goodwin JF (1982) The frontiers of cardiomyopathy. Br Heart J 48: 1—18
9. Hanrath P, Mathey DG, Kremer P, Sonntag F, Bleifeld W (1980) Effect of verapamil on left ventricular isovolumic relaxation time and regional left ventricular filling in hypertrophic cardiomyopathy. Am J Cardiol 45: 1258—1264
10. Kaltenbach M, Hopf R (1985) Treatment of hypertrophic cardiomyopathy: Relation to pathological mechanisms. J Mol Cell Cardiol 17, Suppl 2: 59—68
11. Kuhn H, Krelhaus W, Bircks W, Schulte HD, Loogen F (1978) Indication for surgical treatment in patients with hypertrophic obstructive cardiomyopathy. In: Kaltenbach M, Loogen F, Olsen EGJ (eds) Cardiomyopathy and Myocardial Biopsy. Springer-Verlag, Berlin—Heidelberg—New York, pp 308—315
12. Kuhn H, Thelen U, Köhler E, Lösse B (1980) Die hypertrophische nicht obstruktive Kardiomyopathie (HNCM) — Klinische, hämodynamische, elektro-, echo- und angiokardiographische Untersuchungen. Z Kardiol 69: 457—469
13. Lösse B, Kuhn H, Krönert H, Rafflenbeul D, Kirschner P, Schulte HD, Loogen F (1980) Hämodynamische Auswirkungen konservativer und operativer Therapie bei hypertrophischer obstruktiver Kardiomyopathie. Z Kardiol 69: 470—477
14. Lösse B, Kuhn H, Loogen F, Schulte HD (1983) Exercise performance in hypertrophic cardiomyopathies. Eur Heart J 4, Suppl F: 197—208

15. Lösse B, Loogen F, Schulte HD (1984) Frühe und späte hämodynamische Veränderungen nach operativer Therapie der hypertrophischen obstruktiven Kardiomyopathie. Z Kardiol 73: 654—662

16. Maron BJ, Merrill WH, Freier PA, Kent KM, Epstein SE, Morrow AG (1978) Long-term clinical course and symptomatic status of patients after operation for hypertrophic subaortic stenosis. Circulation 57: 1205—1213

17. Morrow AG, Reitz BA, Epstein SE, Henry WL, Conkle DM, Itscoitz SB, Redwood DR (1975) Operative treatment in hypertrophic subaortic stenosis: Techniques and the results of pre- and postoperative assessments in 83 patients. Circulation 52: 88—102

18. Oakley CM (1974) Clinical recognition of the cardiomyopathies. Circ Res 34/35, Suppl II: 152—167

19. Redwood DR, Goldstein RE, Hirshfeld J, Borer JS, Morganroth J, Morrow AG, Epstein SE (1979) Exercise performance after septal myotomy and myectomy in patients with obstructive hypertrophic cardiomyopathy. Am J Cardiol 44: 215—220

20. Schicha H, Vyska K, Becker V, Seipel L, Feinendegen LE (1970) Minimale kardiale Transitzeiten bei gesunden und herzkranken Personen: Untersuchungen mit Indium-113m und der Gamma-Retina. Atomkernenergie 15: 150—156

21. Schicha H, Vyska K, Knapp W, Becker V, Heck H, Hollmann W, Feinendegen LE (1974) Minimale kardiale Transitzeiten (MTT's) in der Herzdiagnostik — Messungen mit der Gamma-Retina und Indium-113m, IV. MTTs bei Untrainierten und Leistungssportlern in Ruhe und nach Belastung. Z Kardiol 63: 733—744

22. Schulte HD, Bircks W, Körfer R, Kuhn H (1981) Surgical aspects of typical subaortic and atypical midventricular hypertrophic obstructive cardiomyopathy (HOCM). Thorac Cardiovasc Surg 29: 375—380

23. Sigwart U, Schicha H, Schmidt H, Becker V, Mertens HM, Gleichmann U, Feinendegen LE (1978) Vergleich minimaler kardialer Transitzeiten mit invasiv erhaltenen hämodynamischen Parametern. Ergebnisse aus simultaner Isotopen-Herzfunktionsanalyse und Herzkatheteruntersuchung. Herz/Kreisl 10: 15—20

24. Spiller P, Brenner C, Karsch KR, Loogen F, Neuhaus KL (1977) Systolische und diastolische Funktion des linken Ventrikels bei hypertrophischer obstruktiver Kardiomyopathie. Z Kardiol 66: 483—490

25. Spiller P, Brenner C, Neuhaus KL, Sauer G (1978) Disorders of left ventricular performance in congestive and hypertrophic obstructive cardiomyopathy. In: Kaltenbach M, Loogen F, Olsen EGJ (eds) Cardiomyopathy and Myocardial Biopsy. Springer-Verlag, Berlin—Heidelberg—New York, pp 186—195

26. Swanton RH, Brooksby IAB, Jenkins BS, Webb-Peploe MM (1977) Hemodynamic studies of β blockade in hypertrophic obstructive cardiomyopathy. Eur J Cardiol 5/4: 327—341

27. Turina J, Jenni R, Krayenbuehl, Turina M, Rothlin M (1986) Echocardiographic findings late after myectomy in hypertrophic obstructive cardiomyopathy. Eur Heart J 7: 685—692

28. Vyska K, Profant M, Schicha H, Becker V, Freundlieb C, Feinendegen LE (1975) Theoretische Grundlagen der Anwendung der minimalen kardialen Transitzeiten für die Bestimmung der Ejektionsfraktion in der Herzkammer. In: Pabst HW, Hör G, Schmidt HAE (Eds) Nuklearmedizin — Fortschritte der Nuklearmedizin in klinischer und technologischer Sicht; Schattauer-Verlag, Stuttgart—New York, pp 68—72

29. Vyska K, Schicha H, Becker V, Feinendegen LE (1971) Minimale kardiale Transitzeiten (MTTs) in der Herzdiagnostik. Messungen mit der Gamma-Retina und Indium-113m. I. MTT's bei gesunden Personen. Z Kreislaufforsch 60: 192—202

30. Wigle ED, Sasson Z, Henderson MA, Ruddy TD, Fulop J, Rakowski H, Williams WG (1985) Hypertrophic cardiomyopathy. The importance of the site and the extent of hypertrophy. A review. Progr Cardiovasc Dis 28: 1—83

Authors' address:
Prof. Dr. med. Benno Lösse, Medizinische Klinik und Poliklinik der Universität, Abteilung für Kardiologie, Pneumologie und Angiologie, Moorenstr. 5, D-4000 Düsseldorf, F.R.G.

Diagnosis of hypertrophic cardiomyopathies by non-ECG-gated cardiac computed tomography (CCT)

H. Kuhn, R. Blümm, F. Gietzen, K. Böcker and E. Waßmuth

Medical Hospital II and Institute of Radiology of the Municipal Hospital of Bielefeld, Academic Teaching Hospital of the University of Münster, F.R.G.

Introduction

In patients with hypertrophic cardiomyopathies a clear cut diagnosis may be difficult for echocardiographic reasons: General anatomic conditions (e.g. deformities of the chest and/or emphysema) may not lead to sufficient quality of echocardiogram. The location of hypertrophic myocardium may be present predominantly at the apex of the left ventricle which in general cannot be visualized by one- and two-dimensional echocardiography. This is the case in patients with atypical hypertrophic cardiomyopathy and in patients with hypertrophic non-obtructive cardiomyopathy (HNCM) without thickened septum at the basis of left ventricle (7).

Therefore, the study was designed to investigate the diagnostic significance of another non-invasive method, i.e., non-ECG-gated cardiac computed tomography (CCT).

Patients and Methods

A comparative study in consecutive patients with hypertrophic cardiomyopathy was performed (*n* = 55; HOCM, *n* = 38; HNCM, *n* = 15; morbus Fabry (resembling HNCM), *n* = 2). All patients in whom no sufficient quantification of septal thickness was possible by echocardiography were excluded.

The non-ECG-gated CCT was performed within 1 week after echocardiography, with patients in the supine position, intravenous (cubital vein) injection of about 150—200 ml non-ionic contrast medium, flow 4—8 ml/s, gantry tilting 20 °, section intervals, 5—8 mm (see Figs. 1 and 2). For further technical details see refs. (9, 11).

One examination lasted for about 10 to 15 min. The echocardiogram and the CCT were analyzed qualitatively (regarding the form of ventricular deformity) and quantitatively (estimation of septal thickness) respectively, by at least two independent observers.

The septal thickness was quantified using the standards of the American Society of Echocardiography. The septal thickness in CCT was measured at the upper third of the left ventricle and was always related to the section, which showed the maximum size of left ventricular cavity.

In 18 patients, left and right heart catheterization was performed for different reasons (surgical treatment in HOCM, definite proof of HNCM or atypical HOCM). In all pa-

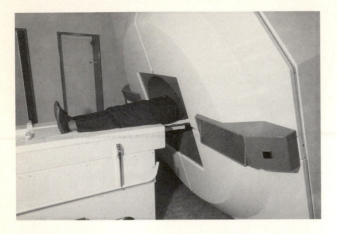

Fig. 1. Typical condition showing a patient in whom CCT is performed (gantry tilting, 20 °).

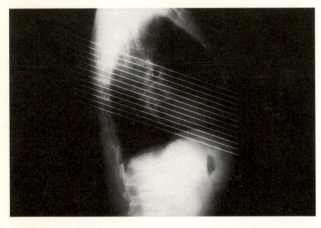

Fig. 2. Several sections can be obtained by CCT.

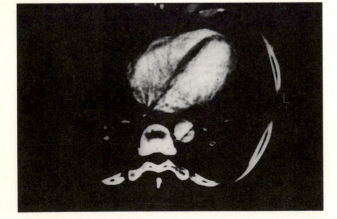

Fig. 3. Contrast medium enhanced cardiac computed tomogram of a 30-year-old man without cardiac disease. Normal right and left ventricles and normal thickness of intraventricular septum are demonstrated. Note the round apex of the left ventricle. The tomogram resembles the apical 4-chamber echocardiogram-view.

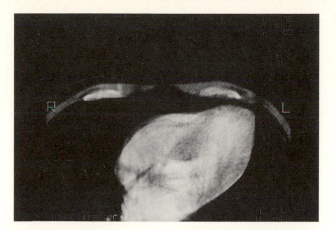

Fig. 4. The same position is shown in a 34-year-old man with hypertrophic obstructive cardiomyopathy. The typical subaortic thickening of intraventricular septum can be seen. The apical site is round.

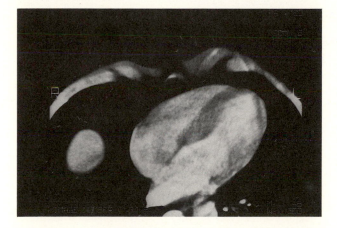

Fig. 5. Cardiac computed tomogram from a 65-year-old man. A shape resembling hypertrophic obstructive cardiomyopathy is shown. The same form was diagnosed by echocardiography and left ventricular angiography. However, no intraventricular gradient was measured. Myocardial biopsy revealed the typical picture of phospholipid storage disease (morbus Fabry).

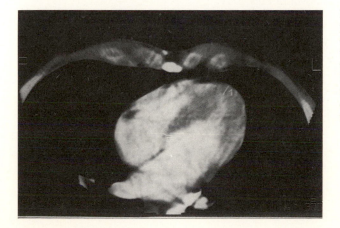

Fig. 6. 40-year-old man with hypertrophic non-obstructive cardiomyopathy (HNCM). The tomogram demonstrates the typical increasing thickening of intraventricular septum and of free wall with funnel-like muscular obliteration of the apex of the left ventricle.

tients with HNCM, endomyocardial catheter biopsy was additionally performed to exclude myocardial storage disease (7).

Results

As can be seen in Fig. 8, in five cases the septal thickness was normal ($n = 3$) or nearly normal ($n = 2$). In these patients HNCM was present, as could be supposed from CCT, and proved by left heart catheterization, which showed the typical funnel-like obliteration of the apex (7). The correlation of septal thickness between echocardiogram and CCT was unexpectedly high ($r = 0,90$, $p < 0.001$ (Fig. 8)).

The mean values of septal thickness were 19.8 ± 5.2 mm ($x \pm SX$) (echocardiogram) and 20.2 ± 6.1 mm (CCT).

To date, normal values of the amount of left ventricular thickness are available from five normal subjects (Fig. 3) and, in addition, from a large number of patients suffering from different disorders (e.g., bronchus carcinoma) without evidence of heart disease. These data are published elsewhere (9). It could be demonstrated that exact measurements of septal tickness and evaluation of ventricular form was possible in the same way as has been seen in patients with hypertrophic cardiomyopathies. The correlation between echocardiogram and CCT proved to be even better.

In Table 1, the diagnosis by CCT was correlated with the definite diagnosis obtained from all information (clinical examination, invasive ($n = 18$) and non-invasive methods, including myocardial biopsy). The diagnosis using CCT was based on the form of left ventricular deformity, i.e., obstruction of the base or middle of the left ventricle in typical and atypical HOCM, obliteration with increasing septal thickness towards the apex of the left ventricle in patients with HNCM.

As can be seen, in all cases, hypertrophic cardiomyopathy was correctly recognized (100 %). In two cases primarily resembling HNCM, myocardial biopsy revealed myocardial storage disease which has to be excluded in all cases of HNCM (7). In addition, good diagnostic differentiation could be made between HOCM (diagnostic specificity, 92 %) and HNCM (80 %). The thickness of the free wall and the left ventricular diameter was not sufficiently quantifiable using CCT, because no sharp shape was visualized at this site. Typical examples are shown in Figs. 3—7.

Table 1. Correlation between the definite diagnosis of hypertrophic obstructive cardiomyopathy (HOCM), hypertrophic non-obstructive cardiomyopathy (HNCM) and morbus Fabry obtained by non-invasive and invasive methods, compared with diagnosis obtained by CCT.

Definite diagnosis		Diagnosis by CCT		
		HCM	HOCM	HNCM
	n	n	n	n
HOCM	38	38 (100%)	35 (92%)	3 (8%)
HNCM	15	15 (100%)	3 (20%)	12 (80%)
M. Fabry	2	2	1	1

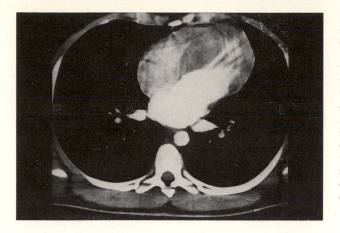

Fig. 7. Hypertrophic non-obstructive cardiomyopathy (HNCM) in a 47-year-old man. Extreme left ventricular hypertrophy predominantly afflicting the apical site of the left and of the right ventricle, as could be detected by CCT. Note the pronounced obliteration of both the right and left ventricle with increasing septal thickening towards the apex. Myocardial storage disease could be excluded by endomyocardial biopsy.

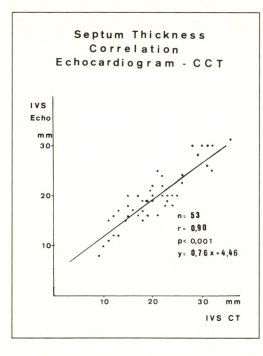

Fig. 8. Correlation (regression line) of septal thickness, measured by echocardiography and CCT.

Discussion

It has been demonstrated by several authors (1—4, 6, 10—12, 14) that CCT may be a method for visualization of thickened pericardium and myocardium. However, this is, to our knowledge the first study which: (1) investigates systematically the diagnostic significance of CCT in patients with different forms of hypertrophic cardiomyopathies and (2) uses the non — ECG — gated CCT (with the advantage of less intensity of radiation and of a less time-consuming technique, by 6—8 fold). Preliminary data have already been published (4, 8).

As was shown, an unexpectedly high correlation was observed regarding septal thickness, as measured by echocardiography and CCT ($r = 0,90$, $p < 0.001$). The reason for this good correlation is unclear. The picture obtained by CCT apparently reflects the enddiastole (11) because of its longer duration compared to systole. It could also be supposed that the reduced movement of intraventricular septum in hypertrophic cardiomyopathies plays an important role. However, this seems not to be the case because identical data have been obtained in normal subjects.

In addition, the diagnostic specificity of non-ECG-gated cardiac computed tomography for HOCM and HNCM was high (92 % and 80 %, respectively). CCT was also easy to perform and did not consume much time (duration of examination was less than 15 min).

Surprisingly, the quality of pictures was nearly the same as that obtained by the ECG-gated CCT (11).

Therefore, these results indicate that the non-ECG-gated CCT seems to be a very helpful non-invasive method for diagnosing hypertrophic cardiomyopathies and differentiating between the obstructive and the non-obstructive form. Because of the high accuracy in estimating the septal thickness, this is mainly true for patients in whom hypertrophic cardiomyopathy could not be exactly diagnosed by commonly used non-invasive methods (mainly ECG and echocardiogram).

Compared to magnetic resonance imaging, CCT is, of course, much less expensive. It is available to nearly all hospitals and is less time-consuming (5). Compared to digital subtraction angiography, CCT is a method for the sectional visualization of the myocardium to quantify left ventricular hypertrophy. Both methods used together may be of special diagnostic help. They may also serve as a suitable method for follow-up studies.

Further studies are needed to evaluate the diagnostic significance in atypical forms of hypertrophic cardiomyopathies, i.e., in cases in which hypertrophied myocardium is situated not in the typical subaortic or apical, but more at the inferior or ventral site of the left ventricle. According to our experience in these regions, tangential sections may "pretend" myocardial thickening. Therefore, correlation studies with normal subjects and with other forms of left ventricular hypertrophy are planned.

Acknowledgements

The authors are very grateful to Prof. Hort and Prof. Frenzel, of the Institute of Pathology, University of Düsseldorf, for performing light and electromicroscopy evaluation of myocardial biopsies.

Summary: In order to study the significance of non-ECG-gated cardiac computed tomography (CCT) for the diagnosis of hypertrophic cardiomyopathies, the method was applied in 55 consecutive patients and the data were correlated with the echocardiogram. In a subset of 18 patients left and right heart catheterization was additionally performed, and in a subset of 17 patients, endomyocardial biopsy was performed.

The CCT turned out to be an easily applicable, non-time-consuming method for obtaining a sectional visualization of the left and right ventricle. Regarding the septal thickness, there was an unexpectedly high correlation between CCT and echocardiogram (r = 0.9). The left ventricular deformity observed by echocardiogram and angiography in patients with hypertrophic cardiomyopathies corresponded well to that visualized by CCT, leading to a good differentiation between HOCM and HNCM (diagnostic specificity: 92 % and 80 %, respectively).

It is concluded that the non — ECG — gated CCT seems to be a very helpful non-invasive method for diagnosing hypertrophic cardiomyopathies and differentiating between the obstructive and non-obstructive forms. From a clinical point of view, this may be important, mainly in patients in whom no clear-cut diagnosis is possible using previously applied non-invasive methods, including echocardiography. It may also be useful for follow-up studiese, providing a sectional insight into the distribution of left ventricular hypertrophy.

References

1. Carlsson E, Lipton M, Skiöldebrand C, Berninger W, Redington R (1980) Erfahrungen mit der Computertomographie bei der in vivo-Herzdiagnostik. Radiologe 20: 44
2. Doppman J, Rienmüller R, Lissner J, Zyran J, Bolte HD, Strauer B, Hellwig H (1981) Computed tomography in constrictive pericardial disease. J Comput Assist Tomogr 5: 1
3. Guthaner D, Wexler L, Harell G (1979) CT demonstration of cardiac structures. Am J Roentgenol 133: 75
4. Gietzen F, Blümm R, Frenzel H, Kuhn H (1985) Diagnose der hypertrophischen Kardiomyopathien mittels Kardiocomputertomographie. Z Kardiol 74 Suppl III: 63
5. Higgins CM, Byrd BF, Stark D, McNamary M, Lanzer P, Lipton M, Botvinick E, Chatterjee K (1985) Magnetic resonance imaging in hypertrophic cardiomyopathy. Am J Cardiol 50: 990
6. Janson R, Lackner K, Grube E, Thurn P (1979) Nichtinvasive Diagnostik der idiopathischen hypertrophischen subvalvulären Aortenstenose (IHSS) mit der Computertomographie (CT). Z Kardiol 68: 270 (Abstr)
7. Kuhn H, Mercier J, Köhler E, Frenzel H, Hort W, Loogen F (1983) Differential diagnosis of hypertrophic cardiomyopathies: Typical (subaortic) hypertrophic obstructive cardiomyopathy, atypical (midventricular) hypertrophic obstructive cardiomyopathy and hypertrophic non obstructive cardiomyopathy. Europ Heart J, 4 Suppl F: 93
8. Kuhn H, Gietzen F, Blümm R, Waßmuth E, Pfeiffer K (1985) Klinische Bedeutung der Kardiocomputertomographie bei Kardiomyopathien. Z Kardiol 74 Suppl 5: 107
9. Kuhn H, Gietzen F, Blümm R, Böcker K, Waßmuth E. Die Diagnose der hypertrophischen Kardiomyopathien mittels nicht EKG-gesteuerter Kardiocomputertomographie (in Vorbereitung)
10. Lackner K, Simon H, Thurn P (1979) Kardiocomputertomographie — neue Möglichkeiten in der radiologischen nicht invasiven Herzdiagnostik. Z Kardiol 68: 667
11. Lackner K (1986) Kardiocomputertomographie. In: Simon H, Schoob W (eds) Diagnostik in der Kardiologie und Angiologie. Thieme Verlag, Stuttgart—New York, pp 272—293
12. Sagel S, Weiss E, Gillard R, Hounsfield G, Jost R, Stanley R, Ter-Pogossian M (1977) Gated computed tomography of the human heart. Invest Radiol 12: 563
13. Ter-Pogossian M, Weiss E, Coleman R, Sobel M (1976) Computed tomography of the heart. Am J Roentgenol 127: 79
14. Thelen M (1982) Kardiocomputertomographie bei Kardiomyopathien. Dtsch Med Wschr 107: 1859

Authors' address:
Prof. Dr. med. H. Kuhn, Medizinische Klinik II der Städtischen Krankenanstalten Bielefeld-Mitte, Teutoburgerstraße, D-4800 Bielefeld 1, F.R.G.

Is regional wall stress a stimulus for myocardial hypertrophy in hypertrophic cardiomyopathy?

P. K. Blanksma

Department of Cardiology, University Hospital Groningen, The Netherlands

Introduction

The question posed in the title of this paper is, of course, a very difficult one to answer, as regional wall stress, especially in the irregularly shaped ventricle in HCM patients, cannot be measured directly. In trying to answer at least some aspects of the question one could analyze the obstructive phenomenon in HCM and see what influence the obstruction has on global systolic wall stress. Furthermore, one should investigate whether some additonal thickening of the wall, especially of the so called non-affected part of it, can be found in obstructive cases.

Dynamic outflow tract obstruction

In obstruction, we may discriminate morphologic factors, dependent on the shape and proportions of the outflow tract of the left ventricle, and functional dynamic factors, among others, dependent on early systolic ejection rate, which could be influenced e.g. pharmacologically or by an extrasystole (2, 7). This is shown in Fig. 1. On the left, it can be seen that the obstruction begins during ejection. After its onset, a sudden decrease of flow and a rise of outflow tract resistance can be seen. After intravenous administration of verapamil, it can be seen (left) that obstruction is less severe; its onset is later during ejection. Also there is a normalization of the flow curve, and a decrease in outflow tract resistance.

Secondly we will look at the influence of obstruction on left ventricular wall stress. For this purpose we investigated 19 patients with clinically proven HCM by cardiac catheterization. None of them had significant mitral regurgitation. The methods we used are extensively described elsewhere (2). In short, we performed simultaneous pressure measurements during left ventricular angiography. Left ventricular volume was calculated frame by frame from the biplane cineangiogram. From these results, we also calculated global wall stress throughout the cardiac cycle.

We could discriminate two types of obstruction. In Fig. 2 (group A) we can see that after the onset of obstruction, wall stress only decreases; its peak occurs before the onset of obstruction. In Fig. 3 (group B) the onset of obstruction is much earlier than in the case shown in Fig. 2. Peak wall stress occurs after the onset of obstruction. In this case, it might be expected that obstruction also has some influence on regional wall stress in

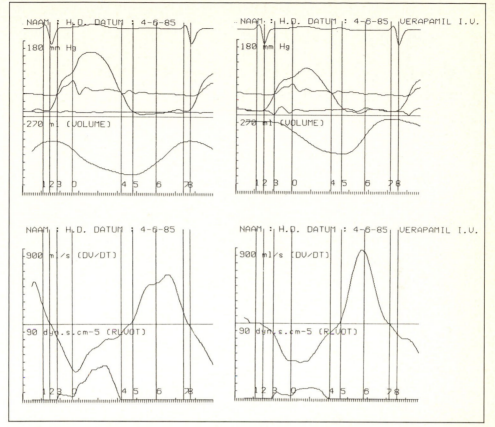

Fig. 1. Pathophysiology of left ventricular outflow tract obstruction in HCM. The effect of verapamil is seen in the right panel, the control situation on the left. From top to bottom: ECG, pressure curves of the left ventricle, ascending aorta and pulmonary wedge position, left ventricular volume curve (obtained from a calibrated nuclear probe) dV/dt curve (LV flow), and outflow tract resistance. The onset of obstruction is indicated with the vertical marker 0.

the "non-affected" parts of the ventricular wall. Comparing the hemodynamic findings in the patients with the two types of obstruction and patients without obstruction we could find almost no differences, except the timing of the peaks of the wall stress curves and the onset of obstruction (Table 1). The level of peak wall stress does not essentially diff. between non-obstructive cases, and type A and B of obstructive cases. Only in type A does there seem to be a somewhat better systolic function as judged from ejection fraction and peak systolic ejection rate. So the influence of obstruction on wall stress may not be that important for ventricular function. Perhaps there may be some influence on relaxation because of the mechanisms, pointed out by Brutsaert et al. (3), who stressed the importance of contraction loading and relaxation loading in the occurrence of relaxation disturbances. However, although verapamil improves relaxation, it has almost no influence on these timing events and on the shape of the wall stress curves (2).

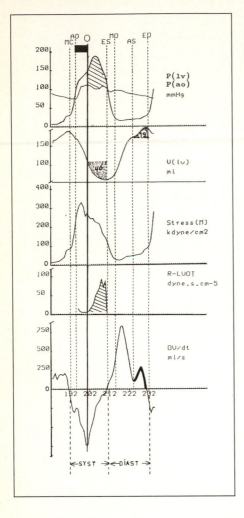

Fig. 2. Type A obstruction. From top to bottom: pressure curves of the left ventricle and ascending aorta, volume curve (obtained by frame by frame analysis of a biplane ventricular cineangiogram), wall stress curve (calculated by the formula of Mirsky), outflow tract resistance, and dV/dt. Obstruction starts late during ejection (marker 0), and the peak of the wall stress curve occurs before onset of obstruction. Note that a large part of the stroke volume is ejected after the onset of obstruction.

Morphology of the left ventricular outflow tract

Now let us look at the morphology of the ventricular wall. It is well known that an abnormal morphology is one of the most prominent factors in HCM (14). Whether the wall thickening found in these patients is real hypertrophy has to be discussed, because hypertrophy must be considered as a reaction of the myocardium to high wall stress, which is not present in HCM patients (12, 13). The site, size and shape of the septal deformity determine the likelihood of occurrence of an outflow tract obstruction (14). The abnormal myocardial morphology has been demonstrated by numerous authors (10, 11), among them Maron et al. (11), who described this by means of 2-D echocardiography and found several types. Recently we found in magnetic resonance imaging a more accurate and comprehensive way of looking at the wall thickness throughout the whole left ventricle (1, 4). We performed it with the method described by Dismore et al. (5). They

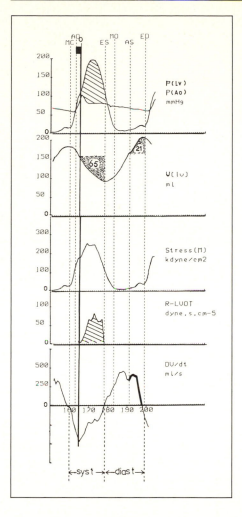

Fig. 3. Type B obstruction. Similar data as in Fig. 2. Now obstruction starts early during ejection and the peak of the wall stress occurs during obstruction. An even greater part of stroke volume is ejected during obstruction, compared to the patient in Fig. 2.

advised using a kind of pseudo-double-angulation technique of cardiac imaging, in which the patient is put on his left side with 30 ° rotation. In this way a simple method is obtained to visualize a long axis view, a four chamber view and four cross sectional views, carried out by the multiple slice technique. By this method we investigated 22 patients with HCM, using a Philips imaging system operating at 0.5 T, with a proton resonance frequency of 21.3 MHz. Images were obtained using the ECG-gated spin echo technique. Acquisition of the image started 50 ms after the R-wave (20 ms trigger delay, TE 30 ms). This yielded an image during late diastole. Images were acquired in a 256 × 256 matrix. The preparation gradient was in a left-to-right direction.

We often found myocardial wall thickening in places that could not be visualized by 2-D echocardiography, especially the apex and the left lateral wall. By our method, we could divide the patients into four groups:

Table 1. Hemodynamic measurements in HCM patients.

		NOCM n = 8	HOCM-A n = 3	HOCM-B 8 = 8
Ved		133± 47	141± 44	121± 9 ml
Ves		55± 31	34± 24	49± 21 ml
EF		60± 12	78± 9	60± 16%
plv (max)	***	123± 20	190± 12	210± 31 mm Hg
LV gradient	**	—	65± 7	103± 19 mm Hg
PW stress		278± 68	257±112	268± 98 kdyne/cm^2
T-PWS	**	181±140	100± 50	319±128 ms
L-LV obstr.		—	217± 77	119± 53 ms
PER	*	482±198	654± 86	382±128 ml/s
PFR		413±163	699±154	412±190 ml/s

Values are means ± 1 S.D. *: $p < 0.05$; **: $p < 0.005$; ***: $p < 0.0005$. Abbreviations: (EF) ejection fraction; (PW) peak wall stress; (T-PWS) time from onset of ejection to peak wall stress; (T-LV obstr.) time from onset of ejecton to onset of obstruction; (PER) peak ejection rate; (PFR) peak filling rate.

Table 2. MRI classification of hypertrophic cardiomyopathy.

	NYHA	Long axis area	P.W.Th.
1. Anteroseptal (chordal SAM)	1.4±0.7	26.4±6.1 cm^2	12.5±4.5 mm
2. High septal (obstruction)	2.5±0.5	42.7±5.6	14.5±3.8
3. Mid septal (no obstruction)	1.8±0.3	46.2±9.9	15.6±5.2
4. Latero-apical (no obstruction)	1.3±0.7	38.8±3.4	15.4±1.4

(NYHA) patients' complaints graded according to the New York Heart Association classification; (P.W.Th.) posterior wall thickness, measured by the four chamber view.

1. The anteroseptal type, in which nothing special is seen on the four chamber view, but in the cross sectional views the anteroseptal part of the left ventricular wall is thikkened. Most of these patients had no, or almost no symptoms. Often a chordal SAM was found on echocardiography, which caused no obstruction (9).
2. The high septal type: this is the classic hypertrophic cardiomyopathy with obstruction. Often serious symptoms were present, requiring operation ultimately. All patients had valvular SAM on echocardiography and obstruction. Sometimes the thickening also extended into the lower parts of the septum.
3. The isolated mid-septal type: some of these patients also had serious symptoms, especially arrhythmias in the older patients. No SAM or obstruction could be found.
4. The apico-lateral type: symptoms differed widely among patients. In this group echocardiographic data were often incomplete because of the localization of the pathology.

A gradual transition was found between the four groups. When we look at these localizations, we can say that the pathologic process does not only differ in an apex-to-base direction (vertically) but also in a transverse direction (horizontally). Main localizations can be found in a tract, spiraling down from the high septal region across the anterior wall towards the lateral and apical region.

In all patients, we measured minimum posterior wall thickness just behind the mitral valve, as an expression of (secondary) hypertrophy in the "non-affected" part of the ventricular wall. We also measured total cross-sectional area in the four chamber view as an expression of the extension of the (primary) pathological process of HCM. These measurements should not be considered absolutely, but as a means for comparing the different patient groups. We found that in the anteroseptal type posterior wall thickness and cross sectional area were less. The anteroseptal type can be considered as a less severely affected group. In the other groups, no differences in these measurements could be found (Table 2).

Conclusions

In conclusion, we can say that in some HCM patients (group B, Fig. 3) some additional afterload is imposed on the ventricular wall by the obstructive phenomenon. However, by magnetic resonance imaging which, for the time being, is the most powerful technique in imaging the ventricular wall throughout the left ventricle, no relation can be found of the presence of obstruction, and the thickness of the least affected part of the myocardium. This might be considered as an argument against the importance of obstruction in the pathophysiology of HCM.

Summary: To answer the question of whether regional wall stress may be a stimulus for myocardial hypertrophy in hypertrophic cardiomyopathy, we have to firstly look at the nature of dynamic outflow tract obstruction and its influence on left ventricular wall stress. We may discriminate two types of outflow tract obstruction: type A, in which peak wall stress occurs before the onset of obstruction and type B, in which it occurs afterwards. Only in type B could one expect that obstruction could have any influence on wall stress. In type B the obstruction is more severe and occurs earlier than in type A. Secondly, to say something about regional wall stress, we should look at the morphology of the left ventricular wall. We have found magnetic resonance imaging to be an accurate and comprehensive way of looking at this. We may discriminate four types of left ventricular wall morphology in hypertrophic cardiomyopathy: (a) the anteroseptal type, (b) the upper septal type, (c) the midseptal type, (d) the apico-lateral type. Only in the upper septal type is outflow tract obstruction found. However, posterior wall thickness, as a measure of hypertrophy, is not different in these patients from posterior wall thickness in types c and d, in which no obstruction is found. Also, no difference is found in cross-sectional area in the long axis plane between types b, c and d. Only in type a, which seems to represent a less seriously affected group, posterior wall thickness and cross-sectional area are less than in the other groups. From these findings, it may be concluded that only in patients with an early onset obstruction could some influence of obstruction be expected on wall stress, but with magnetic resonance imaging no effect of obstruction on wall thickness can be demonstrated.

References

1. Been M, Kean D, Smith MA, Douglas RHB, Best JJK, Muir AL (1985) Nuclear magnetic resonance in hypertrophic cardiomyopathy. Br Heart J 54: 48—52

2. Blanksma PK (1985) Pressure-volume and stress-strain relation-ships in hypertrophic cardio-myopathy. In: van der Wall E, Lie KI (eds) Recent views on hypertrophic cardiomyopathy, Martinus Nijhof pp 63—69

3. Brutsaert DL, Rademakers FE, Sys FU (1984) Triple control of relaxation: implications in cardiac disease. Circulation 69: 190—196

4. Budinger ThF, Lautebur PC. Nuclear magnetic resonance technology for medical studies. Science 184: 226: 288—98

5. Dinsmore RE, Wismer GJ, Levine RA, Okada RD, Brady TJ (1984) Magnetic resonance imaging of the heart. Positioning and gradient angle selection for optimal imaging plane. Am J Radiol 143: 1135—1142

6. Hamer JPM (1985) Problems and pitfalls in the diagnosis of hypertrophic cardiomyopathy by echocardiography. In: van der Wall E, Lie KI (eds) Recent view on hypertrophic cardiomyopathy, Martinus Nijhof pp 9—19

7. Henry WL, Clark CE, Griffith JM, Epstein SE (1975) Mechanism of left ventricular outflow tract obstruction in patients with idiopathic hypertrophic subaortic stenosis. Am J Cardiol 35: 337—345

8. Higgins CB, Byrd III BF, Stark D, McNamara M, Lanzer P, Lipton MJ, Schiller NB, Botvinick E, Chatterjee K (1985) Magnetic resonance in hypertrophic cardiomyopathy. Am J Cardiol 55: 1121—1126

9. Gardin JM, Talino JV, Stephanides L (1981) Systolic anterior motion in the absence of hypertrophic cardiomyopathy. Circulation 63: 181—188

10. Gilbert BW, Pollick C, Adelman AG (1980) Hypertrophic cardiomyopathy, subclassification by M-mode echocardiography. Am J Cardiol 45: 861—872

11. Maron BJ, Gottdiener JS, Epstein SE (1981) Patterns and significance of distribution of left ventricular hypertrophy in hypertrophic cardiomyopathy. Am J Cardiol 48: 418—428

12. Pouleur H, Rousseau MF, van Eyll Chr, Blasseur LA, Charlier LA (1983) Force — velocity — length relations in hypertrophic cardiomyopathy — evidence of normal or depressed myocardial contractility. Am J Cardiol 52: 813—817

13. Strauer BE (1979) Myocardial oxygen consumption in chronic heart disease: role of wall stress, hypertrophy and coronary reserve. Am J Cardiol 44: 730—740

14. van der Wall E (1985) Recent views on left ventricular function in hypertrophic cardiomyopathy: hemodynamic concepts and their clinical implications. In: van der Wall E, Lie KI (eds) Recent views on hypertrophic cardiomyopathy, Martinus Nijhof pp 71—99

15. Wigle ED, Sanon S, Henderson MA, Ruddy TD, Fulop J, Rakowsky H, Williams WG (1985) Hypertrophic cardiomyopathy. The importance of the site and extent of hypertrophy. A review. Progress in Cardiovasc Dis 28:1-83

Author's address:
Dr. P. K. Blanksma, Department of Cardiology, University Hospital Groningen, Postbus 30001, NL-9700 RB Groningen, The Netherlands

Evidence for true obstruction to left ventricular outflow in obstructive hypertrophic cardiomyopathy (muscular or hypertrophic subaortic stenosis)

E. D. Wigle and H. Rakowski

Division of Cardiology, Department of Medicine, Toronto General Hospital and University of Toronto, Canada

1. Introduction

Hypertrophic cardiomyopathy (HCM) is characterized by symmetrical or asymmetrical hypertrophy of the left and/or right ventricles (Table 1). It is a primary disorder of heart muscle in which the site and extent of the hypertrophic process are believed to be of importance in determining the disease manifestations (30). In this discussion we will limit our remarks to the commonest form of HCM, that is associated with ventricular (asymmetrical) septal hypertrophy (Table 1). It has been traditional to hemodynamically classify this form of HCM into obstructive and nonobstructive types, depending on whether or not there is a pressure gradient across the left ventricular outflow tract due to mitral leaflet-septal contact (5, 21, 30). In obstructive HCM this pressure gradient may be persistent (gradient at rest), labile (spontaneously variable), or latent (provocable) (5, 30, 31). In discussing whether there is true obstruction to left ventricular outflow in obstructive HCM, we will focus our attention on the situation in which there is a persistent subaortic pressure gradient at rest.

Table 1. Types of hypertrophic cardiomyopathy.

	Approximate incidence*
Left ventricular involvement	
Asymmetrical hypertrophy	
Ventricular septal hypertrophy	90%
Midventricular hypertrophy	1%
Apical hypertrophy	3%
Posteroseptal and/or lateral wall hypertrophy	1%
Symmetrical (concentric) hypertrophy	5%
Right ventricular involvement	

* at the Toronto General Hospital. The incidence of the different types of hypertrophic cardiomyopathy varies considerably between different centers.

2. Types of systolic pressure difference in HCM

Prior to reviewing the evidence for true obstruction to left ventricular outflow in obstructive HCM, it is necessary to define the four different types of systolic pressure difference that may be encountered in HCM (30, 31) (Table 2, Fig. 1). An early systolic impulse gradient across the aortic valve results from flow acceleration in early systole (18). This gradient may be greater than normal in HCM due to very rapid early systolic ejection, but it ends by mid-systole, when flow acceleration decreases (18). A second type of systolic pressure difference within the left ventricle in HCM is that produced by mid-ventricular obstruction at the level of the papillary muscles (Fig. 1, right). We have en-

Table 2. Differentiation of intraventricular pressure differences that may be encountered in hypertrophic cardiomyopathy.

	Obstructive HCM	Cavity obliteration	Impulse gradient	Midventricular obstruction
Hemodynamics				
Elevated LV inflow pressure	+	−	+	−
Entrapment criteria*	−	+	−	−
Time of peak systolic gradient	Late	Late	Early	Late
Spike–and–Dome aortic pressure	+	−	−	−
Spike–and–Dome aortic flow	+	−	−	−
LV ejection time	Increased	Normal (or short)	Normal (or short)	Increased
Cineangiography				
Mitral–septal contact (radiolucent line)	+	−	−	−
LV end–systolic volume	Variable	Small	Normal	Base small Apex large
Mitral regurgitation	++	±	−	−
LV cavity obliteration	± Late if +	+ Early	−	−
Echocardiography				
1D				
Severe SAM	+	−	−	−
Left atrial enlargement	+	−	−	±
Aortic valve notch	+	−	−	−
2D				
Mitral leaflet–septal contact	+	−	−	−
Clinical				
Apical murmur	3—4/6	0—2/6	±	2—4/6
Reversed split S_2	+	−	−	−

* See Text. LV = Left ventricle; SAM = Systolic anterior motion of mitral leaflet; 1D and 2D = one and two–dimensional echocardiography.

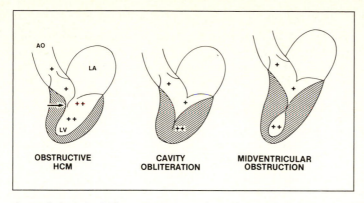

Fig. 1. The left ventricular (LV) inflow tract pressure concept (26). In obstructive HCM all LV pressures proximal to the outflow tract obstruction caused by mitral leaflet-septal contact (arrow) are elevated, including the inflow tract pressure just inside the mitral valve. In cavity obliteration and midventricular obstruction, the pressure at the apex of the LV is elevated, but the inflow tract pressure is not (see text). (AO) Aorta; (LA) left atrium.

countered a number of these cases that have been associated with apical myocardial infarction and aneurysm formation, in whom the apical systolic pressure is elevated, but both the left ventricular inflow and outflow tract pressures are low and equal to aortic systolic pressure (30) (Table 2, Fig. 1, right). Left ventricular cineangiography reveals midcavity obliteration (occlusion) at the level of the papillary muscles. This cineangiographic appearance in midventricular obstruction must be distinguished from end-systolic papillary muscle approximation (without obstruction) that occurs in HCM when there is extensive left ventricular and papillary muscle hypertrophy (30). An impulse gradient and the gradient that occurs in midventricular obstruction are readily recognized (Table 2).

The third type of pressure difference that may be encountered in HCM is the intraventricular pressure difference that may be associated with cavity obliteration (7) (Table 2, Fig. 1, centre). In this situation the apical cavity obliteration occurs early in systole (12) and the catheter recording the elevated apical systolic pressure is often observed to be outside the end-systolic cineangiographic silhouette of the left ventricle (7, 12). The apical left ventricular pressure is elevated (Fig. 1, center), whereas all other pressures in the left ventricle, including the left ventricular inflow tract pressure, are low and equal to the outflow tract and aortic systolic pressures (26). The intraventricular pressure difference of cavity obliteration is not associated with echocardiographic or cineangiographic mitral leaflet-septal contact (30) (Table 2).

The elevated apical systolic pressure in cavity obliteration was originally attributed to the apical catheter being enfolded (7), engulfed (7), or entrapped (26) by isometrically contracting myocardium in the obliterated apex of the ventricle. More recently it has been suggested that the intraventricular pressure difference in cavity obliteration is the result of a high pressure being generated by the rapidly contracting apex, and that this pressure is somehow not transmitted to the less contractile base of the left ventricle (8, 9). However, Doppler velocity signals recorded at the junction between the rapidly contracting apex and the poorly contracting base (13, 23) (D in Fig. 2, right), do not correlate in time or magnitude with the measured intraventricular pressure difference (31). Thus it would seem most likely that the elevated left ventricular systolic pressure in cavity

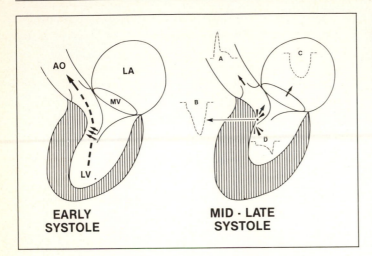

EARLY
SYSTOLE

MID - LATE
SYSTOLE

Fig. 2. Left: In obstructive HCM there is rapid, early systolic ejection (dashed line) through the outflow tract that is narrowed by septal hypertrophy. This results in Venturi forces (three short oblique arrows in the outflow tract) drawing the anterior (upper two arrows) and/or posterior (lower arrow) mitral leaflet(s) towards the septum (systolic anterior motion). Subsequent mitral leaflet-septal contact results in obstruction to left ventricular (LV) outflow and concomitant mitral regurgitation, as seen on the right.

Right: By midsystole, anterior mitral leaflet-septal contact causes obstruction to LV outflow (converging and diverging lines) resulting in decreased forward aortic flow (smaller arrow) and mitral regurgitation (oblique arrow arising from mitral orifice).

(A), (B), (C) and (D) indicate Doppler velocity recordings throughout systole in ascending aorta (8) (A) (flow towards transducer); at the level of mitral leaflet-septal contact (5, 6), (B); in left atrium (5) (C); and near apex LV (5) (D). In (B), (C), and (D), flow is away from transducer. Peak velocities recorded at (B), correlate accurately with simultaneously measured pressure gradient (6) whereas late peaking velocities at (D) do not.

(AO) Aorta; (LA) left atrium; (MV) mitral valve; (LV) left ventricle (see text). (Reproduced with the permission of American Heart Association from (31)).

obliteration is due to the apical catheter being enfolded, engulfed or entrapped by isometrically contracting myocardium as was originally suggested (7). In these circumstances, the high pressure recorded may be a reflection of intramyocardial tissue pressure (26).

The fourth type of intraventricular pressure difference that may be encountered in HCM is the subaortic pressure gradient due to mitral leaflet-septal contact in obstructive HCM (Fig. 1, left, and Fig. 2, Table 2). In this situation (Fig. 1, left) the left ventricular outflow tract pressure distal to mitral leaflet-septal contact (and proximal to the aortic valve) is low and equal to aortic systolic pressure, whereas all ventricular pressures proximal to the obstruction, including the left ventricular inflow tract pressure just inside the mitral valve, are elevated (26). This type of subaortic pressure gradient is associated with echocardiographic and cineangiographic evidence of mitral leaflet-septal contact (30) (Fig. 2, right), and an elevated left ventricular inflow tract pressure (26) (Fig. 1, left), whereas in cavity obliteration or in midventricular obstruction the left ventricular inflow tract pressure is not elevated (26, 30) (Fig. 1, center and right), and there is no evidence of mitral leaflet-septal contact (Table 2) (30). It is essential in the management of patients with HCM to distinguish an obstructive subaortic pressure gradient due to mitral leaflet-septal contact, from the intraventricular pressure difference that may be associated with cavity obliteration or midventricular obstruction (30, 31).

The remainder of this discussion will be directed at deciding whether the subaortic pressure gradient due to mitral leaflet-septal contact in obstructive HCM represents true obstruction to left ventricular outflow.

3. Mechanism of mitral leaflet systolic anteriormotion in obstructive HCM

In 1971 we first suggested that mitral leaflet systolic anterior motion could result from Venturi forces acting on the mitral leaflets, due to the rapid, nonobstructed early systolic ejection jet passing closer to the mitral leaflets than is normal, as a result of the outflow tract being narrowed by the ventricular septal hypertrophy (29) (Fig. 2, left). Subsequently, extensive clinical (30) experimental (1), echocardiographic (30), Doppler (13) and surgical (30) observations have supported this concept (Figs. 2, 3). By decreasing septal thickness, the ventriculomyectomy operation increases the size of the left ventricular outflow tract (LVOT) and results in the early systolic ejection path being displaced away from the mitral leaflets, thus reducing or abolishing the Venturi forces on these leaflets (Fig. 3). As a result, mitral leaflet systolic anterior motion (SAM), the obstruction to outflow and the mitral regurgitation are abolished. The abolition of the obstruction normalizes aortic flow with the result that the spike and dome aortic flow and pressure profiles and aortic valve notch are abolished. Left ventricular ejection time is no longer prolonged and splitting of the second heart sound (S2) becomes normal. The abolition of the obstruction abolishes the early systolic contraction load on the left ventricle which should improve LV relaxation (30) and result in a reduction in LV end-diastolic (LVEDP) and left atrial pressures (LAP). Abolition of the mitral regurgitation would also decrease LVEDP and LAP as well as LA size, thus rendering the patient less liable to atrial arrhythmias. The abolition of the apical systolic murmur results from the abolition of the obstruction and the mitral regurgitation, while these two factors plus the lowering of

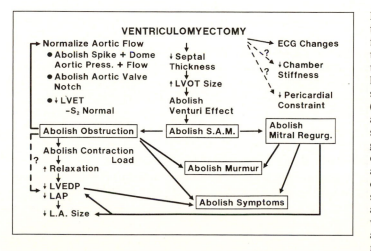

Fig. 3. Ventriculomyectomy enlarges LV outflow tract (LVOT), thereby abolishing Venturi forces on mitral leaflets and mitral leaflet systolic anterior motion (SAM). This results in abolition of LVOT obstruction and mitral regurgitation, which accounts for changes in aortic pressure and flow, decrease in LV end-diastolic (LVEDP) and left atrial pressures (LAP), as well as the decrease or abolition of the apical murmur and the patient's symptoms. Postoperative changes in ECG, chamber stiffness, or degree of pericardial constraint are not essential to the success of this surgery.
(Reproduced with permission from (30)).

LVEDP and LAP result in a lessening or abolition of the patient's symptoms. It is not known whether a decrease in chamber stiffness or in the degree of pericardial constraint could also favour symptomatic benefit following the ventriculomyectomy operation. There is no evidence that surgically induced ventricular conduction defects explain the beneficial effects of the surgery.

Some authors have suggested various myocardial contraction mechanisms (8, 9) as the cause of systolic anterior motion, but these suggestions are considered unlikely, if not untenable, based on the dynamics of development and cessation of mitral leaflet-septal contact (30). Although mitral leaflet systolic anterior motion is believed to result from Venturi forces on the mitral leaflets, it is presently unclear whether mitral leaflet-septal contact is maintained by continuing Venturi forces and/or by the elevated left ventricular systolic pressure proximal to the obstruction (30, 31).

4. Evidence that mitral leaflet-septal contact is the cause of the subaortic pressure gradient and mitral regurgitation in obstructive HCM

a. HCM patients with severe mitral leaflet systolic anterior motion, associated with early and prolonged mitral leaflet-septal contact, have subaortic pressure gradients, whereas patients with moderate, mild or no systolic anterior motion do not (30).

b. Combined hemodynamic-echocardiographic (30) and hemodynamic-cineangiographic (12) studies indicate that the onset of the subaortic pressure gradient (defined as the peak of the aortic percussion wave), occurs just before or simultaneously with the onset of mitral leaflet-septal contact.

c. The time of onset in systole of mitral leaflet-septal contact determines the magnitude of the pressure gradient, the degree of prolongation of left ventricular ejection time, and the percentage of stroke volume that is ejected against the obstruction (30). Thus, early (and prolonged) mitral leaflet-septal contact is associated with a high pressure gradient, marked prolongation of left ventricular ejection time, and a large percentage of left ventricular stroke volume is ejected against the obstruction. In contrast, mitral leaflet-septal contact of late onset (and short duration) is associated with a small pressure gradient, mild prolongation of left ventricular ejection time and only a small percentage of left ventricular stroke volume is ejected against the obstruction. If mitral leaflet-septal contact occurs after 55 % of the systolic ejection period, no pressure gradient develops (30).

d. Recently reported high pulsed repetition frequency (PRF) pulsed Doppler (13, 30), as well as continuous (13, 22) wave and colour Doppler (15, 22) studies provide important new confirmatory evidence that the site of the obstruction, and hence the origin of the pressure gradient in obstructive HCM, is at the level of mitral leaflet- septal contact (Fig. 2, right). In valvular aortic stenosis, the velocity of the jet accelerates just proximal to the stenotic valve (15), and the peak flow velocity at the level of the valve permits calculation of the transvalvular gradient, which correlates closely with the simultaneously determined hemodynamic pressure gradient (13). Similarly, in obstructive HCM, the velocity of the jet accelerates just proximal to the obstruction, i.e., mitral leaflet-septal contact (15), and the peak flow velocity at the level of mitral leaflet-septal contact (13, 22, 30) (B in Fig. 2, right), permits calculation of the subaortic pressure gradient that correlates closely with the simultaneously measured hemodynamic pressure gradient. The fact that virtually identical flow velocity and pressure relationships exist across the valve in valvular aortic stenosis and across the site of mitral leaflet-septal contact in obstructive HCM provides essentially incontrovertible evidence that the site of mitral leaflet-septal contact is the origin of the subaortic pressure gradient in obstructive HCM (22, 31).

e. A number of characteristic features of obstructive HCM occur in close time proximity to the onset of mitral leaflet-septal contact (30). These are: the peak of the aortic percussion wave (12, 30), the onset of flow deceleration in the ascending aorta (10) (A in Fig. 2, right), the point of inflection on the rising left ventricular pressure (3) and on the continuous wave Doppler recording (B in Fig. 2, right), and the onset of partial aortic valve closure. In addition, it has recently been shown in obstructive HCM that there is an abrupt slowing of left ventricular emptying (4) and of inward left ventricular wall motion (20) during systole. This combination of near simultaneous events strongly suggests a sudden alteration of systolic hemodynamics in obstructive HCM, i.e., the onset of obstruction due to mitral leaflet-septal contact (30, 31).

f. Mitral regurgitation, believed to be due to mitral leaflet systolic anterior motion, has been shown by indicator dilution techniques to invariably accompany the subaortic pressure gradient in obstructive HCM, although Doppler and cineangiographic studies do not always detect it (28, 30). In the absence of an independent mitral valve abnormality, the degree of mitral regurgitation in the individual case is directly related to the severity of the obstruction, and hence the severity of mitral leaflet-septal contact (28, 30). Although mitral regurgitation may be detected by cineangiographic (30) or Doppler (13) techniques at the onset of systole, both cineangiographic (30) and colour Doppler (15, 22) studies reveal that the major portion of mitral regurgitation occurs in the last half of systole and is a major determinant of the end-systolic size of the left ventricle. In obstructive HCM, both colour Doppler (15, 22) and cineangiographic (30) studies reveal rapid, unobstructed, early systolic ejection into the aorta, the onset of mitral leaflet-septal contact and the obstruction, followed by predominantly late systolic mitral regurgitation (eject/obstruct/leak) (30) (Fig. 2).

5. Evidence of true obstruction to left ventricular ejection associated with the subaortic pressure gradient, due to mitral leaflet-septal contact in obstructive HCM

a. All ventricular systolic pressures proximal to mitral leaflet-septal contact are elevated

As is the case with valvular aortic stenosis, in obstructive HCM, all ventricular systolic pressures proximal to the obstruction are elevated, including the left ventricular inflow tract pressure (21, 26) (Fig. 1, left). Catheters recording these high pressures can be freely moved about within the left ventricular cavity without altering the high systolic pressures (26) and, indeed, multiple catheters may be placed in the left ventricle proximal to the obstruction and equally elevated pressures recorded (21, 26). When the proximal end of any of these catheters is opened, blood "shoots out" in systole, indicating that the distal tip of the catheter is in a high pressure, blood-filled area of the left ventricle (26).

b. Prolongation of left ventricular ejection time

One of the most characteristic features of any form of obstruction to left ventricular outflow is a prolongation of left ventricular ejection time. We have previously demonstrated that the degree of prolongation of left ventricular ejection time in obstructive HCM is directly related to the magnitude of the pressure gradient (27) and that both are related to the time of onset of mitral leaflet-septal contact in systole (30). This direct relationship between the magnitude of the pressure gradient and the degree of prolongation of left ventricular ejection time is maintained whether the gradient is increased or decreased by pharmacological or surgical means (27). Some authors, who have adopted a nonobstructive viewpoint of obstructive HCM, have suggested that the prolonged ejection time is related to impairment of left ventricular relaxation (9, 11, 18). However, prolongation of left ventricular ejection time does not occur in nonobstructive HCM with impairment of left ventricular relaxation (30, 31). A prolonged ejection time only occurs in obstructive HCM and the degree of prolongation is related to the severity of the obstruction (27, 30, 31), as is the case with valvular aortic stenosis.

c. Percentage of left ventricular stroke volume ejected in the presence of the obstructive subaortic pressure gradient

It is recognized that there is rapid, nonobstructed, early systolic ejection in obstructive HCM (Fig. 2, left). If this were not the case, there would be no Venturi effect to cause mitral leaflet systolic anterior motion. The question to be answered here is: What percentage of left ventricular stroke volume leaves the left ventricle after the onset of mitral leaflet-septal contact and the pressure gradient? No fewer than five different techniques have been used to study this question and the results are very similar. Thus, cineangiographic (30), echocardiographic (10), nuclear angiographic (3), as well as Doppler (17) and electromagnetic flow studies (2, 19, 21), have indicated that between 40% and 70% of left ventricular stroke volume leaves the left ventricle after the onset of mitral leaflet-septal contact and/or the subaortic pressure gradient. With the onset of the obstruction to outflow, the calculated resistance across the outflow tract increases dramatically (2) and this is accompanied by a sudden deceleration in ascending aortic flow (10), a decrease in the rate of left ventricular emptying (4) and a sudden decrease in inward left ventricular wall motion (20). Ascending aortic (2, 10, 13, 14, 16, 17, 19, 24) and left ventricular outflow tract (13, 16, 22, 30, 32) velocity-flow studies indicate continuing but reduced ejection into the left ventricular outflow tract and the aorta (A and B, in Fig. 2, right), during the presence of the subaortic pressure gradient. Cineangiographic (30) as well as colour (15, 22) and continuous wave Doppler studies (C in Fig. 2, right) indicate that the major portion of mitral regurgitation occurs in the last half of systole, after the onset of mitral leaflet-septal contact and the subaortic obstruction. Thus, there is overwhelming evidence (3, 10, 13, 15, 17, 19, 21, 22, 30) to indicate that a very significant percentage of left ventricular stroke volume leaves the left ventricle as forward or regurgitant flow during the presence of the obstructive subaortic pressure gradient. The actual percentage of left ventricular stroke volume that is ejected in the presence of the subaortic obstruction is determined by the time of onset of mitral leaflet-septal contact in systole, which also determines the mangnitude of the pressure gradient, the amount of mitral regurgitation and the degree of prolongation of left ventricular ejection time (30).

This systolic overload is not only of hemodynamic importance in obstructive HCM but is also of metabolic and clinical significance (see below).

d. Myocardial ischemia associated with obstructive subaortic pressure gradients

In patients with obstructive HCM, large pressure gradients are associated with increased myocardial oxygen consumption and metabolic evidence of myocardial ischemia during pacing. Surgical abolition of the pressure gradient results in a marked reduction in myocardial oxygen consumption and alleviation of the myocardial ischemia (6). These observations are consistent with the elevated left ventricular systolic pressure causing increased myocardial oxygen consumption and resulting in myocardial ischemia.

e. Symptoms related to the presence of the obstructive subaortic pressure gradient

Although it is recognized that HCM patients with and without obstructive pressure gradients may have similar symptoms, we have recently reported that patients with obstructive HCM have a significantly higher incidence of Class III-IV NYHA symptomatology, as well as a significantly higher overall incidence of angina and dyspnea (30). Patients with obstructive pressure gradients also have a significantly higher incidence of grade III-IV/VI apical systolic murmurs and reversed splitting of the second heart sound (30). These observations provide evidence that the obstructive pressure gradients in HCM are not only of hemodynamic and metabolic significance, but also of profound clinical significance and are in keeping with the dramatic clinical benefits derived from a successful ventriculomyectomy operation (30) (Fig. 3).

6. A brief comment on the nonobstructive viewpoint in HCM

The nonobstructive viewpoint suggests that left ventricular emptying in HCM occurs faster and more completely than normal (9, 11, 18) that an intraventricular pressure difference develops between the rapidly contracting apex and poorly contracting base of the left ventricle (8, 9), and that forward aortic flow (18) and left ventricular emptying (9) virtually cease well before end-systole, i.e., the left ventricle is essentially isovolumetric (9) during the late systolic period of no forward flow. Mitral leaflet-septal contact is attributed to left ventricular cavity obliteration right up to the submitral area (9).

Although superficially plausible, this nonobstructive viewpoint does not stand up to careful scrutiny:

a. The authors (9, 11) make no attempt to distinguish between the subaortic pressure gradient due to mitral leaflet-septal contact in obstructive HCM from the intraventricular pressure difference that may be encountered in cavity obliteration (Fig. 1).

b. Doppler flow velocity studies (13, 23) (D in Fig. 2, right) do not support the concept that a pressure gradient develops between the rapidly contracting apex and the poorly contracting basal region of the left ventricle, but Doppler studies do provide conclusive evidence that the pressure gradient arises in the subaortic area at the site of mitral leaflet-septal contact (13, 22, 30) (B in Fig. 2, right).

c. Although catheter mounted velocity flow probe studies suggest that in late systole there is no significant forward aortic flow in obstructive and nonobstructive HCM, four other methods of investigating forward aortic flow in obstructive HCM have failed to confirm this finding (10, 14, 16, 17, 19, 24). These other methods indicate that there is a rapid deceleration of ascending aortic flow in early systole that occurs virtually simultaneously with the onset of mitral leaflet-septal contact (10). Subsequently, there is reduced but definite forward aortic flow throughout the rest of systole (10, 14, 16, 17, 19, 24) (A in Fig. 2, right). Both continuous wave (13, 32) and multigated Doppler (16, 24) studies in obstructive HCM reveal that ascending aortic flow is very non-uniform after the onset of the obstruction. Multigated studies (16, 24) reveal cessation of forward aortic flow prior to the end of systole near the posterior aortic wall, whereas forward flow continues near the anterior aortic wall. These observations dictate extreme caution in the interpretation of aortic velocity-flow measurements when they are recorded from a single aortic site by a technique such as catheter mounted velocity flow probe (24, 31).

d. The nonobstructive viewpoint suggests that mitral leaflet systolic anterior motion and subsequent mitral leaflet-septal contact is due to cavity obliteration of the submitral area of the left ventricle, i.e. very little left ventricular emptying occurs after the onset of mitral leaflet-septal contact (8, 9). However, we have shown that mitral leaflet systolic anterior motion bears no relation to the inward motion of the left ventricular posterior wall or to cavity obliteration, and that mitral leaflet-septal contact occurs about 200 ms prior to minimal left ventricular diameter (30). In addition, large obstructive pressure gradients due to mitral leaflet-septal contact have been demonstrated to occur in the absence of any cavity obliteration (30). Finally, a number of studies have documented that a significant percentage of left ventricular emptying into the aorta and left atrium occurs after the onset of mitral leaflet-septal contact and the obstructive pressure gradient (3, 10, 13, 15, 17, 19, 21, 22, 30), i.e., the left ventricle is not isovolumetric during the last half of systole, as suggested by those holding the nonobstructive viewpoint.

7. Conclusion

As a result of the foregoing analysis, one can only conclude that true obstruction to left ventricular outflow does exist in obstructive HCM and it is caused by prolonged mitral leaflet-septal contact. Recent pulsed (13, 30), continuous wave (13, 22, 32), multigated (16, 24), and colour (15, 22) Doppler studies only reinforce this conclusion, which was previously based on clinical (5, 25), phonocardiographic (5, 25), echocardiographic (10, 30), hemodynamic (5, 21, 26, 27, 30) and cineangiographic (12, 30) evidence. Appropriate care must continue to be exercised in distinguished the subaortic pressure gradient in obstructive HCM, from the intraventricular pressure difference encountered in cavity obliteration or in midventricular obstruction (30). Fortunately, there are now both clinical and echo-Doppler criteria that permit clear distinction between these different types of intraventricular pressure difference in HCM without resorting to invasive studies (10, 13, 15–17, 22, 30, 32). The latter should be reserved for diagnostic problems and/ or when surgery is being considered.

To deny the presence of obstruction to left ventricular outflow in obstructive HCM is to deny these patients appropriate medical and/or surgical therapy.

Summary: In obstructive hypertrophic cardiomyopathy (muscular or hypertrophic subaortic stenosis), there is rapid early systolic ejection through an outflow tract that is narrowed by ventricular septal hypertrophy. This results in Venturi forces acting on the mitral leaflets, which cause mitral leaflet systolic anterior motion. Subsequent mitral leaflet-septal contact results in obstruction to left ventricular outflow and concomitant mitral regurgitation. Evidence is provided that the subaortic pressure gradient in obstructive hypertrophic cardiomyopathy reflects true obstruction to left ventricular outflow. It is important to distinguish this truly obstructive subaortic pressure gradient, due to mitral leaflet-septal contact, from an early systolic impulse gradient, as well as from the intraventricular pressure difference that may be encountered in midventricular obstruction or cavity obliteration.

References

1. Bellhouse BJ, Bellhouse FH (1982) The fluid mechanics of subaortic stenosis in a model left ventricle. University of Oxford, Department of Engineering Science, Report No 1032/72
2. Bircks W, Bostroem B, Gleichmann U, Kreuzer H, Loogen F (1968) Electromagnetic flow measurement in the ascending aorta before and after repair of valvular and subvalvular lesions including IHSS. Proceedings of the Vth European Congress of Cardiology (Athens), pp 13—22
3. Bonow RO, Ostrow HG; Rosing DR, Cannon RO, Leon MB, Watson RM, Bacharach SL, Green MV, Epstein SE (1984) Dynamic pressure-volume alterations during left ventricular ejection in hypertrophic cardiomyopathy: Evidence for true obstruction to left ventricular outflow. Circulation 70: II-17 (Abstr)
4. Bonow RO, Crawford-Green C, Betocci S, Rosing DR, Maron BJ (1985) Left ventricular ejection dynamics in hypertrophic cardiomyopathy: Comparison with valvular aortic stenosis. J Am Coll Cardiol 5: 394 (abstract)
5. Braunwald E, Lambrew CT, Morrow AG, Pierce GE, Rockoff SD, Ross J Jr (1964) Idiopathic hypertrophic subaortic stenosis. Circulation 30: IV, 3—119
6. Cannon RO, Rosing DR, McIntosh CL, Epstein SE (1985) Hypertrophic cardiomyopathy (HCM): Improved hemodynamics, metabolism and anginal threshold following surgical relief of obstruction. Circulation 72: III-447 (Abstr)
7. Criley MJ, Lewis KB, White RI, Ross RS (1965) Pressure gradients without obstruction: a new concept of "hypertrophic subaortic stenosis". Circulation 22: 881—887
8. Criley MJ, Lennon PA, Abbasi AS, Blaufuss AH (1976) Hypertrophic cardiomyopathy, In: Levine HJ (ed) Clinical Cardiovascular Physiology. Grune & Stratton Inc., New York, pp 771—827
9. Criley MJ, Seigel RJ (1985) Has 'obstruction' hindered our understanding of hypertrophic cardiomyopathy? Circulation 72: 1148—1154
10. Glasgow GA, Gardin JM, Burns CS, Childs WJ, Henry WL (1980) Echocardiographic and Doppler flow observations in idiopathic hypertrophic subaortic stenosis (IHSS). Circulation 62: III-99 (abstr)
11. Goodwin JF (1982) The frontiers of cardiomyopathy. Br Heart J 48: 1—18
12. Grose RM, Strain JE, Spindola-Franco H (1985) Angiographic and hemodynamic correlations in hypertrophic cardiomyopathy. Circulation 73: III-15 (abstr)
13. Hatle L, Angelsen B (1985) Doppler ultrasound in cardiology. In: Lea & Febiger, Philadelphia, pp 205—217
14. Hernandez RR, Greenfield JC Jr., McCall BW (1964) Pressure-flow studies in hypertrophic subaortic stenosis. J Clin Invst 43: 401—407
15. Holt B, Sahn DJ, Dalton N, Smith SC, Yun Y, Dittrich H (1985) Color Doppler flow mapping studies of jet formation in hypertrophic cardiomyopathy (HCM). Circulation 72: III-447 (abstract)
16. Jenni R, Ruffmann K, Vieli A, Anlinker M, Krayenbuehl HP (1985) Dynamics of aortic flow in hypertrophic cardiomyopathy. Europ Heart J 6: 391—398

17. Maron BJ, Gottdiener JS, Arce J, Rosing DR, Wesley YE, Epstein SE (1985) Dynamic subaortic obstruction in hypertrophic cardiomyopathy: analysis by pulsed Doppler echocardiography. J Am Coll Cardiol 6: 1—15
18. Murgo JP, Alter BR, Dorethy JF, Altobelli SA, McGranahan GM Jr (1980) Dynamics of left ventricular ejection in obstructive and nonobstructive hypertrophic cardiomyopathy. J Clin Invest 66: 1369—1382
19. Pierce GE, Morrow AG, Braunwald E (1964) Idiopathic hypertrophic subaortic stenosis III. Intraoperative studies of the mechanism of obstruction and its hemodynamic consequences. Circulation 30: IV, 152—207
20. Pouleur H, Van Eyll C, Gurne O, Hanet C, Rousseau MF (1985) Regional velocity of shortening in hypertrophic cardiomyopathy: Evidence for true impedance to shortening in the presence of outflow gradients. Circulation 72: III-448 (abstract)
21. Ross J Jr., Braunwald E, Gault JH, Mason DT, Morrow AG (1966) The mechanism of the intraventricular pressure gradient in idiopathic hypertrophic subaortic stenosis. Circulation 34: 558—578
22. Stewart WJ, Schiavone WA, Salcedo EE, Lever HM, Cosgrove DM, Gill CC (1985) Intraoperative Doppler velocity correlates with outflow gradient in HOCM pre- and post-myectomy. Circulation 72: III-447 (abstr)
23. Stewart WJ, Schiavone WA (1986) Doppler echocardiographic evaluation of valvular stenosis. In: Pohost GM, Higgins CB, Morganroth J, Schelbert HR (eds) New Concepts in Cardiac Imaging. Year Book Medical Publishers Inc. Chicago, pp 65—89
24. Vieli A, Jenni R, Anliker M (1986) Spatial velocity distributions in the ascending aorta of healthy humans and cardiac patients. IEEE Transactions on Biomedical Engineering 33: 28—34
25. Wigle ED, Heimbecker RO, Gunton RW (1962) Idiopathic ventricular septal hypertrophy causing muscular subaortic stenosis. Circulation 26: 325—340
26. Wigle ED, Marquis Y, Auger P (1967) Muscular subaortic stenosis: initial left ventricular inflow tract pressure in the assessment of intraventricular pressure differences in man. Circulation 35: 1100—1117
27. Wigle ED, Auger P, Marquis Y (1967) Muscular subaortic stenosis: The direct relation between the intraventricular pressure gradient and left ventricular ejection time. Circulation 36: 36—44
28. Wigle ED, Adelman AG, Auger P, Marquis Y (1969) Mitral regurgitation in muscular subaortic stenosis. Am J Cardiol 24: 698—706
29. Wigle ED, Adelman AG, Silver MD (1971) Pathophysiological considerations in muscular subaortic stenosis. In: Wolstenholme GEW, O'Connor M (eds) Hypertrophic obstructive cardiomyopathy. Ciba Foundation Study Group 47. London, pp 63—76
30. Wigle ED, Sasson Z, Henderson MA, Ruddy, TD, Fulop J, Rakowski H, Williams WG (1985) Hypertrophic cardiomyopathy. The importance of the site and the extent of hypertrophy. A review. Prog Cardiovasc Dis 28: 1—83
31. Wigle ED (1987) Hypertrophic cardiomyopathy. A 1987 Viewpoint. (Editorial). Circulation, 75: 311—322
32. Yock PG, Hatle L, Popp RL (1985) Dispersion of high-velocity left ventricular outflow jets in hypertrophic obstructive cardiomyopathy. J Am Coll Cardiol 5: II-394 (abstr)

Authors' address:

E. D. Wigle, M.D., Toronto General Hospital, 200 Elizabeth Street, Toronto, Ontario, M5G 2C4, Canada

Dynamic obstruction to left ventricular outflow: The case for its existence in hypertrophic cardiomyopathy

B. J. Maron and S. E. Epstein

Cardiology Branch, National Heart, Lung, and Blood Institute, National Institutes of Health Bethesda, Maryland, U.S.A.

Obstruction to left ventricular outflow is a feature of hypertrophic cardiomyopathy (HCM) that has been of great interest to clinicians and students of this disease for over 25 years, and while generally regarded as a prominent and important component of HCM, its clinical and pathophysiologic significance has been the source of periodic and often intense disagreement and controversy (1—20). In the early 1960s, a number of investigators observed that those patients with HCM and a loud systolic heart murmur had markedly increased systolic pressure and a pressure gradient recorded within the left ventricle at cardiac catheterization (5, 21—23). This subaortic gradient could easily be distinguished from gradients artifactually produced by physical entrapment of the catheter between left ventricular trabeculations (3—5). It was therefore concluded that true obstruction to left ventricular outflow existed in these patients with HCM.

In many patients with this disease, the magnitude of the gradient under basal conditions varies considerably from day to day, or even during the course of a cardiac catheterization. Other patients with HCM, while showing little or no obstruction to left ventricular outflow under basal conditions, are nevertheless capable of generating a gradient with certain physiologic or pharmacologic provocations (Fig. 1). Thus, the subaortic gradient appears to reflect a dynamic form of obstruction to left ventricular outflow that can be reduced or augmented by a number of interventions that alter arterial pressure, myocardial contractility or ventricular volume (21—23).

The argument against obstruction

From time to time, however, the importance and even the existence of left ventricular outflow tract obstruction in HCM has been questioned (2, 6—9, 11, 16, 17, 24). Criley (2, 6, 16, 17), Goodwin (8), and Murgo and associates (7, 9) have been most prominent in maintaining this position. Much of this debate has centered around the appropriate-

Puplished previously, in part, in the American Journal of Cardiology (58: 1093—6, 1986) and reproduced with permission of the Journal.

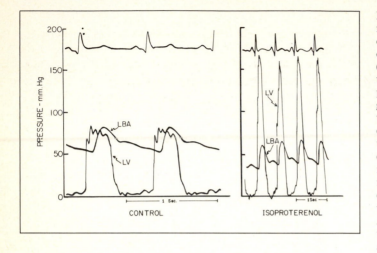

Fig. 1. Effects of an infusion of isoproterenol on simultaneously recorded left ventricular (LV) and left brachial artery (LBA) pressures in a patient with HCM. No gradient is present between body of left ventricle and brachial artery under basal (control) conditions. With administration of isoproterenol, a marked gradient is elicited. Reproduced with permission from the American Heart Association; from Braunwald et al. (21).

ness of the term "obstruction" to describe the systolic pressure difference that is measured between the left ventricular cavity and outflow tract in the catheterization laboratory. The controversy undoubtedly emanates largely from the fact that the features of left ventricular ejection in patients with HCM and a subaortic gradient are complex and probably unique. It has been established, for example, that the ventricle in HCM ejects a considerable proportion of its stroke volume early, rapidly, and at high velocity (about 75 % of forward flow is ejected in the first third of the systolic ejection period), resulting in a relatively small end-systolic volume (1—4, 6, 7—9, 11, 13, 15—20, 23, 25—27).

Those who oppose equating the subaortic pressure gradient with outflow obstruction do not dispute that pressure gradients exist in HCM, nor do they argue that gradients are simply artifacts, produced when the catheter tip is enfolded and entrapped within the contracting myocardium and trabeculations of obliterated portions of the left ventricle. Nevertheless, they regard these gradients as incidental and unimportant to the disease process. They believe that forward flow cannot be impeded or truly obstructed in a ventricle that rapidly ejects a substantial proportion of its stroke volume before the gradient is maximal in mid-systole. To these investigators, the elevated intraventricular pressures are not due to a mechanical impedance to left ventricular emptying caused by systolic anterior motion (SAM) and contact of the mitral leaflets with the ventricular septum during systole. Rather, the elevated pressures are said to be produced by continued isometric contraction of the ventricle in the late phase of systole during which time there is cavity obliteration; Goodwin believes that the papillary muscles, rather than the mitral leaflets, are the cause of SAM (28). Hence, to those with this viewpoint, the subaortic gradient and SAM do not reflect true obstruction to left ventricular outflow but are merely the consequences of premature and excessive emptying of a hyperdynamic ventricle. This distinction is by no means trivial, as approximately 25 % of the overall patient population with HCM exhibit a gradient across the left ventricular outflow tract (20, 29), and this subgroup of patients frequently develop severe symptoms refractory to medical therapy.

The argument for obstruction

We and others, however, hold that the available evidence overwhelmingly favors the concept that when a patient with HCM manifests a subaortic pressure gradient in association with SAM (Fig. 2), the gradient reflects true anatomic and mechanical obstruction to left ventricular outflow and constitutes an important determinant of the clinical course (3—5, 10, 12—15, 18, 22, 23, 25—27, 29—46). This evidence derives from clinical studies utilizing a variety of techniques (hemodynamic, contrast and radionuclide angiographic, Doppler, and echocardiographic (3—5, 10, 12—15, 18, 19, 22, 23, 25—27, 29—46). These studies have shown that the subaortic gradient develops at the same time in mid-systole that the mitral valve initially makes direct contact with the ventricular septum (Fig. 3); the earlier and more prolonged this mitral-septal apposition, the more severe the outflow gradient (10, 12, 23, 38—41). Most importantly, while the hyperdynamic left ventricle does indeed eject a considerable proportion of its stroke volume rapidly and early in systole, and end-systolic volume is reduced (Fig. 3—7), nevertheless a *large proportion of left ventricular emptying (about 50 %) occurs in the presence of the subaortic gradient (and elevated intraventricular systolic pressures) and mitral-septal contact (13, 15, 23, 25, 27, 32—34). Hence, the left ventricle is not truly devoid of blood when the gradient is present (Fig. 8); the gradient and blood flow coexist in mid-systole, ejection does not cease prematurely in mid-systole, and forward flow persists throughout the systolic ejection period in most patients (13, 15, 19, 23, 25—27, 30—34, 54)* (Fig. 3—8). Recent observations supporting this view are those of Grose et al. (18). In a group of ten patients with HCM, these authors showed that the radiolucent line in left anterior oblique cineangio-

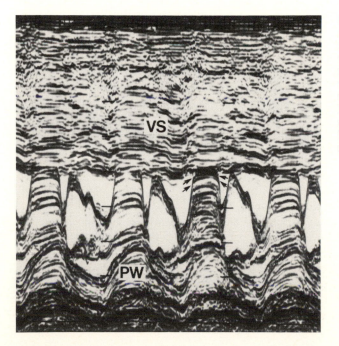

Fig. 2. M-mode echocardiogram showing marked systolic anterior motion of the mitral valve with prolonged contact of anterior mitral leaflet (arrows) with ventricular septum (VS) in a patient with HCM and a 100 mm Hg subaortic gradient measured at cardiac catheterization under basal conditions (PW) = posterior left ventricular wall.

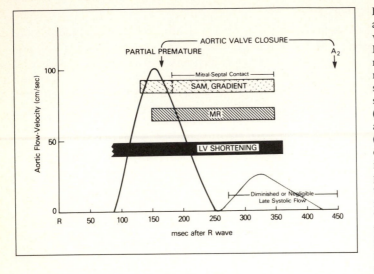

Fig. 3. Timing relation of aortic flow-velocity waveform obtained with Doppler to systolic anterior motion (SAM) of the mitral valve, partial midsystolic aortic valve closure, left ventricular (LV) cavity shortening and mitral regurgitation (MR) in 20 patients with obstructive HCM. Time intervals shown represent mean values for the patient group corrected for heart rate. A "bifid" flow-velocity pattern is depicted because it was detected in all but four patients. (A_2) = the aortic valve closure component of the second heart sound. Reproduced with permission from the American College of Cardiology; from Maron et al. (15).

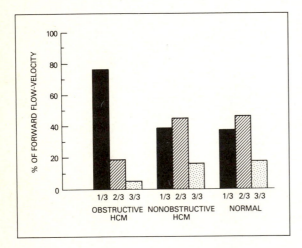

Fig. 4. Fraction of forward flow-velocity detected in the ascending aorta by Doppler in the first, second and last thirds of the systolic ejection period. Comparisons are made between patients with obstructive ($N = 20$) and nonobstructive HCM ($N = 30$) and normal subjects ($N = 20$). Reproduced with permission from the American College of Cardiology; from Maron et al. (15).

grams representing SAM, occurred virtually simultaneously with the onset of the sub-aortic pressure gradient measured by catheter micromanometry, at which time the left ventricle still had a considerable quantity of blood remaining to be ejected.

Echocardiographic studies have also demonstrated that SAM is a primary event (10, 12, 20, 23, 33, 37—44, 46, 47) and not due to posterior wall motion or cavity obliteration. SAM is probably produced when the forces generated by blood ejected by a hyperkinetic ventricle at high velocity into the narrowed left ventricular outflow tract pull the mitral valve leaflets (usually the distal portion) anteriorly across the left ventricular outflow tract until they make contact with the septum (i.e., Venturi phenomenon) (19, 45, 46).

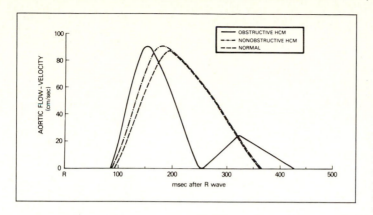

Fig. 5. Representative flow-velocity waveforms obtained in the ascending aorta from 20 patients with obstructive HCM, 30 patients with nonobstructive HCM, and 20 normal subjects. Each curve represents a composite of the contour and timing of all waveforms in that particular subgroup of patients. Reproduced with permission from the American College of Cardiology; from Maron et al. (15).

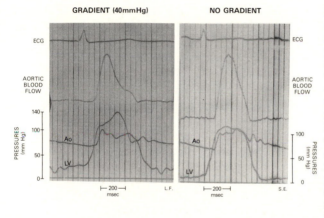

Fig. 6. *Left.* Simultaneous recordings of instantaneous aortic flow (with a Buckberg flow probe affixed to ascending aorta) and pressures in the left ventricle (LV) and aorta (Ao) obtained at time of operation (ventricular septal myotomy-myectomy) in a patient with HCM and a 40 mm Hg basal left ventricular outflow tract gradient. Note that aortic blood flow occurs coexistent with the pressure gradient; early flow is augmented, and at endsystole aortic flow is greatly reduced (but nevertheless present). The aortic flow profile resembles a "spike and dome" configuration.
Right. Aortic flow and pressures obtained in the same fashion at operation in a patient who had no significant subaortic gradient under basal conditions. Note that aortic blood flow is more evenly (normally) distributed throughout the systolic ejection period, and late systolic flow is increased (without the "dome" configuration shown in the left panel).

Doppler investigations (including preliminary color flow mapping studies) confirm that the site of jet formation and elevated velocities is at or near the point of maximum mitral systolic anterior motion (19, 35). In many patients, SAM also appears to interfere with normal closure of the mitral valve, and may lead to mitral regurgitation (which is usually mild) (15, 20, 48, 49) (Fig. 9); however Yock et al. (19) dispute this potential mechanism for mitral regurgitation in HCM based on their observation that mitral regurgitation is detectable by Doppler in early systole before the onset of SAM.

These angiographic, echocardiographic, and Doppler-derived observations indicate that prolonged mitral-septal contact constitutes a mechanical impediment to left ventricular outflow and is the cause of increased intraventricualr systolic pressures and the

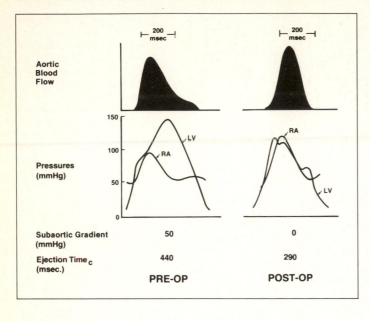

Fig. 7. Aortic blood flow pattern obtained in the operating room before and after ventricular septal myotomy-myectomy in a patient with HCM. *Left.* prior to myotomy-myectomy the subaortic gradient between left ventricle (LV) and radial artery (RA) is 50 mm Hg and left ventricular ejection time (corrected for cycle length) is 440 msec. Aortic flow profile is similar in contour to that shown in Fig. 6 with substantial early rapid ejection of blood from the left ventricle, blood flow co-existent with the gradient in mid-systole, reduced late systolic flow (but nevertheless blood blow persisting throughout the ejection period).
Right. After operative abolition of the gradient, the aortic blood flow contour has normalized and the ejection time has shortened considerably to a normal duration (290 msec).

subaortic gradient in HCM. Indeed, in our experience and that of other investigators (19, 20, 23, 38—44, 46), a substantial left ventricular outflow gradient under basal conditions is virtually always associated with marked SAM and prolonged mitral-septal contact. However, this observation does not exclude the possibility that occasional patients, or subjects without heart disease, may exhibit non-artifactual subaortic gradients that are not associated with marked SAM. These gradients are usually recorded only with provocative maneuvers, and can be due either to mid-cavity muscular obstruction (50, 51) or possibly cavity obliteration (18, 52). Four of the patients recently reported by Grose et al. (18) appear to demonstrate this latter phenomenon.

As Wigle has emphasized (23), left ventricular ejection dynamics are not identical in all patients with obstructive HCM. The percentage of the forward stroke volume that is obstructed, the magnitude of the pressure gradient, and the degree of prolongation of left ventricular ejection time are all related directly to the time of onset of mitral leaflet-ventricular septal contact (i.e., the time in systole when subaortic obstruction is initiated). Hence, the earlier in systole that mitral-septal contact occurs, the less the amount of forward flow that is ejected early, and consequently the greater is the flow that is obstructed (by SAM).

There are other observations substantiating the conclusion that true obstruction to left ventricular outflow exists in the patient with HCM. Evidence that the left ventricle is emptying and working against a mechanical impediment to flow is the prolonged left ventricular ejection time that is consistently identified in patients with a subaortic pressure gradient (compared to the normal ejection time present in patients without a gra-

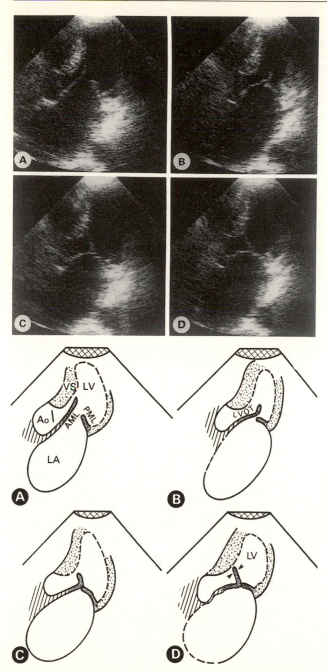

Fig. 8. Sequential stop-frame images obtained with two-dimensional echocardiography during the same cardiac cycle in a patient with obstructive HCM. Apical long-axis view with the transducer rotated laterally to permit visualization of the aorta (Ao), aortic valve and left ventricular outflow tract (LVOT). Shown sequentially with (A) and (B) in diastole and (C) and (D) during the subsequent systole. In (A) the mitral leaflets are separated. In (B) the anterior and posterior mitral leaflets approach each other and the distal portion of anterior leaflet (AML) begins to bend anteriorly; (C) After coaptation, the anterior leaflet moves toward the ventricular septum. (D) In mid-systole, the distal portion of anterior leaflet makes contact with the ventricular septum (VS) (arrows), but the left ventricular (LV) cavity is not greatly reduced in size (either in absolute terms or relative to its enddiastolic size) i.e., there is no evidence of true cavity obliteration at the time when the left ventricular outflow tract gradient occurs. The endocardial border of the left ventricular cavity is delineated by a broken line in each panel. Schematic drawings appear below echocardiograms. (LA) = left atrium; (PML) = posterior mitral leaflet. Reproduced with permission from the American College of Cardiology; from Spirito and Maron (42).

dient) (13, 15, 20, 23, 53) (Fig. 10), as well as the left ventricular shortening that is evident even after markedly increased intraventricular pressures or SAM appear (13, 15, 20, 23, 33) (Fig. 11). Also, concomitant with SAM in mid-systole, the aortic valve closes partially

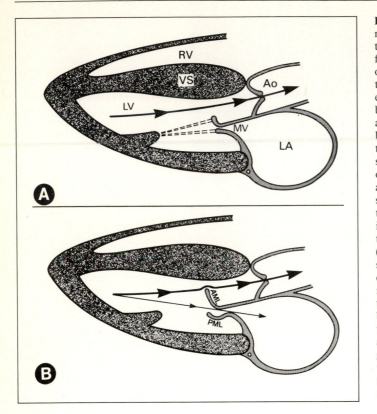

Fig. 9. Diagrammatic representation of directions of systolic blood flow in the left ventricle of patients with obstructive HCM. Shown in early systole (A) when blood is ejected rapidly at high velocity from the left ventricle (LV) through the anatomically small left ventricular outflow tract into the acending aorta (Ao), sucking the anterior mitral leaflet (AML) anteriorly toward the ventricular septum (VS); In (B), in mid-systole, the systolic anterior motion of the mitral valve permits a second small ejection stream of blood to be diverted out of the mitral orifice into the left atrium (LA), as mitral regurgitation. MV = mitral vale; (PML) = posterior mitral leaflet; (RV) = right ventricle.

and aortic blood flow decelerates abruptly, suggesting a sudden interposition of a mechanical impediment to outflow. While in most patients with obstructive HCM studied by transcutaneous Doppler echocardiography, a second late-systolic velocity peak may be detected ("bifid" waveform) (13, 15, 20, 30, 31, 54), some patients may not show evidence of this second velocity peak (15, 19). However, direct measurements at operation of ascending aorta blood flow provide clear evidence that late systolic aortic flow does occur in patients with obstructive HCM (25, 27). This persistence of forward blood flow throughout systole would seem to be the most plausible explanation for the reopening of the aortic valve in late systole after mid-systolic closure and the "dome" component of the "spike and dome" arterial pressure tracing, which are both characteristic findings in patients with HCM and outflow gradients (but which are not present in patients with the nonobstructive form of the disease).

Differences in patients with and patients without obstruction

While Murgo et al. (7) reported that abrupt mid-systolic deceleration of forward flow occurs both in patients with and in patients without outflow obstruction, all other investigators (13, 15, 20, 27, 30, 31, 54) have found this pattern of aortic flow velocity to

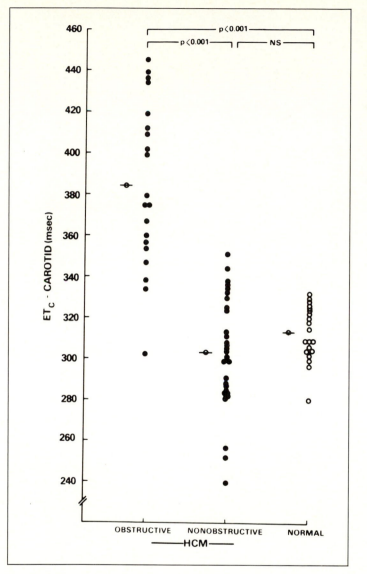

Fig. 10. Corrected ejection time (ET_c) obtained from the external carotid pulse in patients with obstructive ($N = 20$) or nonobstructive ($N = 30$) HCM and in normal subjects ($N = 20$), (θ) = mean values; (NS) = not significant. Reproduced with permission from the American College of Cardiology; from Maron et al. (15).

be confined to patients with subaortic gradients and to be absent in the nonobstructive form of HCM (13, 15, 20, 54) as well as in other cardiac diseases (30, 54). However, careful analysis of the work of Murgo and colleagues reveals several critical flaws which may help explain some of the discrepancies between their observations and those of several other investigators. First, Murgo et al. (7) reported no differences in forward flow time between patients with and patients without gradients, in part, because the authors chose to express these values as a percentage of the total systolic ejection period. This

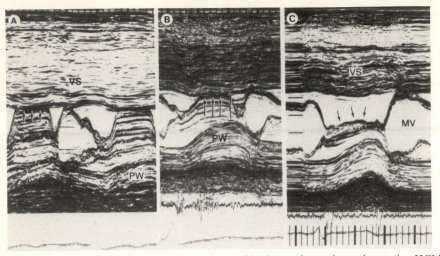

Fig. 11. Mitral valve echocardiograms from patients with obstructive and nonobstructive HCM. In obstructive HCM (A and B), marked systolic anterior motion of the mitral valve is present with prolonged contact between the anterior leaflet (arrows) and ventricular septum (VS), persisting for about 50 % of echocardiographic systole. (B) The broken vertical line denotes the minimum transverse left ventricular cavity dimension which occurs *after* mitral-septal contact; hence, systolic anterior motion of the mitral value occurs while the left ventricle is still actively contracting. Note high frequency mid-systolic sound on simultaneously recorded phonocardiogram, possibly produced by mitral-septal contact. (C) In nonobstructive HCM, systolic anterior motion of the mitral valve is absent (arrows). Simultaneous phonocardiograms and lead II electrocardiograms are shown below. (MV) = mitral value (PW) = posterior left ventricular wall. Reproduced with permission from the American College of Cardiology; from Maron et al. (15).

approach had the effect of minimizing differences in ejection period between the two hemodynamic subgroups. Such differences were undoubtedly further masked by the inclusion of two patients into the obstructive group (of only eight total patients) who had only trivial basal gradients of less than 20 mm Hg and inclusion of two patients into the nonobstructive group of nine patients who had marked SAM. Furthermore, the left ventricular ejection times reported in *absolute* terms by Murgo et al. (7) were longer in patients with gradients than in those without gradients, and these differences did indeed achieve statistical significance when ejection time was assessed angiographically (356 ms versus 303 ms). Finally, the lack of clear differences in normalized forward flow time between patients with and patients without gradients may reflect, in part, the particularly small sample sizes utilized by the authors.

The methodology used by Murgo and colleagues also could have accounted for discrepancies between some of their findings and those of other authors. The multisensor catheter system utilized by Murgo et al. (7) is designed so that while the flow-velocity probe is situated near the tip, it may be as much as 9 cm from the independent pressure sensor. Hence, flow-velocity may be measured in the transverse aorta, or in a much more distal segment of ascending aorta than is the simultaneously recorded pressure. Compounding this problem is the fact that the catheter must often be maneuvered blindly and is difficult to stabilize in the aorta due to fling and whip. Therefore, obtaining reliable and reproducible flow-velocity waveforms, free of artifact and with a minimal and acceptable angle of incidence relative to the direction of blood flow, is frought with considerable technical difficulties. These are important considerations, because in the tortuous distal portions of the ascending aorta (e.g., where the ascending aorta turns leftward and posteriorly into its transverse segment) and near the medial aortic wall-isolated, shortened and abbreviated flow-velocity waveforms may be inadvertently sampled, even in subjects without heart disease (55). These waveforms, distorted in duration and form, appear morphologically similar to those that are characteristic of patients with obstructive HCM (13, 15, 19, 27), and are also similar to the aortic waveforms described by Murgo and associates in patients with nonobstructive HCM (7). In addition, Yock et al. (19) have emphasized that even in patients with obstructive HCM ascending aorta flow patterns at end-systole are complex and inhomogenous, second velocity peaks may not be uniform at all sampling sites, and velocity profiles recorded at any one position may not necessarily reflect net flow in the aorta at that point in time. An understanding of these principles may help to explain the apparent discrepancies between those transcutaneous Doppler studies that demonstrated a second late systolic velocity peak (13, 15, 20, 30, 31, 54) and the invasive studies of Murgo et al. (7) that did not show a second peak in aortic flow.

It should be emphasized that patients with and patients without obstruction show different left ventricular architecture; these structural features may largely account for the different blood flow profiles (in the ascending aorta) exhibited by these two hemodynamic subgroups. For example, Spirito and Maron (56) found that the left ventricular outflow tract cross-sectional area, as measured from the two-dimensional echocardiogram, was significantly larger in patients without gradients as compared to those patients with basal gradients; in patients without gradients the larger outflow tract size often appeared to be related to more distal (apical) distribution of ventricular septal hypertrophy.

Finally, hemodynamic and metabolic studies performed in the catheterization laboratory (57) have shown that patients with HCM and outflow gradients have, as a group, higher coronary blood flow and myocardial oxygen consumption both at rest and during atrial pacing than patients without gradients; the higher coronary flow is undoubtedly caused by the elevated left ventricular systolic pressures and consequently the increased oxygen demand, thus demonstrating that the gradient and resulting high intraventricular systolic pressures have important physiologic consequences.

Relevant data from the results of surgery

There are also considerable data suggesting that the left ventricular outflow tract gradients measured in patients with obstructive HCM are of great clinical importance. Over the past 25 years it has been the approach of a number of institutions, including our own, to reduce or abolish the subaortic gradient by operation (usually by septal myotomy-myectomy, but occasionally by myotomy alone or by mitral valve replacement), primarily in those patients with moderate to severe functional limitation who have marked gradients and who have not benefitted from an adequate trial of drug therapy (58—71). The rationale for this approach was predicated on the assumption that if systolic intraventricular pressures could be normalized, the resulting reduction in myocardial wall stress would have important physiologic effects and thereby lead to symptomatic improvement. The outcome of these operations demonstrates that the surgical treatment of symptomatic patients with obstructive HCM does indeed exert salutary hemodynamic and symptomatic effects. Over 1,500 operations have been performed on patients with obstructive HCM worldwide at ten major institutions having an active surgical experience with this disease (i.e., in which > 50 operations have been performed) (59—69, 71). The vast majority of these procedures involved the septal myotomy-myectomy (Morrow procedure) or myotomy, or minor modifications of these operations. Operative mortality has been about 5%.

Basically, three important effects of operation in obstructive HCM have been defined. Firstly, surgery consistently abolishes or substantially reduces the subaortic gradient and SAM (40, 41, 59—71) without importantly compromising global left ventricular function (72). Secondly, the decrease in left ventricular pressure is associated with a decrease in myocardial oxygen consumption and an improvement in lactate metabolism (73) and restoration of a normal forward ascending aorta blood flow profile (Fig. 7) (25, 27). Thirdly, most operated patients experience long-lasting symptomatic benefit after relief of the subaortic gradient following surgery. In the largest series (64, 65), about 70 % of the patients operated upon at the National Institutes of Health reported important symptomatic improvement for up to 25 years after surgery (average follow-up of 5 years), and the gradient and SAM did not recur postoperatively (59—71). Objective improvement in exercise capacity (74, 75) and increased pacing-induced anginal threshold have also been shown to occur postoperatively (73). The association between symptomatic improvement after operation and relief of obstruction (and normalization of intraventricular systolic pressure) strongly suggests a causal relation between the two. Although unproven, it is also possible that some of the beneficial effects of operation may be related to improvement in diastolic function, another important disease component of HCM. Of note, even though Goodwin and associates have forcefully argued that the subaortic gradient in HCM is "incidental" to the disease process, they have nevertheless periodically advised surgery for patients with marked pressure gradients and symptoms (8).

Summary: The debate and controversy over the hemodynamics of obstruction and left ventricular ejection in HCM is an interesting and complex one in which periodic disagreement has appeared during the last 20 years. We believe that the available data unequivocally support the concept that in those patients with HCM who have left ventricular outflow gradients measured at catheterization (and who have associated marked SAM) a mechanical impediment to forward flow, and thus true obstruction to left ventricular outflow, does exist. Most importantly, the gradient has critical clinical implications by virtue of the markedly elevated intraventricular systolic pressures associated with it. These chronically elevated pressures are potentially detrimental to the left ventricle (a view held even by investigators opposed to the term "obstruction"), by virtue of increasing systolic myocardial wall stress and myocardial oxygen demand. Therefore, surgical abolition of the obstruction and normalization of these pressures remains an important and rational therapeutic objective in those severely symptomatic patients who have obstruction to left ventricular outflow and who have failed to benefit from drug therapy.

References

1. Hernandez RR, Greenfield JC, McCall BW (1964) Pressure-flow studies in hypertrophic subaortic stenosis. J Clin Invest 43: 401—407
2. Criley JM, Lewis KB, White RI, Ross RS (1965) Pressure gradients without obstruction: A new concept of "Hypertrophic subaortic stenosis". Circulation 32: 881—887
3. Ross J Jr, Braunwald E, Gault JH, Mason DT, Morrow AG (1966) Mechanism of the intraventricular pressure gradient in idiopathic hypertrophic subaortic stenosis. Circulation 34: 558—578
4. Ross J, Gault JH, Mason DT (1966) On the question of obstruction in idiopathic hypertrophic subaortic stenosis (editorial). Ann Int Med 65: 859—861
5. Wigle ED, Marquis Y, Auger P (1967) Muscular subaortic stenosis. Initial left ventricular inflow tract pressure in the assessment of intraventricular pressure differences in man. Circulation 35: 1100—1117
6. Wilson WS, Criley JM, Ross RS (1967) Dynamics of left ventricular emptying in hypertrophic subaortic stenosis: a cineangiographic and hemodynamic study. Am Heart J 73: 4—16
7. Murgo JP, Alter BR, Dorethy JF, Altobelli SA, McGranahan GM (1980) Dynamics of left ventricular ejection in obstructive and nonobstructive hypertrophic cardiomyopathy. J Clin Invest 66: 1369—1382
8. Goodwin JF (1982) The frontiers of cardiomyopathy. Br Heart J 48: 1—18
9. Murgo JP (1982) Does outflow tract obstruction exist in hypertrophic cardiomyopathy? N Engl J Med 307: 1008—1009
10. Pollick C, Morgan CD, Gilbert BW, Rakowski H, Wigle ED (1982) Muscular subaortic stenosis. The temporal relationship between systolic anterior motion of the anterior mitral leaflet and the pressure gradient. Circulation 66: 1087—1094
11. Sugrue DD, McKenna WJ, Dickie S, Myers MJ, Lavender JP, Oakley CM, Goodwin JF (1984) Relation between left ventricular gradient and relative stroke volume ejected in early and late systole in hypertrophic cardiomyopathy. Assessment with radionuclide cineangiography. Br Heart J 52: 602—609
12. Pollick C, Rakowski H, Wigle ED (1984) Muscular subaortic stenosis: the quantitative relationship between systolic anterior motion and the pressure gradient. Circulation 69: 43—49
13. Gardin JM, Debestani A, Glasgow GA, Butman S, Burn CS, Henry WL (1985) Echocardiographic and Doppler flow observations in obstructed and nonobstructed hypertrophic cardiomyopathy Am I Cardiol 56: 614—621
14. Levine RA, Weyman AE (1985) Dynamic subaortic obstruction in hypertrophic cardiomyopathy: criteria and controversy (editorial). J Am Coll Cardiol 6: 16—18
15. Maron BJ, Gottdiener JS, Arce J, Rosing DR, Wesley YE, Epstein SE (1985) Dynamic subaortic obstruction in hypertrophic cardiomyopathy: Analysis by pulsed Doppler echocardiography. J Am Coll Cardiol 6: 1—15
16. Siegel RJ, Criley JM (1985) Comparison of ventricular emptying with and without a pressure gradient in patients with hypertrophic cardomyopathy. Br Heart J 53: 283—291
17. Criley JM, Siegel RJ: (1985) Has "obstruction" hindered our understanding of hypertrophic cardiomyopathy? (editorial) Circulation 72: 1148—1154
18. Grose R, Strain J, Spindola-Franco H (1986) Angiographic and hemodynamic correlations in patients with hypertrophic cardiomyopathy and intracavity pressure gradients. Am J Cardiol 58: 1085—1092
19. Yock PG, Hatle L, Popp RL (1986) Patterns and timing of Doppler-detected intracavitary and aortic flow in hypertrophic cardiomyopathy. J Am Coll Cardiol 8: 1047—1058
20. Maron BJ, Epstein SE (1986) Clinical significance and therapeutic implications of the left ventricular outflow tract pressure gradient in hypertrophic cardiomyopathy. Am J Cardiol 58: 1093—1096

21. Braunwald E, Lambrew CT, Rockoff SD, Ross J Jr, Morrow AG (1964) Idiopathic hypertrophic subaortic stenosis. I. A description of the disease based upon an analysis of 64 patients. Circulation 30, suppl IV: IV-2-119

22. Epstein SE, Henry WL, Clark CE, Roberts WC, Maron BJ, Ferrans VJ, Redwood DR, Morrow AG (1974) Asymmetric septal hypertrophy. Ann Int Med 81: 650—680

23. Wigle ED, Sasson Z, Henderson MA, Ruddy TD, Fulop J, Rakowski H, Williams WG (1985) Hypertrophic cardiomyopathy. The importance of the site and the extent of hypertrophy. A review. Prog Cardiovasc Dis 28: 1—83

24. Shabetai R (1983) Cardiomyopathy: How far have we come in 25 years, how far yet to go? J Am Coll Cardiol 1: 252—263

25. Pierce GE, Morrow AG, Braunwald E (1964) Idiopathic hypertrophic subaortic stenosis. III. Intraoperative studies of the mechanism of obstruction and its hemodynamic consequences. Circulation 30, supp IV: IV—152—207

26. Jenni R, Ruffman A, Vieli M, Anliker M, Krayenbuehl HP (1985) Dynamics of aortic flow in hypertrophic cardiomyopathy. Eur Heart J 6; 391—398

27. Maron BJ, McIntosh CL, Seipp HW (1985) Evidence favoring existence of true subaortic obstruction in hypertrophic cardiomyopathy: Intraopertaive aortic flow studies before and after operation (abstract). Circulation 72, suppl III : III-447

28. Gerke J, Goodwin JF (1978) The significance of systolic anterior motion (SAM) on the mitral echo pattern in hypertrophic cardiomyopathy. Clin Cardiol 1: 152—162

29. Maron BJ, Nichols PF, Pickle LW, Wesley YE, Mulvihill JJ (1984) Patterns of inheritance in hypertrophic cardiomyopathy: Assessment by M-mode and two-dimensional echocardiography. Am J Cardiol 53: 1087—1094

30. Joyner CR, Harrison FS, Gruber JW (1971) Diagnosis of hypertrophic subaortic stenosis with a Doppler velocity detector. Ann Int Med 74: 692—696

31. Boughner DR, Schuld RL, Persaud JA (1975) Hypertrophic obstructive cardiomyopathy. Assessment by echocardiographic and Doppler ultrasound techniques. Br Heart J 37: 917—923

32. Morgan CD, Pollick C, Wigle ED (1979) Cineangiographic timing of left ventricular outflow obstruction and systolic emptying in muscular subaortic stenosis (abstract). Circulation 60, suppl II: II-262

33. Glasgow GA, Gardin JM, Burn CS, Childs WH, Henry WL (1980) Echocardiographic and Doppler flow observations in idiopathic hypertrophic subaortic stenosis (IHSS) (abstract). Circulation 62, suppl III: III-99.

34. Bonow RO, Ostrow HG, Rosing DR, Cannon MB, Leon RM, Watson SL, Bacharach MV, Green SE (1984) Dynamic pressure-volume alterations during left ventricular ejection in hypertrophic cardiomyopathy: Evidence for true obstruction to left ventricular outflow (abstract). Circulation 70, suppl II: II-17

35. Hoit B, Sahn DJ, Dalton N, Smith SC, Yun Y, Dittrich H (1985) Color Doppler flow mapping studies of jet formation in hypertrophic cardiomyopathy (abstract). Circulation 72, suppl III: III-447

36. Stewart WJ, Schiavone WA, Salcedo EE, Lever HM, Cosgrove DM, Gill CC (1985) Intraoperative Doppler velocity correlates with outflow gradient in HOCM pre and post myectomy (abstract). Circulation 72, suppl III: III-447

37. Bryg J, Labovitz AJ, Williams GA, Kennedy HL (1986) Systolic anterior motion of the mitral valve is temporally related to peak pressure gradient in hypertrophic obstructive cardiomyopathy. (abstract) J Am Coll Cardiol 7: 138A

38. Henry WL, Calrk CE, Gancy DL, Epstein SE (1973) Echocardiographic measurement of the left ventricular outflow gradient in idiopathic hypertrophic subaortic stenosis. N Eng J Med 288: 989—993

39. Shah PM, Taylor RD, Wong M (1981) Abnormal mitral valve coaptation in hypertrophic obstructive cardiomyopathy: proposed role in systolic anterior motion of mitral valve. Am J Cardiol 48: 258—262

40. Shah PM, Gramiak R, Kramer DH (1969) Ultrasound location of left ventricular outflow obstruction in hypertrophic obstructive cardiomyopathy. Circulation 40: 3—11

41. Spirito P, Maron BJ, Rosing DR (1984) Morphologic determinants of hemodynamic state following ventricular septal myotomy-myectomy in patients with hypertrophic cardiomyopathy: M-mode and two-dimensional echocardiographic assessment. Circulation 70: 984—995

42. Spirito P, Maron BJ (1984) Patterns of systolic anterior motion of the mitral valve in hypertrophic cardiomyopathy: assessment by two-dimensional echocardiography. Am J Cardiol 54: 1039—1046

43. Shah PM, Gramiak R, Adelman AG, Wigle ED (1972) Echocardiographic assessment of the effects of surgery and propranolol on the dynamics of outflow obstruction in hypertrophic subaortic stenosis. Circulation 45: 516—521

44. Popp R, Harrison D (1969) Ultrasound in the diagnosis and evaluation of therapy of idiopathic hypertrophic subaortic stenosis. Circulation 40: 905—914

45. Wigle ED, Adelman AG, Silver MD (1971) Pathophysiological considerations in muscular subaortic stenosis. In: Wolstenholme GEW and O'Connor M (eds) Hypertrophic obstructive cardiomyopathy. CIBA-Foundation Study Group Monograph 37, London, J & A Churchill, pp 63—75

46. Henry WL, Clark CE, Griffith JM, Epstein SE (1975) Mechanism of left ventricular outflow obstruction in patients with obstructive asymmetric septal hypertrophy (idiopathic hypertrophic subaortic stenosis). Am J Cardiol 35: 337—345

47. Gilbert BW, Pollick C, Adelman AG, Wigle ED (1980) Hypertrophic cardiomyopathy: Subclassification by M-mode echocardiography. Am J Cardiol 45: 861—872

48. Wigle ED, Adelman AG, Auger P, Marquis Y (1969) Mitral regurgitation in muscular subaortic stenosis. Am J Cardiol 24: 698—706

49. Kinoshita N, Nimura Y, Okamoto M, Miyatake K, Nagata S, Sakakibara H (1983) Mitral regurgitation in hypertrophic cardiomyopathy. Noninvasive study by two-dimensional Doppler echocardiography. Br Heart J 49: 574—583

50. Eslami B, Aryanpur I, Tabaeezadeh M, Alipour M, Nazarian I, Shakibi JG (1979) Midventricular obstruction. Jap Heart J 20: 117—126

51. Falicov RE, Resnekov L (1977) Mid-ventricular obstruction in hypertrophic obstructive cardiomyopathy. New diagnostic and therapeutic challenge. Br Heart J 39: 701—705

52. Grose R, Maskin C, Spindola-Franco H, Yipintsoi T (1981) Production of left ventricular cavitary obliteration in normal man. Circulation 64: 448—455

53. Wigle ED, Auger P, Marquis Y (1967) Muscular subaortic stenosis. The direct relation between the intraventricular pressure difference and the left ventricular ejection time. Circulation 36: 36—44

54. Gault JH, Ross J Jr, Mason DT (1966) Patterns of brachial arterial blood flow in conscious human subjects with and without cardiac dysfunction. Circulation 34: 833—848

55. Louie EK, Maron BJ, Greene KJ (1986) Variations in flow-velocity waveforms obtained by pulsed Doppler echocardiography in the normal human aorta. Am J Cardiol 58: 821—826

56. Spirito P, Maron BJ (1983) Significance of left ventricular outflow tract cross-sectional area in hypertrophic cardiomyopathy: A two-dimensional echocardiographic assessment. Circulation 67: 1100—1108

57. Cannon RO, Leon MB, Rosing DR, Epstein SE (1985) Comparison of coronary flow and myocardial metabolism at rest and during pacing-induced ischemia between patients with obstructive and non-obstructive hypertrophic cardiomyopathy (abstract). Circulation 72, suppl III: III-446

58. Wigle ED, Trimble AS, Adelman AG, Bigelow WG (1968) Surgery in muscular subaortic stenosis. Prog Cardiovasc Dis 11: 83—112

59. Bigelow WG, Trimble AS, Wigle ED, Adelman AG, Felderhof CH (1974) The treatment of muscular subaortic stenosis. J Thorac Cardiovasc Surg 68: 384—392

60. Bolton MR, King JF, Polumbo RA, Mason DT, Pugh DM, Reis RL, Dunn MI (1974) The effects of operation on the echocardiographic features of idiopathic hypertrophic subaortic stenosis. Circulation 50: 897—900

61. Morrow AG, Reitz BA, Epstein SE, Henry WL, Conkle DM, Itscoitz SB, Redwood DR (1975) Operative treatment in hypertrophic subaortic stenosis: Techniques, and the results of pre and post-operative assessment in 83 patients. Circulation 52: 88—102

62. Reis RL, Hannah H, Carley JE, Pugh DM (1977) Surgical treatment of idiopathic hypertrophic subaortic stenosis (IHSS). Postoperative results in 30 patients following ventricular septal myotomy and myectomy (Morrow procedure). Circulation 56, suppl II: II-128—132
63. Agnew TM, Barratt-Boyes BC, Brandt PWT, Roche AHG, Lowe JB, O'Brien KG (1977) Surgical resection in idiopathic hypertrophic subaortic stenosis with a combined approach through aorta and left ventricle. J Thorac Cardiovasc Surg 74: 307—316
64. Maron BJ, Merrill WH, Freier PA, Kent KM, Epstein SE, Morrow AG (1978) Long-term clinical course and symptomatic status of patients after operation for hypertrophic subaortic stenosis. Circulation 57: 1205—1213
65. Maron BJ, Epstein SE, Morrow AG (1983) Symptomatic status and prognosis of patients after operation for hypertrophic obstructive cardiomyopathy: Efficacy of ventricular septal myotomy and myectomy. Eur Heart J 4, Suppl F: 175—185
66. Schapira JN, Stemple DR, Martin RP, Rakowski H, Stinson EB, Popp RL (1978) Single and two-dimensional echocardiographic visualization of the effects of septal myectomy in idiopathic hypertrophic subaortic stenosis. Circulation 58: 850—860
67. Binet JP, David P, Piot JD (1983) Surgical treatment of hypertrophic obstructive cardiomyopathies. Eur Heart J 4, suppl F: 191—195
68. Beahrs MM, Tajik AJ, Seward JB, Giuliani ER, McGoon DC (1983) Hypertrophic obstructive cardiomyopathy: 10—21 year follow-up after partial septal myectomy. Am J Cardiol 51: 1160—1166
69. Bircks W, Schulte HD (1983) Surgical treatment of hypertrophic obstructive cardiomyopathy with special reference to complications and to atypical hypertrophic obstructive cardiomyopathy. Eur Heart J 4, suppl F: 187—190
70. Fighali S, Krajcer Z, Leachman RD (1984) Septal myomectomy and mitral valve replacement for idiopathic hypertrophic subaortic stenosis: short- and long-term follow-up. J Am Coll Cardiol 3: 1127—1134
71. Rothlin ME, Gobet D, Haberer T, Krayenbuehl HP, Turina M, Senning A (1983) Surgical treatment versus medical treatment in hypertrophic obstructive cardiomyopathy. Eur Heart J 4, suppl F: 215—223
72. Borer JS, Bacharach SL, Green MV, Kent KM, Rosing DR, Seides SF, Morrow AG, Epstein SE (1979) Effect of septal myotomy and myectomy on left ventricular systolic function at rest and during exercise in patients with IHSS. Circulation 60, suppl I: I-82—87
73. Cannon RO, Rosing DR, McIntosh CL, Epstein SE (1985) Hypertrophic cardiomyopathy (HCM): Improved hemodynamics, metabolism, and anginal threshold following surgical relief of obstruction (abstract). Circulation 72, suppl III: III-447
74. Redwood DR, Goldstein RE, Hirshfeld J, Borer JS, Morganroth J, Morrow AG, Epstein SE (1979) Exercise performance after septal myotomy and myectomy in patients with obstructive hypertrophic cardiomyopathy. Am J Cardiol 44: 215—220
75. Losse B, Kuhn H, Loogen F, Schulte HD (1983) Exercise performance in hypertrophic cardiomyopathies. Eur Heart J 4, Suppl F 197—208

Authors' address:
Barry J. Maron, M.D., National Institutes of Health National Heart, Lung, and Blood Institute, Building 10, Room 7B-15, Bethesda, Maryland 20892 U.S.A.

Diastolic filling properties in different forms of left ventricular hypertrophy, assessed by 2-D echocardiography

K. Ruffmann, H. Kücherer, A. Mandelbaum, W. Kübler

Department Internal Medicine (Cardiology) Heidelberg University, F.R.G.

Introduction

Left ventricular hypertrophy is known to alter left ventricular function. As invasive studies have shown, it is especially the diastolic function that responds most sensitively to the increment in muscle mass (3). Doppler echocardiography offers a non-invasive means of monitoring the diastolic function of the left ventricle by assessing left ventricular filling pattern. Because of its ease of use and ready availability, this method was chosen to investigate left ventricular filling patterns in different forms of hypertrophy. Dilative cardiomyopathy, arterial hypertension and hypertrophic cardiomyopathy were chosen for comparison in order to ensure a wide range of LV hypertrophy. The study was undertaken to find out how left ventricular filling responds to various degrees of increment in muscle mass, alteration of LV dimensions and change in LV systolic function.

Materials and Methods

Ultrasonic studies were performed in 20 patients (nine female, 11 male; dilative cardiomyopathy, $n = 5$; arterial hypertension, $n = 5$; end-stage renal disease, $n = 5$; hypertrophic cardiomyopathy, $n = 5$), and in five normals without signs of heart disease. In all patients, except those with end-stage renal failure, the diagnosis had been established previously by left heart catheterization. All patients were examined by standard M-mode echocardiography. Left ventricular filling parameters were monitored non-invasively by Doppler echocardiography. Ultrasonic studies were performed with a Hewlett-Packard phased array 2-D echocardiography system that interfaces 2-D echocardiography with pulsed Doppler measurements. The system uses a phased array transducer with a center frequency of 2.5 MHz. For a sampling depth of up to 16 cm, the system allows a pulse repetition frequency of 23 Hz, permitting velocity measurements of 1.0 m/s at an assumed angle of 0° between the incident Doppler ultrasound beam and the direction of intracardiac blood flow. The path of the Doppler ultrasound beam is indicated by a cursor line in the 2-D image display. Patients were examined in the left lateral decubitus position, while the transducer was held at the cardiac apex. The heart was displayed in a conventional four-chamber view. The Doppler sample volume, the location of which is

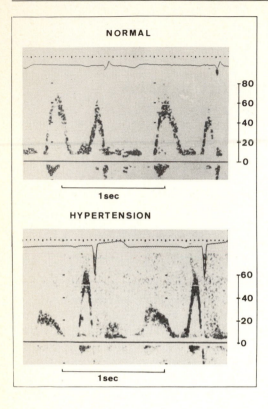

Fig. 1. Example of mitral inflow velocity in a normal person (upper panel) and in a patient with arterial hypertension (lower panel).

indicated by a marker along the cursor line, was positioned at the level of the mitral valve anulus. M-mode echo scans and Doppler flow velocity spectra were recorded on paper at 100 mm/s, along with a standard lead of a surface electrocardiogram. The mitral inflow velocity was recorded and averaged over five successive heart beats. In sinus rhythm, mitral inflow is characterized by an early diastolic peak at the end of the T-wave in the ECG, and a second peak following the P-wave ((Fig. 1). For evaluation, the enveloping curve of the biphasic velocity spectrum was drawn by hand, and the area under the curve assessed by planimetry. The total area under the curve represents blood entering the left ventricle during diastole, at the location of the sample volume, i.e. stroke volume per unit area of the mitral valve anulus. The initial phase of the velocity spectrum was termed early diastolic filling (EDF), the second phase atrial contraction (AC). Mean values for EDF, fractional EDF (i.e., EDF as a percentage of stroke volume) AC, fractional AC and stroke volume were averaged and compared between the groups. In previous experiments, beat-by-beat variation was found to be low (variation coefficients for EDF and AC: 6.6 % and 6.7 %, respectively). Interobserver variability was in the same range. M-mode scans were evaluated, confirming to ASE criteria (6). Left ventricular volumes and LV mass/volume ratio were calculated from M-mode echocardiography parameters (5). For statistical comparison of group differences, analysis of variance was employed. Median value and range are given where values were not normally distributed.

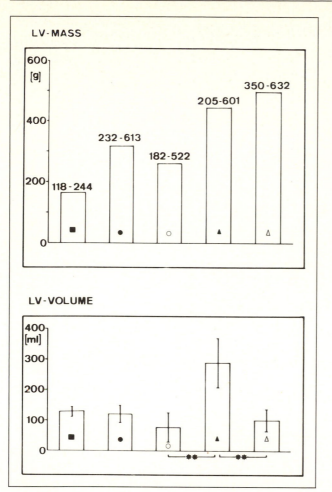

Fig. 2. Upper panel: Left ventricular mass in normals and in different forms of left ventricular hypertrophy. Median values and range are given, since values are not normally distributed. Lower panel: Left ventricular enddiastolic volume; DCM, dilated cardiomyopathy; HCM, hypertrophic cardiomyopathy. Symbols: (■) normal ($n = 5$); (●) arterial hypertension ($n = 5$); (○) end-stage renal disease ($n = 5$); (▲) DCM ($n = 5$); (△) HCM ($n = 5$).

Results

With respect to normals, left ventricular mass was elevated in patients with hypertension and end-stage renal disease, but it was highest in dilated cardiomyopathy and hypertrophic cardiomyopathy (Fig. 2). Left ventricular mass/volume ratio in dilated cardiomyopathy (1.5 ± 0.3) was lower than in normals (Fig. 3); it was increasingly higher for patients with arterial hypertension (2.1 ± 0.6), patients with end-stage renal disease (4.5 ± 1.2), and patients with hypertrophic cardiomyopathy (5.4 ± 1.0). For the patient groups considered, the contribution of early diastolic filling (EDF) to stroke volume (normals, 62 ± 5 %) was highest in dilative cardiomyopathy (54 ± 3 %), lower in hypertensive heart disease (45 ± 6 %), and lower still in end-stage renal disease (42 ± 8 %). It was 43 ± 15 % in hypertrophic cardiomyopathy (Fig. 3). Fractional shortening, as a measure of systolic left ventricular function, was low in dilative cardiomyopathy

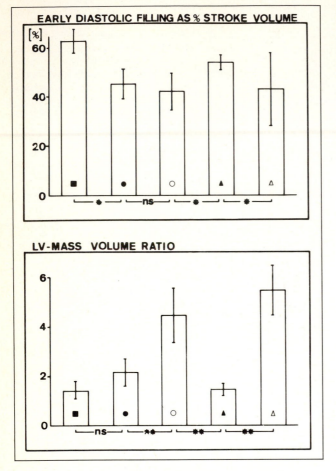

Fig. 3. Upper panel: Early diastolic filling as a percentage of stroke volume. Lower panel: Left ventricular mass/volume ratio. Abbreviations and symbols as in Fig. 2.

$(25 \pm 5\%)$, normal in patients with hypertension $(39 \pm 5\%)$, and at the upper limit of normal in patients with end-stage renal disease $(43 \pm 5\%)$ and hypertrophic cardiomyopathy $(48 \pm 6\%)$, Fig. 4). The relationship of early vs. late maximal velocity of mitral inflow (E/L ratio), as a measure of the diastolic function of the left ventricle, showed a ranking in the reverse order: whereas E/L (normals, 1.4 ± 0.3) was highest in dilated cardiomyopathy (1.1 ± 0.1), it was diminished in hypertension (0.6 ± 0.3), lower in end-stage renal disease (0.5 ± 0.3), and was 0.8 ± 0.3 in hypertrophic cardiomyopathy. An inverse correlation exists between the left ventricular volume/mass ratio and the amount of early diastolic filling (Fig. 5): the smaller and the more hypertrophied the left ventricle is, the greater is the impairment of left ventricular diastolic filling. There was no statistically significant correlation between early diastolic filling and left ventricular mass, nor between early diastolic filling and left ventricular volume.

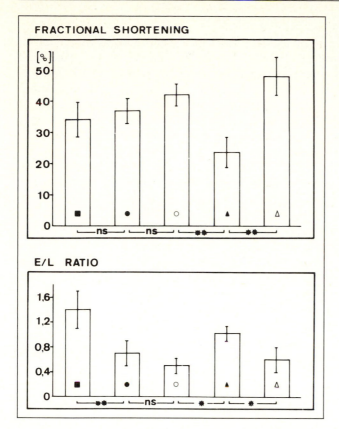

Fig. 4. Upper panel: Fractional shortening, as a measure of left ventricular systolic function. Lower panel: Ratio of maximal velocities during early diastolic filling and following atrial contraction. Velocities were assessed by 2D-Doppler echocardiography. Abbreviations and symbols as in Fig. 2.

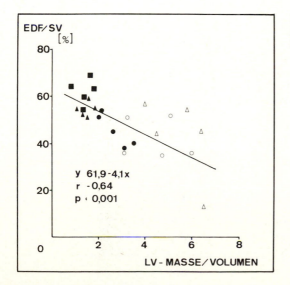

Fig. 5. Correlation between early diastolic filling as a percentage of stroke volume and left ventricular mass/volume ratio.

Discussion

In patients with arterial hypertension and left ventricular hypertrophy, distortion of left ventricular diastolic filling frequently occurs. Early diastolic filling, which is passive, is greatly reduced — perhaps as a consequence of impaired left ventricular relaxation in early diastole and a reduced rate of left ventricular pressure decay — and late diastolic filling, subsequent to atrial contraction, is augmented. This filling pattern may not belong to hypertensive heart disease alone. Small alterations can be found in persons of an older age, and its has been recognized in left ventricular hypertrophy of different origin (2). In patients with hypertrophic cardiomyopathy, where LV mass/volume ratio was highest, both severe reduction of early diastolic filling and unimpaired diastolic function were found. Since the distribution of left ventricular hypertrophy, which was not taken into account, is responsible for different forms of left ventricular ejection dynamics in hypertrophic cardiomyopathy (4), it is possible that different forms of left ventricular hypertrophy influence diastolic filling parameters as well. Furthermore, M-mode echocardiography, which bisects the left ventricle along a single line, may not accurately assess left ventricular hypertrophy when it is not uniformly distributed. M-mode echocardiography has, however, been established as a reliable means of estimating LV-mass in other forms of heart disease (1). In dilative cardiomyopathy, arterial hypertension and end-stage renal disease, impaired systolic performance of the left ventricle apparently does not result in impairment of left ventricular diastolic function. An increase in left ventricular mass does not have this effect either. It is rather the altered left ventricular geometry it induces, i.e., the reduction in chamber size and the augmentation of LV mass/volume ratio, which seems to be the determinant for a reduction in early diastolic filling, i.e., altered left ventricular diastolic function. Thus, cardiac therapy which aims at lowering preload or afterload and accepts a reduction in chamber size, may, in fact, adversely affect left ventricular function (7).

Summary: In order to study the influence of various kinds of left ventricular hypertrophy on left ventricular filling pattern, 20 patients (five dilated cardiomyopathy, five hypertension, five end-stage renal disease, five hypertrophic cardiomyopathy), and five normals were studied by M-mode and pulsed 2D-Doppler echocardiography. Left ventricular dimensions, volumes and mass were derived from standard M-mode echocardiograms. Doppler velocity measurements of mitral inflow provided calculation of left ventricular diastolic filling parameters. While left ventricular diastolic function bore no relation to the impairment of left ventricular systolic function, there was a statistically significant correlation of left ventricular mass/volume ratio and impairment of left ventricular diastolic function. In patients with hypertrophic cardiomyopathy, the parameters varied widely, and additional factors seem to determine left ventricular diastolic function in this group.

References

1. Devereux RB (1987) Detection of Left Ventricular Hypertrophy by M-mode Echocardiography. Anatomic Validation, Standardization, and Comparison to Other Methods. Hypertension 9, No. 2, Part 2, Suppl II: 19—26

2. Hanrath P, Mathey DG, Siegert R et al (1980) Left Ventricular Relaxation and Filling Pattern in Different Forms of Left Ventricular Hypertrophy: An Echocardiographic Study. Am J Cardiol 45: 15—23

3. Hoshino PK, Zile MR, Gaasch WH (1985) Diastolic Dysfunction in Left Ventricular Hypertrophy. Heart Failure 1, No 5: 220—230

4. Jenni R, Ruffmann K, Vieili A, et al (1985) Dynamics of Aortic Flow in Hypertrophic Cardiomyopathy. Eur Heart J 6, No 5: 391—398

5. Reichek N, Devereux RB (1981) Left Ventricular Hypertrophy: Relationship of Anatomic, Echocardiographic and Electrocardiographic Findings. Circ 63, No 6: (1978) 1391—1398

6. Sahn DJ, De Maria A, Kisslo J, Weyman A (1978) Recommendations Regarding Quantitation in M-mode Echocardiographic Measurements. Circ 58: 1072—1083

7. Topol EJ, Traill TA, Fortuin NJ (1985) Hypertensive Hypertrophic Cardiomyopathy of the Elderly. N Engl J Med 312; No 5: 277—283

Authors' address:
Dr. K. Ruffmann, Abteilung Innere Medizin III (Kardiologie), Medizinische Universitätsklinik, Bergheimer Str. 58, D-6900 Heidelberg, F.R.G.

Influence of verapamil on diastolic left ventricular function in myocardial hypertrophy of different origin

O. M. Hess, T. Murakami, and H. P. Krayenbühl

Medical Polyclinic, Cardiology, University Hospital, Zurich, Switzerland

Introduction

An improvement in diastolic filling has been reported after administration of calcium-blocking agents in patients with hypertrophic cardiomyopathy. This effect was attributed to improved left ventricular relaxation and increased early diastolic filling (1, 4—8). The mode of action of the calcium-blockers is, however, not clear, but certainly involves an inhibition of the calcium influx into the muscle cell. A reduction in intracellular cytosolic calcium is thought to be responsible for an improved rate of relaxation in patients with hypertrophic cardiomyopathy. An increase in intracellular calcium is known to be associated with increased contractility and decreased rate of relaxation, as has been reported in the papillary muscle (10). The purpose of the present study was, therefore, to evaluate the effect of verapamil on left ventricular relaxation and diastolic filling in patients with hypertrophic cardiomyopathy and to compare these effects with the response to verapamil in patients with secondary myocardial hypertrophy due to aortic stenosis.

Patients and Methods

Twenty-three patients were included in the present analysis (6). Ten patients with hypertrophic cardiomyopathy and 13 patients with aortic stenosis underwent diagnostic cardiac catheterization. Two patients with hypertrophic cardiomyopathy had a non-obstructive form and two patients with aortic stenosis had pure stenosis. Eleven patients with aortic stenosis had mild to moderate aortic regurgitation (mean regurgitant fraction: 20%, as determined by thermodilution techniques). Ten patients with normal left ventricular function served as controls. The mean age was 45 years in patients with hypertrophic cardiomyopathy, 51 years in patients with aortic stenosis and 36 years in control patients. Functional classification, according to the New York Heart Association (NYHA), was 2 (median) in both groups. All patients were in sinus rhythm and the QRS-complex did not exceed 0.11 s in any of the patients.

Left ventricular high-fidelity pressure was measured with a 7 F-Millar-micromanometer-angiocatheter which was introduced transseptally into the left ventricle. The micromanometer was calibrated by superimposing the high-fidelity pressure curve on the conventional left ventricular pressure tracing (2). The M-mode echocardiogram, a peripheral lead of the standard electrocardiogram and the phonocardiogram were recorded simultanously, together with the high-fidelity pressure tracing (6) at a paper speed of 100 mm/s. M-mode echocardiography was performed with an echocardiograph "Electronics for Medicine" V3280 which was interfaced to a VR-12 oscillograph. The echocardiographic and pressure tracings were digitized manually on an electronic digitizer (Numonics Corp.) interfaced to a PDP 11/34 computer equipped with a printer-plotter (Versatec). Left ventricular internal chamber diameter, left ventricular posterior wall thickness, left ventricular high-fidelity pressure and the first derivative of left ventricular pressure versus time (dP/dt) were calculated every 5 to 10 ms and plotted on the printer-plotter for further analysis. In four patients (two from each group) the quality of the M-mode echocardiogram was not sufficient for quantitative analysis and these echocardiograms were therefore not included in the present analysis.

In each patient, the left ventricular pressure- internal chamber diameter loop was plotted and cycle efficiency was calculated according to the technique of Gibson and Brown (3). Cycle efficiency is defined as the ratio of the loop area to that area of the rectangle which the pressure-diameter loop encloses. In control patients, cycle efficiency ranged between 76% and 92% (mean: 85%±6%).

Indices of left ventricular relaxation

Left ventricular relaxation was determined from the time constant of isovolumic pressure decay (2, 6). The time constant (T) was calculated as the negative reciprocal of the slope of the linear regression of pressure and negative dP/dt coordinates between peak negative dP/dt and mitral valve opening (6). The left ventricular pressure decay is characterized not only by its slope but also by its pressure asymptome (P_B) at dP/dt = 0 mm Hg/s.

Indices of left ventricular filling and diastolic function

Left ventricular filling was determined from simultaneous echo-pressure measurements using early and mean diastolic lengthening rate as filling parameters. Early diastolic lengthening rate (l_e) was calculated between mitral valve opening and the lowest diastolic pressure; mean diastolic lengthening rate (l_m) was obtained between mitral valve opening and end-diastole.

Left ventricular diastolic function was evaluated from simultaneous echo-pressure curves from the lowest diastolic pressure to end-diastole. Quantitative analysis was carried out for three reference points during diastolic filling (lowest diastolic pressure, mid-diastole and end-diastole).

Statistics

Statistical comparisons of data before and after verapamil were carried out by a paired student's *t*-test. Comparisons between controls and patients with hypertrophic cardiomyopathy and aortic stenosis were performed by a one-way analysis of variance. If the analysis was significant, the Scheffé procedure was applied. Comparisons between hypertrophic cardiomyopathy and aortic stenosis were done by an unpaired student's *t*-test. In all tables, mean values ± one standard deviation are given.

Results

Hemodynamic data are summarized in Table 1. Heart rate, left ventricular peak systolic pressure and the maximal rate of left ventricular pressure rise (dP/dt$_{max}$) remained unchanged in both groups before and after verapamil administration. Peak systolic pressure was, however, significantly higher in patients with aortic stenosis than in patients with hypertrophic cardiomyopathy. Left ventricular end-diastolic pressure also remained unchanged in patients with hypertrophic cardiomyopathy before and after verapamil, but increased significantly from 15 to 17 mm Hg in patients with aortic stenosis following verapamil.

Echocardiographic data are summarized in Table 2. Left ventricular end-diastolic internal chamber diameter, left ventricular systolic shortening of the chamber diameter and left ventricular posterior wall thickness remained unchanged in both groups before and after verapamil administration. The chamber diameter was, however, significantly larger and systolic shortening significantly smaller in aortic stenosis than in hypertrophic cardiomyopathy. Cycle efficiency (Fig. 1) however, increased significantly in patients with hypertrophic cardiomyopathy after intravenous verapamil but remained unchanged in patients with aortic stenosis. Cycle efficiency at rest was significantly smaller in hy-

Table 1. Hemodynamic data in hypertrophic cardiomyopathy (HCM) and aortic stenosis (AS) before (C) and after (V) intravenous verapamil.

		HR	LVEDP	LVSP		dP/dt$_{max}$	n
HCM	C	70±10	18±8	138±27		1453±357	10
	V	75±13	18±8	135±26	***	1350±242	10
AS	C	77±7	15±7	200±35	***	1733±344	13
	V	76±6	17±7	200±38		1669±444	13

HR: heart rate (bpm); LVEDP: left ventricular end-diastolic pressure (mm Hg); LVSP: left ventricular peak systolic pressure (mm Hg); dP/dt$_{max}$: maximal rate of left ventricular pressure rise (mm Hg/s); n: number of patients; * $P < 0.05$; *** $P < 0.001$.

Table 2. Echocardiographic data in hypertrophic cardiomyopathy (HCM) and aortic stenosis (AS) before (C) and after (V) intravenous verapamil

		n	D$_{ed}$	Sh	Wth	CE
HCM	C	8	4.0±0.9	37±8	1.04±0.2	71±8
	V	8	4.2±1.0	37±7	1.10±0.2	77±8
AS	C	11	6.0±1.2	28±7	1.09±0.2	80±6
	V	11	5.9±1.0	28±5	1.06±0.2	80±5

n: number of patients; D$_{ed}$: left ventricular internal chamber diameter at end-diastole (cm); Sh: systolic shortening of the internal chamber diameter (%); Wth: left ventricular posterior wall thickness (cm); CE: left ventricular cycle efficiency (%); * $P < 0.05$; ** $P < 0.01$.

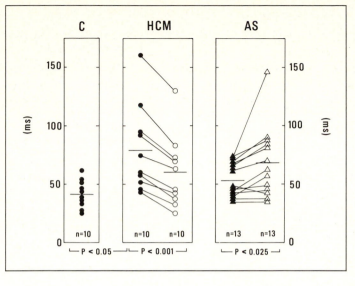

Fig. 1. Cycle efficiency in ten controls (C), eight patients with hypertrophic cardiomyopathy (HCM) and 11 patients with aortic stenosis (AS). Data at rest are given by the closed symbols and data after 0.1 mg/kg intravenous verapamil, by the open symbols. Cycle efficiency is significantly decreased in patients with hypertrophic cardiomyopathy before administration of verapamil when compared to control patients. Following intravenous administration of verapamil cycle efficiency is significantly increased in hypertrophic cardiomyopathy but remains unchanged in aortic stenosis. Thus, verapamil administration is associated with an improvement in asynchronous wall motion in patients with hypertrophic cardiomyopathy. *P*: probability (analysis of variance).

pertrophic cardiomyopathy than in aortic stenosis or controls (Fig. 1) but was normalized after verapamil administration.

Indices of left ventricular relaxation and diastolic filling are summarized in Table 3. The time constant T (Fig. 2) decreased significantly in hypertrophic cardiomyopathy after intravenous verapamil, but increased significantly in aortic stenosis. The time constant T was significantly prolonged at rest in hypertrophic cardiomyopathy when compared to control patients (Fig. 2) but was no longer different from controls after verapamil administration. Early diastolic lengthening rate (Fig. 3) incrased significantly in hyper-

Table 3. Left ventricular relaxation and filling data in hypertrophic cardiomyopathy (HCM) and aortic stenosis (AS) before (C) and after (V) intravenous verapamil.

		n	T		P_B		l_e	l_m	
HCM	C	10	79 ± 37	]] ***	-28 ± 34	] **	5.3 ± 3.5] *	3.0 ± 1.2]]	
	V	10	60 ± 30	] *	-12 ± 24	]]	7.4 ± 4.3	4.3 ± 1.9] ◇	] *
AS	C	13	53 ± 14	]] **	-25 ± 15	] *	7.7 ± 2.0	4.3 ± 1.9	]
	V	13	68 ± 30	]	-46 ± 35	]] *	7.6 ± 2.3	4.2 ± 1.0	

n: number of patients; T: time constant (ms); P_B: pressure intercept (mm Hg); l_e: early diastolic lengthening rate (between mitral valve opening and the lowest diastolic pressure) (cm/s); l_m: mean diastolic lengthening rate (between mitral valve opening and end-diastole) (cm/s); *$P < 0.05$; ** $P < 0.01$; *** $P < 0.001$; ◇$P < 0.06$.

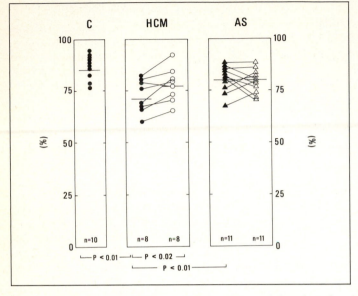

Fig. 2. Time constant (T) of left ventricular isovolumic pressure decay in 10 controls (C), ten patients with hypertrophic cardiomyopathy (HCM) and 13 patients with aortic stenosis (AS). Data at rest are given by the closed symbols and data after intravenous administration of verapamil by the open symbols. Time constant T is significantly prolonged in patients with hypertrophic cardiomyopathy at rest but decreases significantly following verapamil administration. In patients with aortic stenosis time constant T is not different from controls but increases significantly after intravenous administration of verapamil. Thus, verapamil has an opposite effect on relaxation in primary and secondary myocardial hypertrophy because it improves relaxation in hypertrophic cardiomyopathy but delays relaxation in aortic stenosis. *P*: probability (analysis of variance).

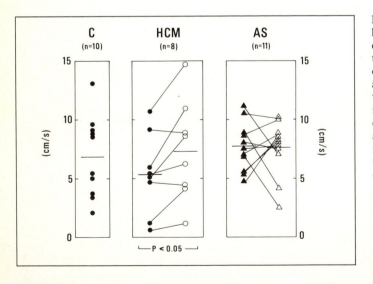

Fig. 3. Early diastolic lengthening rate in ten controls (C), eight patients with hypertrophic cardiomyopathy (HCM) and 11 patients with aortic stenosis (AS). Data at rest are given by the closed symbols and data after intravenous administration of verapamil by the open symbols. Early diastolic lengthening rates are similar in all three groups at rest, but show considerable variations. After administration of verapamil early diastolic lengthening rate increases significantly in patients with hypertrophic cardiomyopathy, but remains unchanged in patients with aortic stenosis. Thus, verapamil has a beneficial effect on early diastolic filling in patients with hypertrophic cardiomyopathy, but not in patients with aortic stenosis. *P*: probability (analysis of variance).

trophic cardiomyopathy after intravenous verapamil, but remained unchanged in aortic stenosis following verapamil. Mean diastolic lengthening rate also increased ($P < 0.06$) in hypertrophic cardiomyopathy after verapamil but was unaffected in aortic stenosis. There were, however, considerable variations in early and mean diastolic lengthening rate before and after verapamil.

Left ventricular diastolic function showed no effect of verapamil on diastolic chamber properties in both groups, because the pressure-diameter relationship remained unchanged before and after verapamil (6). The pressure-diameter curve in hypertrophic cardiomyopathy was, however, located to the left of the curve of patients with aortic stenosis, suggesting an increased chamber stiffness in patients with hypertrophic cardiomyopathy.

Discussion

Several studies of hypertrophic cardiomyopathy have indicated (4—8) that delayed re-laxation, impaired left ventricular filling and diminished left ventricular compliance may be favorably modified by the administration of calcium blocking agents. Hanrath and coworkers (4) reported an increase in wall thinning and chamber diameter lengthening following administration of verapamil. Paulus and coworkers (8) demonstrated that ad-ministration of nitroprusside was accompanied by systemic vasodilation with a decrease in end-diastolic pressure and end-diastolic dimensions, whereas administration of nife-dipine was accompanied not only by systemic vasodilation but also by improved muscle inactivation with a decrease in end-diastolic pressure but with an increase in end-diastolic dimensions. In a previous study from our laboratoy (5), we reported an improvement in left ventricular relaxation with enhanced early diastolic filling but we were not able to show any beneficial effect of verapamil on diastolic chamber properties, as was observed by Paulus and coworkers (8). Thus, in accordance with most studies published in the literature, the salutary effect of calcium channel blockers on diastolic mechanics seems to be related to improved muscle inactivation with increased speed of relaxation and increased diastolic filling. Asynchronous contraction and relaxation has been reported to occur in patients with hypertrophic cardiomyopathy (9) and to represent one of the characteristic features of this entity due to its irregular shape and its severe septal hy-pertrophy. Thus, we evaluated the effect of verapamil on asynchronous left ventricular contraction and relaxation using the cycle efficiency as a measure of synchronous or asynchronous wall motion (3).

Parallel to the improvement in relaxation and diastolic filling, a significant increase in cycle efficiency was observed in patients with hypertrophic cardiomyopathy following intravenous administration of verapamil. Asynchrony of left ventricular contraction and relaxation might explain a prolonged time constant of relaxation with impaired left ven-tricular filling because asymmetric hypertrophy of the left ventricle is likely to be asso-ciated with regional differences in relaxation in normal and hypertrophied muscle areas. Calcium channel blockade might, therefore, act differently on the normal and the hy-pertrophied muscle, for instance verapamil prolongs relaxation of the normal muscle but enhances relaxation of the hypertrophied muscle, resulting in a more uniform relaxation with a decrease in time constant (Fig. 2). An improvement in cycle efficiency could not only explain the improvement in relaxation but also the difference in the response to verapamil in hypertrophic cardiomyopathy and aortic stenosis. Since patients with aortic stenosis had a normal cycle efficiency in 9 out of 11 patients, there was no change in cycle efficiency after verapamil. The two patients with a reduced cycle efficiency improved their cycle efficiency from 73% to 80% in the first patient and from 67% to 74% in the second. Thus, asynchronous wall motion was only present in a small percentage of all patients with aortic stenosis, probably due to the fact that left ventricular hypertrophy was more equally distributed in aortic stenosis than in hypertrophic cardiomyopathy. Administration of verapamil was, therefore, not accompanied by an improvement in relaxation and diastolic filling but was followed by an increase in the rate of relaxation, probably due to the negative inotropic effect of verapamil. Left ventricular passive elastic properties were not affected by the drug because the diastolic pressure-diameter relationship remained completely unchanged before and after verapamil administration.

Thus, we can conclude that verapamil improves relaxation in hypertrophic cardiomyopathy, but delays relaxation in secondary myocardial hypertrophy due to aortic stenosis. Parallel to the improvement in relaxation, an increase in early diastolic filling was observed in hypertrophic cardiomyopathy. The improvement in relaxation and diastolic filling can be explained by an improvement in cycle efficiency with an improvement in asynchronous wall motion after intravenous verapamil. This improvement in cycle efficiency was not observed in patients with aortic stenosis following intravenous administration of verapamil.

Summary: The effect of 0.1 mg/kg verapamil on left ventricular (LV) diastolic mechanics was evaluated in ten patients with hypertrophic cardiomyopathy and 13 patients with aortic stenosis. LV diastolic function was assessed from simultaneous M-mode echocardiograms and high-fidelity pressure measurements at rest and 10 to 15 min after intravenous administration of verapamil. The time constant of LV pressure decay (T), LV early and mean diastolic filling rate as well as diastolic pressure-diameter relations, were determined before and after verapamil administration.

Heart rate, LV peak systolic pressure, maximum and minimum dP/dt remained unchanged in both groups after verapamil administration. LV end-diastolic pressure increased slightly although significantly from 15 to 17 mm Hg ($P < 0.02$) in aortic stenosis but remained unchanged in hypertrophic cardiomyopathy. T decreased significantly from 79 to 60 ms ($P < 0.001$) in hypertrophic cardiomyopathy but increased from 53 to 68 ms ($P < 0.025$) in aortic stenosis. Parallel to the decrease in T, early and mean diastolic lengthening rate increased significantly in hypertrophic cardiomyopathy, but remained unchanged in aortic stenosis before and after verapamil. The diastolic pressure-diameter relation was not affected in both groups by verapamil administration. However, cycle efficiency improved significantly from 71% to 77% ($P < 0.02$) in cardiomyopathy but remained unchanged in aortic stenosis (80% versus 80%).

Thus, it is concluded that verapamil improves relaxation in hypertrophic cardiomyopathy but delays relaxation in aortic stenosis. The beneficial effect of verapamil in hypertrophic cardiomyopathy is related to improved relaxation and diastolic filling rather than to changes in passive elastic chamber properties. The improvement can be explained by an increase in cycle efficiency, with a decrease in LV asynchrony which is not observed in patients with secondary myocardial hypertrophy due to aortic stenosis.

References

1. Bonow RO, Rosing DR, Bacharach SL, Green MV, Kent KM, Lipson LC, Maron BJ, Leon MB, Epstein SE (1981) Effects of verapamil on left ventricular systolic function and diastolic filling in patients with hypertrophic cardiomyopathy. Circulation 64: 787—796
2. Eichhorn P, Grimm J, Koch R, Hess OM, Carroll JD, Krayenbuehl HP (1982) Left ventricular relaxation in patients with myocardial hypertrophy secondary to aortic valve disease. Circulation 65: 1395—1404
3. Gibson DG, Brown DJ (1976) Assessment of left ventricular systolic function in man from simultaneous echocardiographic and pressure measurements. Br Heart J 38: 8—17
4. Hanrath P, Mathey DG, Kremer F, Sonntag F, Bleifeld W (1980) Effect of verapamil on left ventricular isovolumic relaxation time and regional left ventricular filling in hypertrophic cardiomyopathy. Am J Cardiol 45: 1258—1263
5. Hess OM, Grimm J, Krayenbuehl HP (1983) Diastolic function in hypertrophic cardiomyopathy: effects of propranolol and verapamil on diastolic stiffness. Europ Heart J 4 (Suppl F): 47—56
6. Hess OM, Murakami T, Krayenbuehl HP (1986) Does verapamil improve left ventricular relaxation in patients with myocardial hypertrophy? Circulation 74: 530—543
7. Lorell BH, Paulus WJ, Grossman W, Wynne J, Cohn PF (1982) Modification of abnormal left ventricular diastolic properties by nifedipine in patients with hypertrophic cardiomyopathy. Circulation 65: 499—507
8. Paulus WJ, Lorell BH, Craig WE, Wynne J, Murgo JP, Grossman W (1983) Comparison of the effects of nitroprusside and nifedipine on diastolic properties in patients with hypertrophic cardiomyopathy: altered left ventricular loading or improved muscle inactivation? J Am Coll Cardiol 2: 879–886
9. Sanderson JE, Gibson DG, Brown DJ, Goodwin JF (1977) Left ventricular filling in hypertrophic cardiomyopathy. An angiographic study. Br Heart J 39: 661—670
10. Parmley WE, Sonnenblick EH (1969) Relation between mechanics of contraction and relaxation in mammalian cardiac muscle. Am J Physiol 216: 1084—1091

Authors' address:
Otto M. Hess, M.D., Medical Polyclinic, Cardiology, University Hospital, Raemistrasse 100, 8091 Zurich, Switzerland

Systolic anterior movement of the mitral valve and the Venturi effect: an in vitro study

R. Lemke and M. Kaltenbach

Zentrum der Inneren Medizin, Klinikum der J.-W. Goethe-Universität, Frankfurt/Main, F.R.G.

Introduction

Since the introduction of echocardiography, systolic anterior movement (SAM) has been considered to be a typical sign of HOCM. There are several different explanations for the mechanism which causes systolic anterior motion of the mitral valve (1—11).

Valve models for in vitro examinations are very effective in testing complex valve movements, even though their application in vivo may be limited (12).

In order to test the influence of the Venturi effect on the SAM of an experimental „mitral valve", we constructed two different models (13).

The first model will demonstrate a high grade dynamic subvalvular stenosis and mild outflow tract obstruction in the region of the anterior mitral valve. The second model will demonstrate only a high fixed gradient in the region of the anterior mitral valve.

Material and Methods

Several 50 ml plastic syringes, glue, thin latex rubber and thin threads were used.

Model 1 (Fig. 1)

A syringe was cut at the distal end. Into the opening we glued an anterior and a posterior leaflet which consisted of thin latex rubber. The free edges of the valves were attached with thin threads representing the chordae tendineae to the posterior part of the syringe. Anatomically the body of the syringe represented the ventricle and the anterior part of the syringe the ventricular septum. This part of the construction was considered the inflow tract. The outflow tract was constructed in the following way: a oval hole was cut into the upper part of the body of the syringe.

Another syringe, cut open on both ends, was adapted and glued to cover the oval hole in a Y-shaped fashion. The second syringe had an indentation covered with a plastic membrane imitating a mild outflow tract obstruction in the area of the anterior mitral leaflet. Proximal to the mitral valve, a second hole was cut into the original syringe anteriorly. This hole was covered with latex rubber, so that by exerting pressure on the rubber-covered hole, a dynamic subvalvular obstruction would be caused. Two catheters

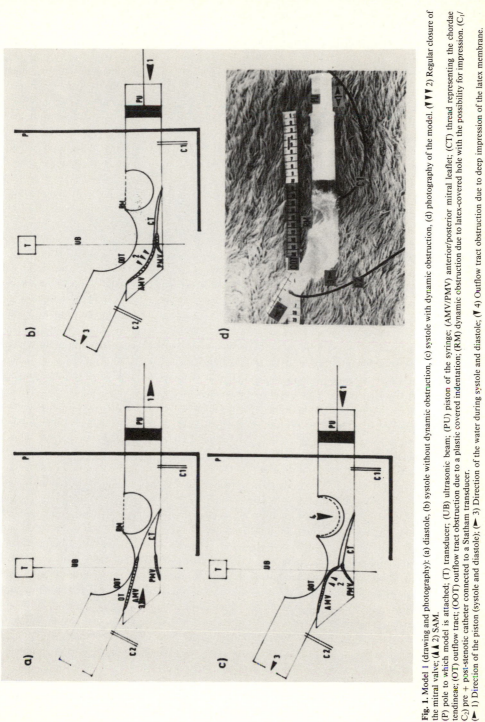

Fig. 1. Model 1 (drawing and photography): (a) diastole, (b) systole without dynamic obstruction, (c) systole with dynamic obstruction, (d) photography of the model. (▼▼▼ 2) Regular closure of the mitral valve; (▲▲ 2) SAM.

(P) pole to which model is attached; (UB) ultrasonic beam; (T) transducer; (PU) piston of the syringe; (AMV/PMV) anterior/posterior mitral leaflet; (CT) thread representing the chordae tendineae; (OT) outflow tract; (OOT) outflow tract obstruction due to a plastic covered indentation; (RM) dynamic obstruction due to latex-covered hole with the possibility for impression. (C₁/ C₂) pre + post-stenotic catheter connected to a Statham transducer.

(➤ 1) Direction of the piston (systole and diastole); (➤ 3) Direction of the water during systole and diastole; (▼ 4) Outflow tract obstruction due to deep impression of the latex membrane.

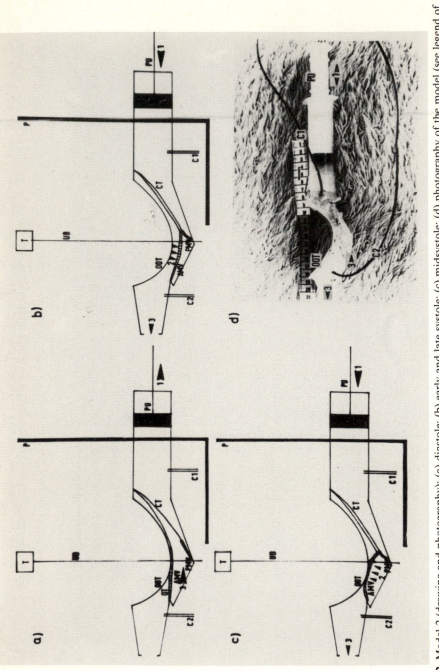

Fig. 2. Model 2 (drawing and photography): (a) diastole; (b) early and late systole; (c) midsystole; (d) photography of the model (see legend of Fig. 1).

in front of and behind the valve were inserted and connected to Statham transducers to measure pre- and postvalvular pressures.

The model was inserted into a water container. By pumping the piston of the syringe a ventricular systole and diastole could be imitated.

Model 2 (Fig. 2)

This model was similar. The outflow tract obstruction was very severe in this case, and there was no possibility of creating a dynamic subvalvular obstruction.

Unlike those in Model 1, the chordae tendineae were inserted anteriorly in the body of the syringe.

Results
Model 1

a. By moving the piston of the syringe a systolic — diastolic valve movement resembling a regular "mitral valve" could be caused. There was no gradient proximal and distal to the valve documented by pressure registration (Fig. 3a, b).

b. In addition to the movement of the piston, a subvalvular gradient was caused by exerting pressure on the hole covered with latex rubber during systole. An obstruction was caused with a poststenotic flow increase. The valve now demonstrated a typical SAM. A pressure gradient of approximately 12 mm Hg could be registered (Fig. 4a, b).

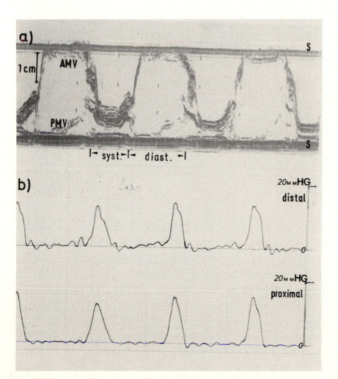

Fig. 3. (a) Systolic — diastolic movement of the anterior and poterior mitral valve. There is no SAM. (b) Pressure tracing distal and proximal to the valve. Because of the moderate outflow tract obstruction, there is no pressure gradient.

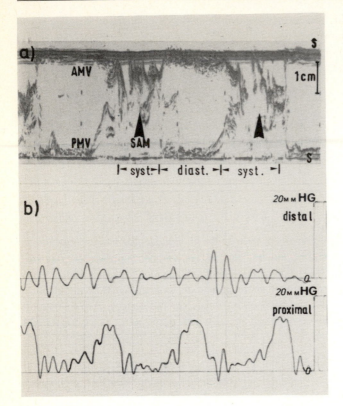

Fig. 4. (a) Systolic — diastolic movement of the anterior and posterior mitral valve. There is a pronounced SAM due to the dynamic obstruction during systole. (b) The pressure tracing shows a gradient of approximately 12 mm Hg distal to the valve.

Model 2

a. By moving the piston of the syringe, a typical SAM of the valve could be caused during systole. The pressure tracing demonstrates a gradient of approximately 10 mm Hg. The poststenotic pressure curve demonstrates a typical dicrotic shape (Fig. 5a, b).

b. After removal of the valve there was still a slight gradient, but the pre- and post-stenotic tracings are almost identical (Fig. 5c).

Discussion

The two models demonstrate that the Venturi effect sufficiently explains the SAM of our experimental "mitral valve". In model 1, a subvalvular dynamic obstruction with a poststenotic increase of flow velocity, causes a typical SAM. The insertion of the chordae tendineae seems to be of minor importance. The posterior insertion of the chordae opposite the obstruction pulls the valve away from the obstruction. But the Venturi effect is obviously stronger so an anterior movement is the result. The pressure tracing confirms an obstruction, demonstrating a gradient of approximately 12 mm Hg during the presence of SAM. No obstruction is present when the movement of the mitral valve is normal and the subvalvular obstruction is released. So, in model 1, the subvalvular obstruction which causes a Venturi effect produces SAM of the mitral valve.

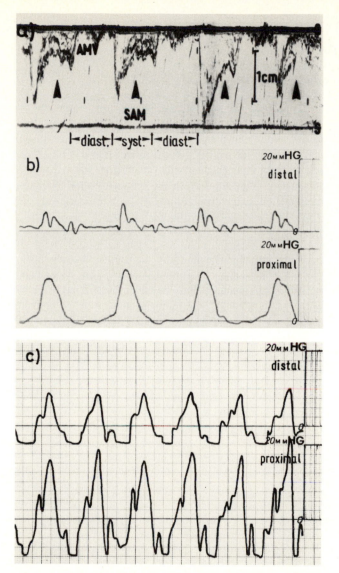

Fig. 5. (a) Systolic — diastolic movement of the anterior mitral valve. There is a pronounced midsystolic SAM. (b) Pressure tracing with a gradient of approximately 10 mm Hg distal to the valve with a typical dicrotic shape of the pressure curve compared with the proximal curve. (c) Pressure tracing after resection of the valve, there is still a gradient due to the remaining high grade obstruction but the shape of the curves is almost identical.

In model 2 there is a constant high grade outflow tract obstruction in the region of the valve. This causes high flow, a typical SAM and a typical poststenotic pressure tracing with a dicrotic curve. The dicrotic curve disappears after resection of the valve but there is still some residual gradient. The insertion of the chordae tendineae is, in model 2, on the same side as the obstruction. During the low-flow condition in early and endsystole, the valve moves away from the obstruction. In midsystole, during high-flow conditions, the valve moves towards the obstruction due to the Venturi effect. So again the Venturi effect is more important than the direction in which the chordae tendineae pull the valve.

In conclusion in our models the Venturi effect is the only reason for the SAM of the mitral valve. In model 1, SAM does not create an obstruction itself, but is caused by an obstruction at a different place. In model 2, SAM itself creates an obstruction, which does not entirely disappear after resection of the valve.

The application of these models in in vivo conditions are limited. But it seems to confirm the thesis that it is not a single anatomically-defined cardiac abnormality, but similar flow conditions which cause SAM of the mitral valve in vivo.

Summary: We constructed two different "mitral valve" models in order to investigate the influence of the Venturi effect on SAM. According to our results, SAM can be caused as a result of a subvalvular obstruction. In this case, the valve itself does not contribute to the degree of outflow tract obstruction (first model). In the second model, the valve itself contributes to the degree of outflow tract obstruction. In both models only the Venturi effect is the cause of SAM. We conclude that different anatomic abnormalities causing a Venturi effect can induce SAM.

References

1. Henry WL, Clark CE, Epstein SE (1973) Asymmetric septal hypertrophy (ASH). Echocardiographic identification of the pathognomonic anatomic abnormality of IHSS. Circulation 47: 225
2. Popp RL, Harrison DC (1969) Ultrasound in the diagnosis and evaluation of therapy of IHSS. Circulation 40: 905
3. Sha PM, Gramiak R, Kramer DH (1969) Ultrasound localization of left ventricular outflow obstruction in HOCM. Circulation 40: 3
4. Shah PM, Gramiak R, Adelman AG, Wigle ED (1971) Role of echocardiography in diagnostic and hemodynamic assessment of HOCM. Circulation 44, 891
5. Cohen MV, Teichholz LE, Gorlin R (1976) B-scan ultrasonography in idiopathic hypertrophic subaortic stenosis. Study of left ventricular outflow tract and mechanism of obstruction. Br Heart J 38, 595
6. Henry WL, Clark CE, Griffith JM, Epstein SE (1975) Mechanism of left ventricular outflow obstruction in patient with obstructive asymmetric septal hypertrophy (Idiopathic hypertrophic subaortic stenosis). Am J Cardiol 35, 337
7. Rodger JD (1976) Motion of mitral apparatus in hypertrophic cardiomyopathy with obstruction. Br Heart J 38, 732
8. Gehrke J (1977) Critical appraisal of one- and two-dimensional echocardiography in hypertrophic cardiomyopathy. Ann Radiol 20 (3—4), 409
9. King FK, DeMaria AN, Miller RR, Hilliard GK, Zelis R, Mason DT (1974) Markedly abnormal mitral valve motion without simultaneous intraventricular pressure gradient due to uneven mitral-septal contact in idiopathic hypertrophic subaortic stenosis. Cardiology 34: 360
10. Naron BJ, Gottdiener JS, Roberts WC, Henry WL, Savages DD, Epstein SE (1978) Left ventricular outflow tract obstruction due to systolic anterior motion of the anterior mitral leaflet in patients with concentric left ventricular hypertrophy. Circulation 57, 527
11. Feigenbaum H (1976) Echocardiography. Philadelphia, p 121
12. Lemke R, Braun B, Klumpp F, Zehner J, Klaus D (1977) Mitralklappen- und Mitralringbewegung bei Mitralstenose anhand von verschiedenen Klappenmodellen. Basis Res Cardiol 72, 57
13. Lemke R, Kaltenbach M (1979) Die Bedeutung der systolischen Vorwärtsbewegung der Mitralklappe für die Ausflußtraktobstruktion bei der hypertrophen obstruktiven Kardiomyopathie (HOCM). Untersuchungen anhand eines Klappenmodells. Z Kardiol 68, 694

Authors' address:

Dr. R. Lemke, Krankenhaus Bethanien, Innere Abteilung, Virchowstraße, 4600 Dortmund 30, F.R.G.

Morphologic evidence for "small vessel disease" in patients with hypertrophic cardiomyopathy

B. J. Maron, J. K. Wolfson, S. E. Epstein, and W. C. Roberts

Cardiology and Pathology Branches, National Heart, Lung, and Blood Institute, National Institutes of Health, Bethesda, Maryland, U.S.A.

Introduction

Many patients with hypertrophic cardiomyopathy (HCM) manifest clinical, hemodynamic or morphologic evidence of myocardial ischemia or damage, including angina pectoris or atypical chest pain (1—3), certain electrocardiographic abnormalities (4—7), myocardial fibrosis at necropsy (8—10), impaired coronary vasodilator reserve and production or decreased consumpton of lactate during stress (11, 12). In this investigation, we considered the possibility that structural alterations in the intramural coronary arteries (IMCA) (13—15) contribute to myocardial ischemia in patients with HCM. Hence, we examined histologic sections of ventricular myocardium from patiens with HCM and from patients with acquired cardiac disease or normal hearts, to determine the prevalence and severity of abnormal IMCA and their relation to areas of fibrosis.

Methods

Selection of patients

The cardiovascular registry of the Pathology Branch of the National Heart, Lung, and Blood Institute was reviewed and 154 hearts of children and adults with HCM were identified and considered for inclusion into the study. Of this number, 106 were excluded for one or more of the following reasons: (1) associated cardiovascular diseases such as systemic hypertension, aortic valvular stenosis, mitral valve prolapse or coronary heart disease (> 50% narrowing of the cross-section lumen of one or more extramural coronary arteries) (37 patients) or systemic diseases, including insulin-dependent diabetes mellitus (seven patients); (2) previous ventricular septal myotomy-myectomy operation with survival more than 1 month postoperatively (19 patients); (3) the specimen was in poor condition and tissue suitable for histologic analysis could not be obtained from the standard three sites in the septum and left ventricular free wall, as described below (18 patients); and (4) the heart was considered to be a particularly good example of HCM that

This study has been previously published, in part, in the Journal of The American College of Cardiology (8: 545—57, 1986) and is reprinted with permission from the American College of Cardiology.

we wished to preserve intact (25 patients). The remaining 48 patients constitute the study group. Each patient met our definition of HCM by virtue of having a hypertrophied, non-dilated left ventricle in the absence of another cardiac or systemic disease that could produce left ventricular hypertrophy (16). Also, eight infants who died of HCM (17, 18) (seven live-born and one stillborn) were examined separately as part of this investigation.

In addition, 68 patients without HCM were selected as controls, including 14 without evidence of cardiac disease and 54 with a variety of relatively common acquired cardiac diseases characterized by an increase in left ventricular mass (Table 1). Each of the 54 control patients with cardiac disease had clinically or hemodynamically significant lesions and died either suddenly, of complications of surgery or cardiac catheterization, or of congestive heart failure. This particular control group was intentionally designed to constitute a population of adult patients with heart diseases that are relatively common in cardiologic practice; as a result, several of the congenital cardiac or systemic diseases in which abnormal IMCA have been reported occasionally (19, 20) are not represented. Certain demographic, clinical and morphologic data in patients with HCM and controls are summarized in Table 2.

Preparation of tissue

Each of the 124 hearts utilized in this study (48 children or adults with hypertrophic cardiomyopathy, eight infants with HCM, and 68 controls) was fixed in formalin. Tissue blocks were taken from the full thickness of the ventricular wall in a plane perpendicular to the long axis of the left ventricle (i.e., transverse plane), about one-half the distance between the aortic valve and left ventricular apex. Tissue sections were obtained from three locations: ventricular septum, anterior left ventricular free wall (about 2 cm lateral to the left anterior descending coronary artery), and posterior left ventricular free wall (between the papillary muscles) (Fig. 1) (21). Each tissue block was embedded in paraffin, sectioned at 6 μm and stained with Movat's pentachrome stain (22).

Table 1. Cardiac diseases in 68 control patients

Disease	No. of Patients	No. with Abnormal IMCA
Coronary heart disease #	18	1
Aortic valvular disease	15*	2[†]
Systemic hypertension	13	1
Dilated cardiomyopathy	8	0
Normals	14	2
Totals	68	6

Symbols: * Includes 11 patients with predominant or pure aortic stenosis as well as two with combined aortic stenosis and regurgitation, one with associated coronary heart disease, and one with an associated atrial septal defect.
[†] Includes one patient with combined aortic stenosis and atrial septal defect and one patient with aortic stenosis and associated coronary heart disease.
heart weight > 400 g.

Table 2. Demographic, clinical and morphologic data in patients with HCM and controls*

	No. of Patients	Age at death (yrs)	Sex (% male)	VS† (mm)	PW† (mm)	VS/PW	No. (%) with Abnormal IMCA	Heart weight (g)
HCM	48 #	29 (11—60)	44	26 (15—44)	16 (9—26)	1.7 (0.8—4.2)	40/48 (83%)	542 (270—1250)
Controls	68	48 (13—80)	69	16 (10—34)	15 (9—23)	1.1 (0.8—2.0)	6/68 (9%)	526 (250—900)
		< 0.001		< 0.001	NS	< 0.001	< 0.001	NS

Abbreviations: NS = non-significant; PW = posterior left ventricular free wall; VS = ventricular septum; VS/PW = ventricular septal to free wall thickness ratio.

Symbols: * Data presented as mean and range, where applicable.

† Ventricular septal measurements were made at the point of maximum thickness, usually about one-half the distance between the aortic valve and left ventricular apex. Left ventricular posterior wall measurements were taken behind the midpoint of the posterior mitral leaflet, at a level corresponding to the tips of the mitral leaflets; trabeculae, papillary muscles, and crista supraventricularis muscle were, by convention, excluded from these measurements.

Does not include eight infants with HCM who were analyzed separately; ventricular septal thicknesses were 8—30 mm (mean 16), posterior free wall thicknesses were 3—15 mm (mean 9) and septal-free wall ratios were 1.4—2.7 (mean 1.9).

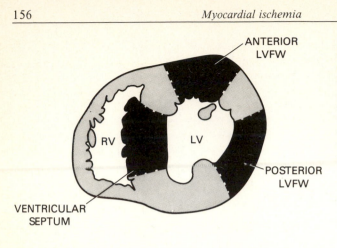

Fig. 1. Section of left ventricle (LV) in the anteroposterior (transverse) plane about one-half the distance between base and apex, showing the location of the three tissue sections that were analyzed quantitatively in each study patient. RV = right ventricle; LVFW = left ventricular free wall.

Analysis of intramural coronary arteries

Assessment of intramural coronary arteries was confined to those arteries ($< 1500 \, \mu m$ in diameter), that were viewed in cross-section (transverse cut) without obvious obliquity and did not appear to be a branch of another intramural vessel, or portions of a "tunnelled" epicardial vessel. Intramural coronary arteries in trabeculae or papillary muscles were excluded from analysis.

The extent to which abnormal IMCA occurred in each tissue section was graded semi-quantitatively based on the number of abnormal arteries and also on an estimation of the degree of wall thickening and luminal narrowing. The grading system used to express the magnitude of these abnormalities was as follows. First, the *frequency* with which altered IMCA were observed in a tissue section was assessed; the number of abnormal IMCA was described by a numerical score based on increments of 0.25 per abnormal intramural coronary artery. These scores ranged from 0.5 to 9.5. Sections with only a single altered intramural coronary artery were not considered abnormal, and in subsequent statistical analyses were treated as if they had a score of zero. Second, for each intramural coronary artery judged to be abnormal the *severity* of wall thickening and apparent luminal narrowing was graded qualitatively as mild (1+), moderate (2+) or severe (3+). Grades for frequency and severity were then averaged to yield an overall assessment of abnormal IMCA morphology for each section. These values were then summed giving a single overall "abnormal IMCA tissue section grade" for all three sections taken from each patient.

Prior knowledge of whether or not the tissue sections studied were from patients with HCM or controls was often inavoidable because particularly large tissue section size or the presence of marked cardiac muscle cell disorganization suggested the presence of HCM (21).

Analysis of myocardial fibrosis

The extent of fibrous tissue formation was assessed qualitatively in each tissue section: none (0), 1+ (mild), 2+ (moderate), and 3+ (severe). Mild fibrosis was judged to be present when an isolated small scar and/or only interstitial fibrous tissue formation was identified; severe fibrosis was characterized by extensive replacement scarring occupying substantial portions of the section. Moderate fibrosis consisted of degrees of replacement scarring, intermediate in extent between that observed with the mild or severe grades. Transmural infarction was defined as scarring involving at least the inner two-thirds of the ventricular wall.

Measurement of tissue section area

The area of the 348 tissue sections analyzed in this study was calculated utilizing a previously described method (21). The boundaries of each section (exclusive of trabeculae and papillary muscles) was traced on ordinary tablet paper with a fine-point marking pen and the area was then measured utilizing a video planimeter.

Interobserver variation

To assess interobserver variability in the identification of abnormal IMCA, 36 tissue sections (12 each of ventricular septum, anterior and posterior free wall) from 12 study patients (10 with HCM and two with other cardiac diseases) were analyzed independently by two observers. Each investigator determined whether or not individual tissue sections showed ≥ 2 abnormal arteries.

Statistical methods

Data were expressed as the mean ± standard error of the mean. Differences between means were assessed with the Student's *t*-test. Differences between proportions were evaluated with the chi-square test.

Clinical features

Of the 48 patients with HCM, death occurred suddenly and unexpectedly in 26, from progressive congestive congestive heart failure in nine, at operation in ten, and from cerebrovascular accident, complications of cardiac catheterization and suicide in one each. Sixteen patients (34%) had been asymptomatic or minimally symptomatic; the remaining 32 (66%) had experienced substantial functional limitation, including ten with moderate symptoms (New York Heart Association functional class II) and 22 with marked symptoms (classes III or IV). Of the 48 patients, 19 (40%) had chest pain.

Of 33 patients having cardiac catheterization, 18 had subaortic gradients of ≥ 30 mm Hg under basal conditions (40—160 mm Hg; average 88), and the remaining 15 patients had no basal gradient or small gradients of ≤ 15 mm Hg. Of the latter 15 patients, ten had provocative maneuvers performed in the cardiac catheterization laboratory (Valsalva maneuver, isoproterenol infusion or amyl nitrite inhalation) which induced gradients of ≤ 20 mm Hg in eight patients and ≥ 50 mm Hg in the other two. Five other patients with no or small basal gradients did not have provocative maneuvers performed.

The eight infants with HCM ranged in age at the time of death from stillborn to 11 months (mean 4 months); six were male and two female. Of the seven live-born infants,

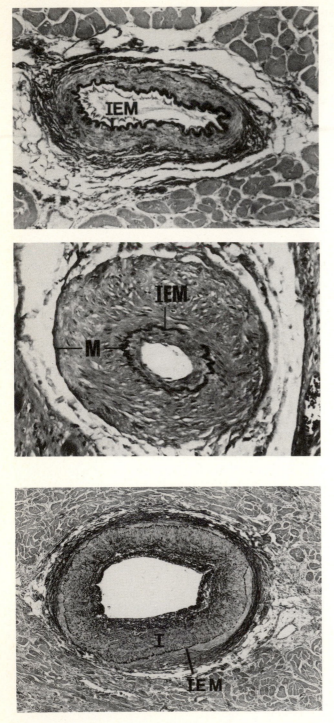

Fig. 2. Normal intramural coronary artery in the ventricular septum. Internal elastic membrane (IEM) is well seen adjacent to the sizeable lumen. Original magnification × 200.

Fig. 3. A single large abnormal intramural coronary artery (IMCA) is seen in a portion of left ventricular wall from a patient with HCM. The arterial wall thickening is due primarily to proliferation of medial (M) components, although the intima is also mildly thickened. Internal elastic membrane (IEM) is well defined. Original magnification × 200.

Fig. 4. A single intramural coronary artery (IMCA) in which the wall thickening is due primarily to an increase in intimal (I) components, from a patient with HCM. Internal elastic membrane (IEM) is well defined. Original magnification × 100.

four died of progressive congestive heart failure, one died suddenly and two died post-operatively.

Results

Histologic features of IMCA

Compared to normal (Fig. 2), abnormal IMCA were characterized by increased size and thickened walls (Fig. 3—7); usually the lumen was narrowed, although some of these arteries had normal-sized or apparently dilated lumen. Thickening of the arterial wall was due to proliferation of medial (Fig. 3) or intimal (Fig. 4) components, particularly smooth muscle cells and collagen. Also, increased numbers of elastic fibres were often present in the intima and mucoid deposits (acid mucopolysaccharide) were occasionally identified in the intima or media. In some arteries isolated intimal proliferation was

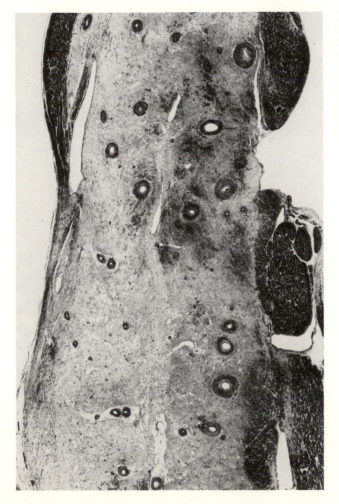

Fig. 5. Low-power photomicrograph showing transmural scarring of the ventricular septum and numerous altered intramural coronary arteries (IMCA) from a patient with HCM; several of these IMCA have thickened walls and narrowed lumens. Original magnification × 8.

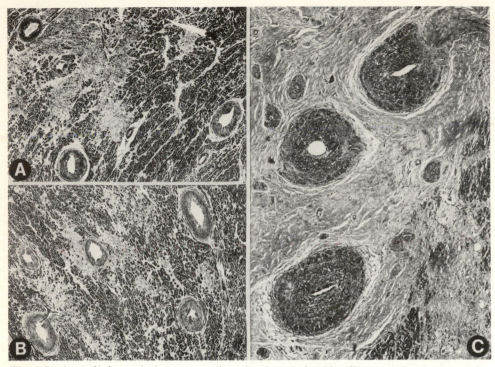

Fig. 6. Sections of left ventricular moyocardium showing relationship of intramural coronary arteries (IMCA) to fibrosis from three patients with HCM. (A) and (B) show patchy areas of fibrous tissue closely associated with several abnormal IMCA: Original magnification ×20. (C) Higher power photomicrograph showing three abnormal IMCA within an area of scarring. Original magnification × 100.

localized to only a portion of the luminal circumference. The internal elastic membrane was frequently distorted or obscured, making it difficult or impossible to discern the relative contribution of the intima or media to thickening of the arterial wall.

Control patients

Of the 68 control patients with normal hearts or cardiac disease other than HCM, six (9%) had abnormal IMCA present in at least one tissue section, including ventricular septum (five patients) or posterior free wall (one patient) (Fig. 8 and 9). Therefore, abnormal arteries were present in only six (3%) of the 204 individual tissue sections analyzed, and the vast majority of these patients (62 or 91%) did not show altered IMCA in any of the tissue sections examined.

A total of 15 abnormal IMCA were identified in the 204 sections, an average of 0.1 ± 0.03 per section and 0.04 per cm^2 of myocardium analyzed (Table 3). The maximum number of abnormal arteries present in any single section was three.

Altered IMCA ranged in external diameter from 90 to 390 μm (mean 215). Most abnormal arteries (13 out of 15, 87%) were mildly or moderately narrowed with localized

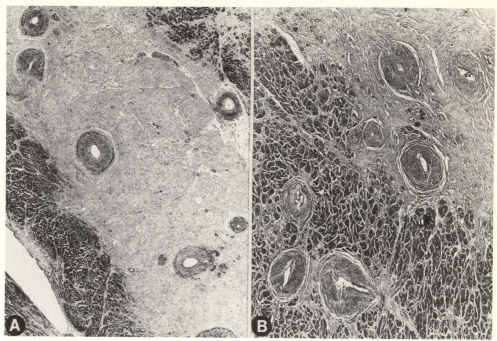

Fig. 7. (A) Area of substantial scarring in which several abnormal intramural coronary arteries (IMCA) are present. Original magnification × 20. (B) Numerous abnormal IMCA are present in a region of fibrosis, as well as in an adjacent area of myocardium which is not scarred. Original magnification × 55.

or modest intimal or medial thickening; only two out of 15 (13%) were considered to be markedly thickened and narrowed. The overall abnormal IMCA tissue section grade, refelcting the frequency as well as the severity of intramural arterial abnormalities for combined ventricular septum and free wall, was 0.08 ± 0.03 (Fig. 10; Table 3).

Patients with hypertrophic cardiomyopathy (HCM)

Of the 48 patients with HCM, 40 (83%) had abnormal IMCA in at least one tissue section; hence, the prevalence of abnormal sections was signifcantly greater in the patients with HCM than in controls (six out of 68; 9%; $p < 0.001$) (Fig. 8). In patients with HCM, altered IMCA were identified in the ventricular septum (33 patients), anterior free wall (20 patients) or posterior free wall (nine patients) (Fig. 9). Therefore, abnormal IMCA were present in 62 (43%) of the 144 individual tissue sections analyzed and most commonly appeared in ventricular septum. Of the 40 patients with abnormal IMCA, such arteries were identified in one tissue section in 23 patients, in two sections in 12 patients and in all three sections in five patients.

In patients with HCM, a total of 433 abnormal IMCA were identified in the 144 tissue sections, an average of 3.0 ± 0.7 per section and 0.9 per cm^2 of myocardium analyzed.

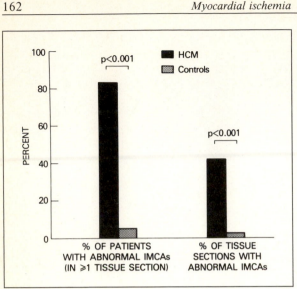

Fig. 8. Prevalence of abnormal intramural coronary arteries (IMCA) in patients with HCM and controls.

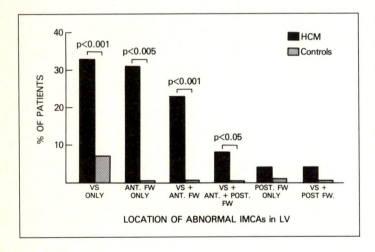

Fig. 9. Distribution of abnormal intramural coronary arteries (IMCA) in the left ventricle (LV) of patients with HCM and controls. ANT. FW = anterior free wall; POST. FW = posterior free wall; VS = ventricular septum.

The maximum number of altered arteries present in any single section was 76. The frequency of abnormal IMCA was significantly greater in patients with HCM than in controls ($p < 0.001$) (Table 3).

Occasionally, numerous abnormal IMCA appeared in clusters, but the distribution of abnormal arteries throughout the tissue section showed no particular predilection for the subendocardial of subepicardial regions. There was no significant relationship between the frequency of abnormal arteries and thickness of either ventricular septum ($r = 0.18$) or posterior free wall ($r = 0.43$).

Abnormal IMCA in patients with HCM were also larger (range 50—1330 μm in external diameter; mean 300) than those in controls (90—390 μm; mean 215). Most altered

Table 3. Frequency of IMCA in patients with HCM and controls

Parameter	HCM	Controls
No. of patients	48	68
Total no. of abnormal IMCA	433	15
Avg. no. of abnormal IMCA/tissue section	3.0±0.7*	0.1 ±0.5*
Maximum no. of abnormal IMCA/tissue section	76	3
Avg. tissue section area (cm²)†	3.5±0.2*	2.3 ±0.1*
Avg. no. of abnormal IMCA/cm² of myocardium #	0.9±0.2	0.04±0.02*
IMCA tissue section grade +	2.1±0.1*	0.08±0.03*

Abbreviations: Avg. = average.
Symbols: * Comparison of these parameters in patients with HCM and controls achieved statistical significance, $p < 0.001$.
† Expressed here for ventricular septum, anterior free wall and posterior free wall combined.
# Analysis on only those tissue sections with abnormal IMCA.
+ Reflects the frequency as well as the severity of abnormal IMCA; data presented here combine ventricular septal and both tissue sections from the free wall in each patient (see text for details).

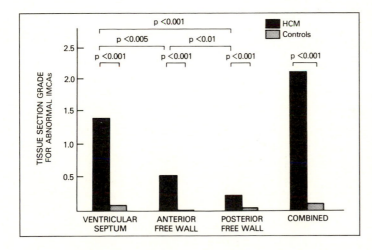

Fig. 10. Semiquantitative expression of magnitude of intramural coronary artery (IMCA) abnormalities in the 48 patients with HCM and 68 controls. Tissue section grade utilized here takes into account both the *frequency* of abnormal IMCA and the apparent *severity* of wall thickening and luminal narrowing (see text for details).

arteries (288 of 452, 64%) were markedly narrowed and thickened while the remainder (164 or 36%) were judged only mildly or moderately narrowed with mild or localized intimal or medical thickening.

The overall abnormal IMCA tissue section grade (for septum and free wall combined) was substantially greater in patients with HCM (2.1±0.1) than in controls (0.08±0.03; $p < 0.001$) (Fig. 10; Table 3). Furthermore, in patients with HCM, the magnitude of IMCA abnormalities was significantly greater in ventricular septum than in anterior free wall and also was greater in anterior free wall than in posterior free wall (Fig. 10).

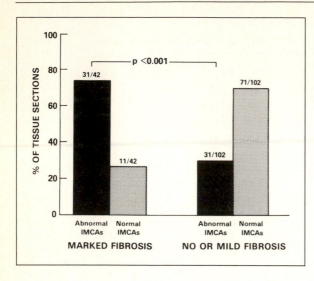

Fig. 11. Relation between occurrence of abnormal intramural coronary arteries (IMCA) and myocardial fibrosis in 144 tissue sections obtained from the ventricular septum and anterior and posterior left ventricular free wall in 48 patients with HCM. Marked fibrosis includes those tissue sections graded as "moderate" or "severe".

Abnormal intramural coronary arteries were identified in ventricular septum from three of the eight infants with HCM. In two of these three infants, numerous altered IMCA had moderate to marked thickening of the vessel wall and luminal narrowing; in the remaining infant, milder arterial abnormalities were present. Fibrosis was not associated with these abnormal IMCA in these three infants.

Relation between and myocardial fibrosis

In the 48 patients with HCM, myocardial scarring was absent or mild in 102 tissue sections and moderate to severe in 42 sections. Abnormal IMCA were significantly more common in those tissue sections with moderate or severe fibrosis (31 out of 42, 74%) than in sections with no or mild fibrosis (31 out of 102, 30%; $p < 0.001$) (Fig. 11). The association between altered IMCA and fibrosis was most significant in ventricular septal sections; abnormal IMCA were present in 19 (90%) of 21 septal sections with moderate to marked fibrosis, but in only 14 (52%) of 27 septal sections with no or mild fibrosis ($p < 0.025$). In 24 of the 31 sections in which both abnormal IMCA and substantial fibrosis were present, a particularly close spatial relationship between the two was apparent, with abnormal arteries located either within or at the margins of areas of replacement fibrosis (Fig. 5—7).

Transmural scarring was present in tissue sections of eight patients, including ventricular septum in seven and anterior free wall in one. In each of these sections, clusters of large number of abnormal IMCA were present either within or adjacent to the large scar (Fig. 5 and 7a). Most of these arteries had a small, narrowed lumen, although in some vessels the arterial lumen appeared normal or even dilated. The relation between abnormal IMCA and myocardial fibrosis was not influenced by patient age or sex.

Of the six tissue sections with abnormal IMCA in the control group, only one showed moderate fibrosis while the remainder had either no or mild fibrosis.

Correlation of IMCA with other clinical or morphologic findings

Various clinical, hemodynamic and morphologic findings in the 48 patients with HCM were compared with the prevalence and severity of abnormal IMCA. There was no correlation between the occurrence or magnitude of IMCA abnormalities and certain clinical and demographic variables such as age of the patient, sex distribution, presence or absence or severity of symptoms, mode of death (sudden versus chronic decompensation) or left ventricular end-diastolic pressure, nor morphologic features such as heart weight or ventricular septal and posterior left ventricular free wall thickness.

Although there was no statistically significant relationship between the presence or absence, or magnitude of left ventricular outflow obstruction and IMCA abnormalities, the abnormal IMCA tissue section grade in patients with nonobstructive HCM (2.8 ± 0.6) exceeded, but did not differ significantly from that of patients with obstructive HCM (1.6 ± 0.4; $p < 0.2$). Altered IMCA were present in each of the 15 patients with nonobstructive HCM and in 12 of 17 patients with obstructive HCM.

Of the 48 patients with HCM, 19 had experienced recurrent episodes of clinically significant chest pain. Of these 19 patients, 15 (79%) had abnormal IMCA in at least one tissue section; however, altered IMCA were also commonly identified in patients without chest pain (25 out of 29, 86%). Furthermore, there was no relationship between the occurrence of chest pain and extent of myocardial fibrosis; chest pain was present in 12 out of 19 patients (63%) with moderate to marked fibrosis and in 14 (48%) of 29 patients with no or mild fibrosis.

As would be expected, patients with HCM had greater ventricular septal and posterior free wall thicknesses and septal-free wall ratios than did the control patients analyzed in this study. However, heart weights in the two groups did not differ significantly and, hence, the greater frequency of IMCA in patients with HCM compared to the controls cannot be explained solely on the basis of differences in left ventricular mass.

Interobserver variation

There was agreement between two observers with regard to the presence or absence of abnormal IMCA in 88% of the observations made (i.e., 32 of 36 tissue sections analyzed).

Discussion

Occurrence and pathogenesis of IMCA in hypertrophic cardiomyopathy (HCM)

The findings of this study demonstrate that many patients (80%) with HCM have structural abnormalities of the intramural coronary arteries. There was great variation in the magnitude of these abnormalities, which were striking an distributed diffusely throughout the left ventricle in some patients and relatively mild in others. Altered IMCA were most common in the ventricular septum, but were also frequently identified in the anterior left ventricular free wall. These findings of abnormal IMCA in HCM are similar to those described in a small number of patients by James and Marshall (14) and in a preliminary study by McReynolds and Roberts (13). The present study extends their observations, however, as our results allow a quantitative expression of the prevalence, distribution and severity of abnormal IMCA in patients who died of HCM, as well as in control patients with a variety of other cardiac diseases.

Our observations indicate that the presence *per se* of abnormal IMCA is not unique for HCM, but that such arteries were also present on a few control patients with left ventricular hypertrophy due to a variety of other cardiac diseases. However, the altered IMCA identified in control patients were much less frequent and severe than those observed in patients with HCM. In particular, abnormal IMCA were infrequently present in patients with systemic hypertension or valvular aortic stenosis. Since these diseases lead to a pressure load on the left ventricular myocardium, our findings suggest that altered myocardial wall stress alone is not suf₉ficient to produce abnormal IMCA in the frequency with which they are found in HCM. In addition, our observation that IMCA abnormalities were as severe in patients without left ventricular outflow obstruction as in patients with obstruction, and the lack of any relationship between left ventricular wall thickness and the frequency or location of abnormal IMCA, further substantiate the conclusion that these abnormal arteries are not solely related to elevated intramyocardial wall tension.

Although we have no definitive data regarding the pathogenesis of abnormal IMCA in patients with HCM, the fact that these altered arteries cannot be ascribed to high ventricular pressures *per se* suggests that they may be a component of the underlying cardiomyopathy and may be present at birth (three of the eight infants with HCM we studied had abnormal IMCA). Alternatively, it is possible that in some patients abnormal IMCA are not present early in life and myocardial scarring occurs first (through some, as yet, undefined mechanism) and hence abnormal IMCA arise secondary to substantial fibrous tissue formation.

It was not possible in this study to systematically relate the location and prevalence of abnormal IMCA to areas of myocardial disorganization. This is due to the fact that assessment of cellular disorganization is generally confined to those regions of myocardium in which cardiac muscle cells are sectioned longitudinally (rather than transversely) (21) and IMCA were commonly observed both in areas of longitudinally and transversely sectioned cardiac muscle cells.

Prior observations on IMCA in other diseases

Previous investigators have reported alterations in small left ventricular intramural coronary arteries (as well as in small arteries in the sinoatrial and atrioventricular nodes) similar to those described in this report (19, 20, 23–29). These observations, which were made in patients with diseases *other than HCM*, included systemic or metabolic diseases in which hypertrophy was absent or mild, such as diabetes mellitus (19), progressive muscular dystrophy (20), Friedreich's ataxia (20, 23), scleroderma (24), homocystinuria (25) and the Marfan syndrome (20). Abnormal IMCA also have been described in a diverse group of primary cardiovascular diseases with or without left ventricular hypertrophy such as tunnel subaortic stenosis (26), primary pulmonary hypertension (20), Newfoundland dogs with discrete fibrous subaortic stenosis, (27, 28) newborns with aortic or pulmonic atresia (29), and the syndrome of congenital deafness, syncope and sudden death associated with QT interval prolongation (20). In addition, small arteries with similar morphologic features have been observed in specialized sinoatrial or atrioventricular conduction tissue of apparently healthy young individuals (including competitive athletes) who died suddenly and either had left ventricular hypertrophy (30) or had no gross evidence of structural heart disease (31, 32). While none of these studies attempted to quantitate the frequency and severity of altered IMCA, it is our impression (based on a review of the published papers) that these arteries occurred in relatively small numbers, and therefore did not constitute the widespread and potentially significant lesion that we observed in most patients with HCM.

Relation between IMCA and myocardial fibrosis

In our study there was no clear relation between the presence of abnormal IMCA and the clinical history of chest pain in patients with HCM. Whereas about 80% of patients who had chest pain had altered IMCA, about 85% of patients who had no chest pain also showed IMCA. It is conceivable that this lack of specificity of abnormal IMCA for patients with chest pain may be due, in part, to the fact that clinical assessment of chest pain in a retrospective analysis such as ours is a difficult and subjective judgement. Most importantly, however, our study identified an important association between abnormal IMCA and objectively determined evidence of severe prolonged ischemia, i.e., myocardial fibrosis. Altered IMCA were more commonly present near or within areas of substantial fi
brosis, and clusters of increased numbes of these arteries were often identified in transmural scars. In our view, these findings suggest that the IMCA abnormalities identified in HCM are probably of pathophysiologic significance. We hypothesize that narrowed small intramural arteries compromise coronary blood flow, resulting in myocardial ischemia which, if prolonged and severe, produces myocardial necrosis and fibrous tissue formation.

Conclusions

In conclusion, the "small vessel" intramural coronary artery disease identified in this study in patients both with and without left ventricular outflow obstruction indicates that this abnormalitiy constitutes a common morphologic component of the disease process in patients with HCM. The presence of abnormal IMCA in some infants who died of HCM implies that these abnormal arteries may be present from birth as part of the developmental abnormality in HCM. The close association of abnormal IMCA with areas of scarring suggests that these vessels may contribute to the formation of myocardial fibrosis.

Summary: Many patients with hypertrophic cardiomyopathy (HCM) have signs and symptoms or metabolic and hemodynamic evidence of myocardial ischemia and dysfunction in the absence of extramural coronary atherosclerosis. To investigate the possibility that a form of "small vessel disease" could account for these findings, a histologic analysis of left venticular myocardium obtained at necropsy was carried out in 48 patients with hypertophic cardiomyopathy and in 68 controls with either normal hearts or acquired heart disease.

In HCM, abnormal intramural coronary arteries (IMCA) were characterized by thikkening of the vessel wall and an apparent decrease in luminal size (external arterial diameter < 1500 μm; average 300 μm). The wall thickening was due to proliferation of medial and/or intimal components, particularly smooth muscle cells and collagen. Of the 48 patients with HCM, 40 (83%) had abnormal IMCAs located in the ventricular septum (33 patients), anterior left ventricular free wall (20 patients) or posterior free wall (nine patients); an average of 3.0 ± 0.7 IMCA were identified per tissue section. Altered IMCAs were also significantly more common in tissue sections having considerable myocardial fibrosis (31 out of 42, 74%) than in those with no or mild fibrosis (31 or 102, 30%; $p < 0.001$). Abnormal IMCA wera also identified in 3 out of 8 infants who died of HCM before 1 year of age.

In contrast, only rare altered IMCA were identified in six (9%) of the 69 control patients, and those arteries showed only mild thickening of the wall and minimal luminal narrowing (abnormal IMCA per section: 0.1 ± 0.05: $p < 0.001$). Moreover, of those patients who did show abnormal IMCA, such vessels were about twenty times more frequent in patients with HCM ($0.9 \pm 0.2/cm^2$ myocardium) than in controls ($0.04 \pm 0.02/ cm^2$ myocardium).

Hence, abnormal IMCA with markedly thickened walls and narrowed lumens are present in increased numbers in most patients with HCM at necropsy, and may represent a congenital component of the underlying cardiomyopathic process. Although the clinical significance of "small vessel coronary artery disease" in HCM is unclear, the occurrence of structurally altered IMCA within or adjacent to areas of substantial myocardial fibrosis suggests a causal role for these arteries in producing ischemia.

References

1. Braunwald E, Lambrew CT, Rockoff SD, Ross J Jr, Morrow AG (1964) Idiopathic hypertrophic subaortic stenosis. I. A description of the disease based upon an analyis of 64 patients. Circulation 30: Suppl IV: 3—217
2. Epstein SE, Henry WL, Clark CE, Roberts WC, Maron BJ, Ferrans VJ, Redwood DR, Morrow AG (1974) Asymmetric septal hypertrophy. Ann Intern Med 81: 650—680
3. St. John Sutton MG, Tajik AJ, Smith HC, Ritman EL (1980) Angina in idiopathic hypertrophic subaortic stenosis. A clinical correlate of regional left ventricular dysfunction: A videometric and echocardiographic study. Circulation 61: 561—568
4. Estes EH Jr, Whalen RE, Roberts SE Jr, McIntosh HD (1963) The electrocardiographic and vectorcardiographic findings idiopathic hypertrophic subaortic stenosis. Am Heart J 65: 155—161
5. Braudo M, Wigle ED, Keith JD (1964) Distinctive electrocardiogram in muscular subaortic stenosis due to ventricular septal hypertrophy. Am J Cardiol 14: 599—607
6. Prescott R, Quinn JS, Littman D (1963) Electrocardiographic changes in hypertrophic subaortic stenosis which simulate myocardial infarction. Am Heart J 66: 43—48
7. Maron BJ, Wolfson JK, Ciro E, Spirito P (1983) Relation of electrocardiographic abnormalities and pattern of left ventricular hypertrophy identified by two-dimensional echocardiography in patients with hypertrophic cardiomyopathy. Am J Cardiol 51: 189—194
8. Maron BJ, Epstein SE, Roberts WC (1979) Hypertrophic cardiomyopathy and transmural myocardial infarction without significant atherosclerosis of the extramural coronary arteries. Am J Cardiol 43: 1086—1102
9. Tanaka M, Fujiwara H, Onodera T, Wu D-J, Hamashima Y, Kawai C (1986) Quantitative analyis of myocardial fibrosis in normal, hypertensive hearts, and hypertrophic cardiomyopathy. Br Heart J 55: 575—581
10. St John Sutton MG, Lie JT, Anderson KR, Frye RL (1980) Histopathological specificity of hypertrophic obstructive cardiomyopathy. Myocardial fibre disarray and myocardial fibrosis. Br Heart J 44; 433—443

11. Pasternac A, Noble J, Streulens Y, Elie R, Henschke C, Bourassa MG (1982) Pathophysiology of chest pain in patients with cardiomyopathies and normal coronary arteries. Circulation 65: 778—789

12. Cannon RO, Rosing DR, Maron BJ, Leon MB, Bonow RO, Watson RM, Epstein SE (1985) Myocardial ischemia in hypertrophic cardiomyopathy: Contribution of inadequate vasodilator reserve and elevated left ventricular filling pressures. Circulation 71: 234—243

13. McReynolds RA, Roberts WC (1975) The intramural coronary arteries in hypertrophic cardiomyopathy (abstract). Am J Cardiol 35: 154

14. James TN, Marshall TK (1975) De Subitaneis Mortibus. XII. Asymmetrical hypertrophy of the heart. Circulation 51: 1149—1166

15. Adachi K, Tanaka H, Ogata M, Yamashita Y, Sugi K, Terasawa M, Ohta K, Koga Y, Toshima H, Umezu T, Morimatsu M, Takahashi N (1985) An advanced form of familial hypertrophic cardiomyopathy showing massive myocardial fibrosis with intramural small arterial thickening. Jpn Heart J 26: 867—877

16. Maron BJ, Epstein SE (1979) Hypertrophic cardiomyopathy: A discussion of nomenclature. Am J Cardiol 43: 1242—1244

17. Maron BJ, Edwards JE, Henry WL, Clark CE, Bingle GJ, Epstein SE (1974) Asymmetric septal hypertrophy (ASH) in infancy. Circulation 50: 809—820

18. Maron BJ, Tajik AJ, Ruttenberg, HD, Graham TP, Atwood GF, Victorica BE, Lie JT, Roberts WC (1982) Hypertrophic cardiomyopathy in infants: Clinical features and natural history. Circulation 65: 7—17

19. James TN (1977) Small arteries of the heart. Circulation 56: 2—14

20. James TN (1964) An etiologic concept concerning the obscure myocardiopathies. Prog Cardiovasc Dis 7: 43—64

21. Maron BJ, Anan TJ, Roberts WC (1981) Quantitative analyis of the distribution of cardiac muscle cell disorganization in the left ventricular wall of patients with hypertrophic cardiomyopathy. Circulation 63: 882—894

22. Movat HZ (1955) Demonstration of all connective tissue elements in a single section. Arch Pathol 60: 289—295

23. James TN, Fisch C (1963) Observations on the cardiovascular involvement in Friedreich's ataxia. Am Heart J 66: 164—175

24. James TN (1974) De Subitaneis Mortibus. VIII. Coronary arteries and conduction system in scleroderma heart disease. Circulation 50: 844—856

25. James TN, Carson NAJ, Froggatt P (1974) De Subitaneis Mortibus. IV. Coronary vessels and conduction system in homocystinuria. Circulation 49: 367—374

26. Maron BJ, Redwood DR, Roberts WC, Henry WL, Morrow AG, Epstein SE (1976) Tunnel subaortic stenosis. Left ventricular outflow tract obstruction reproduced by fibromuscular tubular narrowing. Circulation 54: 404—416

27. Flickinger GL, Patterson DF (1967) Coronary lesions associated with congenital subaortic stenosis in the dog. J Pathol Bacteriol 93: 133—140

28. Muna WFT, Ferrans VJ, Pierce JE, Roberts WC (1978) Discrete subaortic stenosis in Newfoundland dogs: Association of infective endocarditis. Am J Cardiol 41: 746—754

29. Bulkley BH, Weisfeldt ML, Hutchins GM (1977) Isometric cardiac contraction. A possible cause of the disorganized myocardial pattern of idiopathic hypertrophic subaortic stenosis. N Engl J Med 296: 135—139

30. Maron BJ, Roberts WC, McAllister HA, Rosing DR, Epstein SE (1980) Sudden death in young athletes. Circulation 62: 218—229

31. James TN, Froggatt P, Marshall TK (1967) Sudden death in young athletes. Ann Intern Med 67: 1013—1021

32. James TN, Marshall TK (1976) De Subitaneis Mortibus. XVII. Multiple stenoses due to fibromuscular dysplasia of the sinus node artery. Circulation 53: 736—742

Author's address:
Dr. Barry J. Maron, National Institutes of Health, National Heart, Lung, and Blood Institute, Building 10, Room 7B—15, Bethesda, Maryland, 20892, U.S.A.

Myocardial ischemia in hypertrophic cardiomyopathy

R. O. Cannon, III

Cardiovascular Diagnosis Section, Cardiology Branch, National Heart, Lung and Blood Institute, National Institutes of Health, Bethesda, Maryland, U.S.A.

Chest pain is a common symptom reported by patients with hypertrophic cardiomyopathy, even in the absence of epicardial coronary artery disease (4). Although the chest pain often has atypical features (occurring at rest as well as during effort, prolonged duration, variable response to nitrates), several lines of evidence suggest that myocardial ischemia may occur and cause chest pain in this disease. These include: (1) chest pain and abnormal lactate metabolism during pacing (1, 9, 14), (2) reversible defects in perfusion during exercise by thallium-201 scintigraphy (5, 11), (3) abnormal regional left ventricular function (12) and (4) autopsy demonstration of left ventricular necrosis and fibrosis, often in the presence of morphologically abnormal intramural coronary arteries (6, 8). Although it seems likely that some of the chest pain syndromes experienced by patients with hypertrophic cardiomyopathy reflect myocardial ischemia, the exact mechanisms are obscure. Our studies were designed to investigate the mechanism of myocardial ischemia in patients with hypertrophic cardiomyopathy, by examining factors that modified myocardial hemodynamics and coronary blood flow during pacing-induced increases in myocardial oxygen demand.

Patients with hypertrophic cardiomyopathy compared to controls (1)

Echocardiographic criteria for the diagnosis of hypertrophic cardiomyopathy (7) and for the quantitation of hypertrophy (13), as well as techniques for estimating anterior circulation left ventricular coronary flow via the great cardiac vein, have been discussed by us previously (1, 2). Hemodynamic data from the first 20 patients with hypertrophic cardiomyopathy were compared to 28 patients with normal left ventricles; all had angiographically normal coronary arteries. Figure 1 shows that great cardiac vein flow was significantly higher (as was myocardial oxygen consumption) and coronary resistance lower in patients with basal obstruction to left ventricular outflow (≥ 30 mmHg) than in patients without obstruction and in controls.

During the stress of pacing at 130 bpm, most patients with hypertrophic cardiomyopathy began experiencing chest pain, despite a higher coronary flow than controls. At higher paced heart rates, all but two patients with hypertrophic cardiomyopathy complained of chest pain. Measurements of great cardiac vein flow showed an actual decline

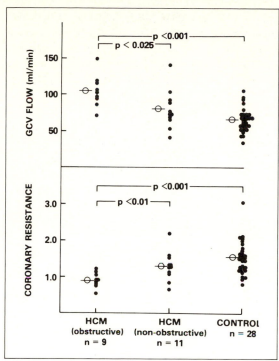

Fig. 1. Great cardiac vein (GCV) flow and resistance at rest in 20 patients with hypertrophic cardiomyopathy (HCM) and in 28 control subjects. Nine patients with hypertrophic cardiomyopathy had resting left ventricular outflow tract gradients of 30 mm Hg or more (0 represents mean value). Reprinted from (1) by permission of the American Heart Association, Inc.

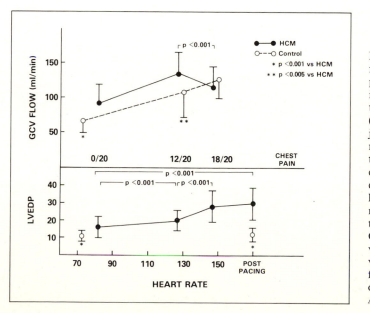

Fig. 2. Top. Great cardiac flow at rest, intermediate pacing, and peak pacing in patients with hypertrophic cardiomyopathy (HCM) and control subjects. Number at bottom represents number of patients with hypertrophic cardiomyopathy experiencing chest pain at each heart rate. **Bottom.** Corresponding LVEDP for the heart rates above. Circles represent mean values with standard deviation bars. Reprinted from (1) by permission of the American Heart Association, Inc.

increases in left ventricular filling pressures. These higher filling pressures might have exerted a compressive effect on the subendocardial microcirculation, causing a fall in flow (Fig. 2) with aggravation of ischemia (Fig. 3). Of interest, despite severe ischemia, is that most patients with hypertrophic cardiomyopathy demonstrated a paradoxical narrowing of myocardial oxygen extraction, similar to the nonischemic controls (Fig. 4).

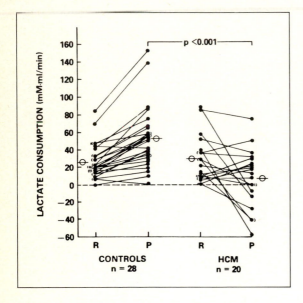

Fig. 3. Lactate metabolism at rest (R) and peak pacing (P) in control subjects and in patients with hypertrophic cardiomyopathy (HCM). Values below the dashed line at 0 represent lactate production. Circles with bars represent mean values. Reprinted from (1) by permisssion of the American Heart Association, Inc.

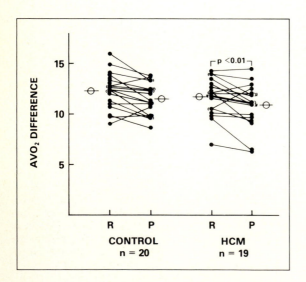

Fig. 4. AVO_2 difference (arterial — great cardiac vein O_2 content; ml O_2/100 ml) in control subjects and in patients with hypertrophic cardiomyopathy (HCM). R = rest; P = peak pacing. Reprinted from (1) by permission of the American Heart Association, Inc.

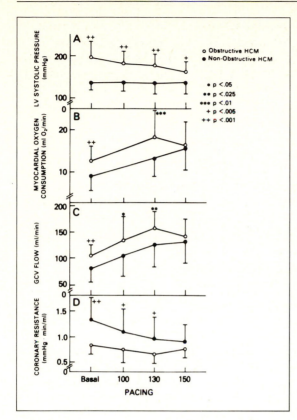

Fig. 5. (A) Left ventricular (LV) systolic pressure; (B) myocardial oxygen consumption in the anterior coronary circulation; (C) great cardiac vein (GCV) flow; and (D) coronary resistance in the anterior circulation for patients with hypertrophic cardiomyopathy. With (○) and without (●) obstruction to left ventricular outflow. Mean values with 1 SD are plotted in the basal state and during pacing. * $p < 0.05$, ** $p < 0.025$, *** $p < 0.005$, + + $p < 0.001$ versus patients without obstruction to left ventricular outflow. Reprinted from (2) with permission from the American College of Cardiology.

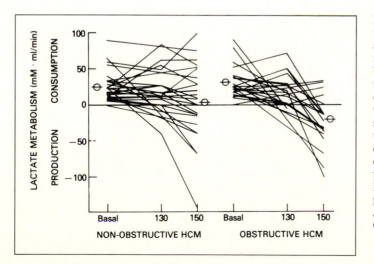

Fig. 6. Lactate consumption in the basal state and during pacing at rates of 130 and 150 beats/min in patients with hypertrophic cardiomyopathy (HCM) with and without obstruction to left ventricular outflow. Lactate consumption < 0 indicates production of lactate by the myocardium. Reprinted from (2) with permission from the American College of Cardiology.

Comparison of patients with and without obstruction (2)

In a larger series of 50 patients with hypertrophic cardiomyopathy (36 men, 14 women, with an average age of 43 years), coronary and myocardial hemodynamics of the 23 patients with basal obstruction (average left ventricular outflow gradient 77 ± 33 mg, left ventricualr systolic pressure 196 ± 33 mm Hg, mean ± 1 SD) were compared to 27 patients without basal obstruction (mean left ventricular systolic pressure 134 ± 18 mm Hg, $p < 0.001$). There was no significant difference in quantity and distribution of hypertrophy between the two groups. As shown in Fig. 5, patients with obstruction had higher great cardiac vein flow and myocardial oxygen consumption, associated with a lower coronary resistance at rest and during pacing to a heart rate of 130, the onset of chest pain for most patients. At paced heart rates of 150, the patients with obstruction demonstrated a decline in flow and an increase in coronary resistance. Evidence of ischemia (decreased lactate extraction, lactate production) was present in both groups (Fig. 6), as was an overall inability to extract more oxygen, despite ischemia (Fig. 7).

Mechanism of ischemia in hypertrophic cardiomyopathy

We interpret our studies as indicating a limitation in appropriate flow reserve, but for different reasons, in patients with and without obstruction to left ventricular outflow. As shown in Fig. 8, most patients with obstruction had higher basal and stess-related coronary flow, related to higher left ventricular systolic pressures and wall stress, with rapid exhaustion of peak flow capacity (which in absolute terms may be relatively normal) as flow requirements increase further with stress. Patients without obstruction appeared to have significantly lower peak coronary flow capacity at the onset of ischemia, suggesting greater impairment in flow delivery, perhaps related to "small vessel" intramural coronary artery disease. During stress, flow reserve may be compromised by greater impairment in the capacity for augmenting coronary flow delivery, resulting in ischemia at lower

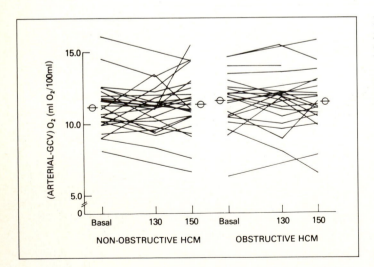

Fig. 7. Arterial minus great cardiac vein (GCV) oxygen content in the basal state and during pacing in patients with and without obstruction to left ventricular outflow. HCM = hypertrophic cardiomypathy. Reprinted from (2) with permission from the American College of Cardiology.

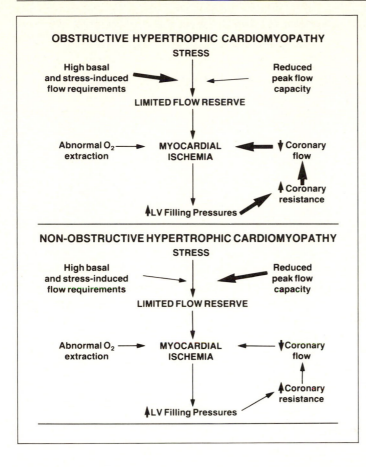

Fig. 8. Proposed mechanisms of myocardial ischemia in hypertrophic cardiomyopathy (large arrows indicate mechanisms of greater importance than those indicated by small arrows). **Top panel:** Patients with significant basal left ventricular (LV) outflow obstruction. **Lower panel:** Patients with little or no obstruction and lower left ventricular systolic pressure have lower basal flow requirements (although higher than that of patients without structural heart disease). Reprinted from (2) with permission from the American College of Cardiology.

coronary flow and myocardial oxygen consumption than in patients with obstruction. In support of the importance of elevated left ventricular systolic pressures on coronary flow and reserve in patients with obstruction, studies from our laboratory have shown a significant reduction in basal and pacing-stimulated coronary flow, with improved anginal threshold and less metabolic evidence of ischemia in patients, following successful operative relief of obstruction, compared to studies performed prior to surgery (3). Elevated filling pressures resulting from ischemia have a deleterious compressive effect on the maximally vasodilated transmural coronary bed resulting in increased coronary resistance and a decrease in flow. Other factors undoubtedly play a role in the induction of ischemia as well, such as septal perforator artery compression (10), altered capillary/myocellular relationships, and effects of abnormal diastolic relaxation on filling of the coronary reservoir, in addition to small vessel disease, previously mentioned. Abnormal oxygen extraction capacity may also contribute to or aggrevate ischemia. The paradoxical decrease in oxygen extraction despite ischemia may be due to altered myocellular/capillary relationships, decreased oxygen extraction capability at high flow velocities, or intramural shunting with oxygenated blood directly entering venous drainage, bypassing ischemic myocardium.

Summary: To investigate the presence, mechanism, and hemodynamic significance of myocardial ischemia in hypertrophic cardiomyopathy, 50 patients underwent a pacing study with measurement of great cardiac vein flow, lactate and oxygen content, and left ventricular filling pressure. Compared to patients without hypertrophic cardiomyopathy, their basal coronary flow, myocardial oxygen consumption, and left ventricular end-diastolic pressure were significantly higher. Further, the 23 patients with basal obstruction to left ventricular outflow had a significantly higher basal great cardiac vein flow and oxygen consumption than the 27 patients without basal obstruction. During pacing to heart rates of 100 and 130 bpm (the anginal threshold for 41 of 50 patients), those with basal obstruction still demonstrated significantly higher coronary flow and oxygen consumption. Most patients, regardless of the presence or absence of obstruction, had metabolic evidence of ischemia, often severe. At a heart rate of 150, most patients with basal obstruction demonstrated an actual decline in coronary flow, which correlated with an increase in left ventricular filling pressures and more severe metabolic evidence of ischemia. In those without obstructon, ischemia occurred at a lower coronary flow, suggesting more impaired coronary flow delivery than those with obstruction. Abnormalities in oxygen extraction were noted in both groups.

Thus, obstruction to left ventricualr outflow results in higher basal and stress-induced coronary flow and oxygen requirements, related to elevated left ventricular systolic pressures, resulting in rapid exhaustion of coronary flow reserve during stress. Patients without obstruction, with lower left ventricular systolic pressures, may have greater impairment of flow delivery during stress as a cause of myocardial ischemia.

References

1. Cannon RO, Rosing DR, Maron BJ, Leon MB, Bonow RO, Watson RM, Epstein SE (1985) Myocardial ischemia in patients with hypertrophic cardiomyopathy: contribution of inadequate vasodilator reserve and elevated left ventricular filling pressures. Circulation 71: 234—243
2. Cannon RO, Schenke WH, Maron BJ, Tracy CM, Leon MB, Brush JE, Rosing DR, Epstein SE (1987) Differences in coronary flow and myocardial metabolism at rest and during pacing in patients with obstructive and patients with nonobstructive hypertrophic cardiomyopathy. J Am Coll Cardiol 10: 53—62
3. Cannon RO, Rosing DR, McIntosh CL, Epstein SE (1985) Hypertrophic cardiomyopathy: improved hemodynamics, metabolism, and anginal threshold following surgical relief of outflow obstruction (abstr.). Circulation 72: III—447
4. Frank S, Braunwald E (1968) Idiopathic hypertrophic subaortic stenosis: clinical analysis of 126 patients with emphasis on the natural history. Circulation 37: 759—788
5. Hanrath P, Mathey D, Montz R, Thiel U, Vorbringer H, Kupper W, Schneider C, Bleifeld W (1981) Myocardial thallium-201 imaging in hypertrophic obstructive cardiomypathy. Eur Heart J 2: 177—185
6. Maron BJ, Epstein SE, Roberts WC (1979) Hypertrophic cardiomyopathy and tramsmural myocardial infarction without significant atherosclerosis of the extramural coronary arteries. Am J Cardiol 43: 1086—1102
7. Maron BJ, Epstein SE (1979) Hypertrophic cardiomypathy: a discussion of nomenclature. Am J Cardiol 43: 1242—1244

8. Maron BJ, Wolfson JK, Epstein SE, Roberts WC (1986) Intramural ("small vessel") coronary artery disease in hypertrophic cardiomyopathy. J Am Coll Cardiol 8: 545—557
9. Pasternac A, Noble J, Streulens Y, Elie R, Henschke C, Bourassa MG (1982) Pathophysiology of chest pain in patients with cardiomypathies and normal coronary arteries. Circulation 65: 778—789
10. Pichard AD, Meller J, Tiecholz LE, Lipnick S, Gorlin R, Herman MV (1977) Septal perforator compression (narrowing) in idiopathic hypertrophic subaortic stenosis. Am J Cardiol 40: 310—314
11. Pitcher D, Wainwright R, Maisey M, Curry P, Sowton E (1980) Assessment of chest pain in hypertrophic cardomyopathy using exercise thallium-201 myocardial scintigraphy. Br Heart J 44: 650—656
12. St. John Sutton MG, Tajik AJ, Smith HC, Ritman EL (1980) Angina in idiopathic hypertrophic subaortic stenosis: a clinical correlate of regional left ventricular dysfunction: a videometric and echocardiographic study. Circulation 61: 561—568
13. Spirito P, Maron BJ, Chiarella F, Bellotti P, Tramarin R, Pozzoli M, Vecchio C (1985) Diastolic abnormalities in patients with hypertrophic cardomyopathy: relation to magnitude of left ventricular hypertrophy. Circulation 72: 310—316
14. Thompson DS, Nagvi N, Juul SM, Swanton RH, Coltart DJ, Jenkin BS, Webb-Peploe MM (1980) Effects of propranolol on myocardial oxygen consumption, substrate extraction, and hemodynamics in hypertrophic obstructive cardiomyoapathy. Br Heart J 44: 488—498

Author's address:
Richard O. Cannon III, M.D., Building 10, Room 7B14, National Institutes of Health, Bethesda, Maryland 20892, U.S.A.

Effects of nifedipine and propranolol combined therapy in patients with hypertrophic cardiomyopathy

R. Hopf and M. Kaltenbach

Zentrum der Inneren Medizin, Klinikum der J.-W. Goethe-Universität, Frankfurt/Main, F.R.G.

Introduction

Hypertrophic cardiomyopathy is characterized by specific features of systolic and diastolic ventricle dynamics caused by myocardial hypertrophy (1, 7, 18, 19, 38, 41, 43, 54, 57). The predominant characteristic is the impaired diastolic function of the left ventricle. Filling pattern is markedly impaired, due to reduced relaxation of the hypertrophic myocardium, extended isovolumic relaxation time and a reduced maximal volume increase. A mitral insufficiency in about half the patients and an increased filling pressure are responsible for pulmonary congestion and, in part, also for patient symptoms (5, 6, 19, 20, 24, 26, 44, 50, 57). In most cases, systolic features of hypertrophic cardiomyopathy are high contractility at rest with a decreased contractility-reserve. In addition, obstructive cardiomyopathy exhibits an intraventricular pressure gradient depending on the sympathetic tone. The existence, or at least the functional role, of an intraventricular obstruction has been recently discussed and is controversial (7, 9, 13, 14, 17, 21, 31, 44, 46).

In addition to surgery, medical treatment with beta-blockers can have beneficial effects on systolic malfunction, whereas calcium antagonists bring about an improvement in ventricular diastolic dynamics (2, 5, 6, 8, 12, 14, 17, 25, 35, 37, 39, 47, 50, 51, 53). Detailed examination of data on long-term treatment with beta-blockers has been disappointing (22, 26, 34, 36). Furthermore, satisfactory improvement in all patients cannot be expected from therapy with calcium antagonists. Thus, this study was designed to examine whether combining a calcium antagonist with a beta-blocker might be a better regimen of therapy for the majority of patients.

Patients and Methods

The study comprised 15 patients with echocardiographic- and angiographic-hemodynamically confirmed hypertrophic cardiomyopathy. There were 14 male and one female patients, ranging in age from 22 to 67 years (mean: 45.5 years). Five patients suffered from non-obstructive hypertrophic cardiomyopathy with left ventricular gradients below 30 mm Hg, even following provocation (the gradient was measured postextrasystolically before and after administration of nitroglycerin, during Valsalva maneuver or ergometry or following the injection of orciprenaline. Listed are always the maximal gradients). The other ten patients presented with obstructive cardiomyopathy, four without a gradient at rest, whereas the other six had gradients between 20 and 80 (mean: 45) mm Hg. In these ten patients, the maximum pressure gradient following provocation was 35—260 (mean: 107) mm Hg. The left ventricular filling pressures for the total patient population ($n = 15$) ranged from 5 to 32 (mean: 16) mm Hg (Table 1). Twelve patients had undergone initial therapy with verapamil. Individual treatment periods had been 60 to 93 (mean: 78.5) months and the oral verapamil dose had been 480 to 640 (mean: 560) mg per day. It seemed advisable to change this therapeutic approach since the treatment results with verapamil were clinically less pronounced when compared to other patients. Of the three remaining patients, two had undergone no previous therapy, and one had been treated with 480 mg propranolol per day for 14 months. During this period his subjective feeling of well-being had deteriorated, as did clinical parameters.

At the beginning of the nifedipine-propranolol treatment, ten patients belonged to classes I and II according to the New York Heart Association (NYHA) classification, three belonged to class II to III and two to class III. Thus, most patients exhibited good stress tolerance. Therapy was discontinued for 10—14 days in patients previously treated with verapamil or propranolol. Then the new medication program was initiated, with a daily oral dose of 30 mg nifedipine and 240 mg propranolol for all patients. A follow-up ECG was performed approximately 90 to 120 min after the initial administration, to detect immediately any unwanted side effects such as bradycardia or conduction disturbances. On the basis of our experience with verapamil, whereby therapeutic effects could be identified and quantified after more than 12 months, we tried to carry out the nifedipine — propranolol treatment for a least 18 months. The patients were checked on all non-invasive findings prior to the onset of therapy and underwent follow-up investigations 1 month thereafter and then at 3—6-month intervals, if no problems demanded an earlier check-up. At all stages of the study, in addition to clinical examination, the following data were registered: one- and two-dimensional echocardiogram, 12-lead ECG at rest, conventional chest X-ray at two projections in an upright position, and radiologic heart volume determination with the patient sitting and the legs elevated. The same electrocardiograph was always used, with exact calibration and no filter. The Sokolow-index was calculated on the basis of the greatest S- and R-wave in the precordial leads. To assess left ventricular wall thickness, a two-dimensional echocardiogram was employed to localize the region of pronounced hypertrophy. Measurements with the help of one- and two-dimensional monitorings at these locations were then performed.

In order to evaluate and document the course of the disease during combined therapy, the following procedure was carried out: whilst without medication prior to nifedipine-propranolol therapy, in all patients ECG, heart volume and echocardiogram were recorded up to three times. Thus it could be shown that the intraindividual spread of measurements was up to 0.4 mV for ECG, up to 2 mm for echocardiogram and was less than 7% for heart volume determination. In addition, there were reliable measurement for comparison with the follow-up data. For each patient, the mean values of all data acquired during treatment were initially calculated, i.e. for ECG, heart volume, and echocardiogram and then compared with the mean individual values prior to treatment (therefore there is little difference between the calculated mean values during verapamil therapy and measured values at the onset on nifedipine-propranolol treatment in some cases). The mean values ± standard deviation were then calculated for the entire patient group. With regard to the total observation period with verapamil and the nifedipine-propranolol therapy, differences were analyzed by a two-way analysis of variance (Friedman test). In addition, the Wilcoxon-test, or in cases of normal distribution the paired *t*-test, was calculated for further comparison. A probability value of $p < 0.05$ was considered statistically significant.

Results

Duration of treatment and drug tolerance

The 15 patients were treated with nifedipine and propranolol for 6 to 24 (mean: 18) months. Termination of treatment became necessary in three patients after only 6 months, due to dizziness and stomach troubles (Patient 8), dizziness and weakness (Patient 6), or the occurrence of syncope and extreme diaphoresis (Patient 14). In two patients, treatment was discontinued after 12 months due to nifedipine allergy (Patient 1) or dizziness and weakness (Patient 13). The other ten patients tolerated the combined treatment well. The study was stopped when eight patients had been treated for 24 months and two for 18 months. Additional therapy became necessary in three patients; in two due to ankle- and crural edema and one was treated with antiarrhythmic medication because of syncopal episodes due to underlying objective severe rhythm disturbances (Table 1).

Symptomatic status

At the onset of therapy, 12 patients presented with typical complaints and findings, particularly dyspnea ($n = 7$), angina pectoris ($n = 7$) and other symptoms such as increased

Table 1. Left ventricular filling pressure (LVEDP), outflow tract gradient at rest and following provocation (provoc.) of all 15 patients, and duration of verapamil and nifedipine-propranolol therapy.

Patient No.	LVEDP (mmHg)	LV-gradient (mmHg) rest	provoc.	Verapamil-treatment (months)	Nifed.-Propr.-treatment (months)	Tolerance
1	14	0	28	—	12	Nifed. allergy
2	16	0	0	84	24	good
3	12	45	110	—	18	good
4	22	0	0	87	24	good
5	32	80	150	90	18	good
6	5	0	35	81	24	good
7	20	0	0	87	24	good
8	23	0	144	66	6	dizzines, stomach ache
9	22	0	0	75	24	good
10	10	0	100	69	6	dizzines, weakness
11	16	20	40	93	24	good
12	10	70	260	66	24	good
13	13	36	96	—	12	dizziness, weakness
14	12	16	72	60	6	syncope, perspiration
15	11	0	60	84	24	good

Table 2. Symptoms in 15 patients with hypertrophic cardiomyopathy (HCM) before and during therapy with nifedipine-propranolol.

Complaints before Nif./Prop.-therapy		During therapy				
		disappeared	improved	unchanged	worsened	newly appeared
dyspnea	n = 7	1	4	2	1	
angina pectoris	n = 7	1	4	2	1	
syncope/collapse	n = 1			1		2
arrhythmias	n = 0					3
weakness/vertigo/ diaphoresis	n = 9	1	2	6		6
edema	n = 0					3
no complaints	n = 3			1	2	

tendency to diaphoresis, dizziness and weakness (*n* = 9). One patient had a history of collapse and syncope. Three other patients, however, were symptom-free. During treatment with nifedipine and propranolol, only two patients reported improvement in their subjective wellbeing. Five patient reported no change in symptoms and eight patients, two of whom had previously been symptom-free, complained of deterioration and the development of symptoms, respectively.

Two patients exhibited syncope for the first time while under therapy. An increase in weakness, dizziness and diaphoresis occurred (Tables 1 and 2).

The symptomatic status, according to the NYHA classification, improved from 2 to 1.7 in the subgroup of 12 patients during pretreatment with verapamil. During treatment with nifedipine and propranolol a tendency to deterioration was seen in the mean of the entire patient population. The mean functional class was 1.9 before and 2.1 at the end of this therapy period (Fig. 1).

Objective status

Blood pressure was not changed by nifedipine-propranolol therapy and was 120.3 $\pm$11.7 over 78.3 $\pm$ 7.9 before and 121.3 $\pm$ 19.2 over 79.3 $\pm$ 11.3 mm Hg during therapy. In no case the systolic pressure was reduced by more than 15 mm Hg or fell below 100 mm Hg.

In contrast, heart rate was reduced in ten patients. The mean heart rate in all patients was 69.5 $\pm$ 12.2 before and 64.7 $\pm$ 23.5 during therapy with nifedipine and propranolol ($p < 0.05$).

ECG findings

The Sokolow-index for the 12 patients pretreated with verapamil had decreased insignificantly from a mean value of 5.3 $\pm$ 1.6 to 5.0 $\pm$ 1.1 mV during the mean treatment period of 78.5 months. The Sokolow-index increased in eight patients, remained unchanged in one and decreased in six during nifedipine-propranolol treatment. The total patient population showed no significant change (5.2 $\pm$ 1.6 vs. 5.3 $\pm$ 1.7 mV) during the 18-month nifedipine-propranolol period (Fig. 2).

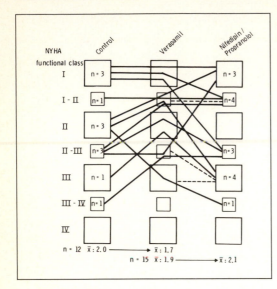

Fig. 1. Symptomatic status of the subgroup of 12 patients, pretreated with verapamil and of the entire group of 15 patients, treated with nifedipine and propranolol, according to the NYHA classification.

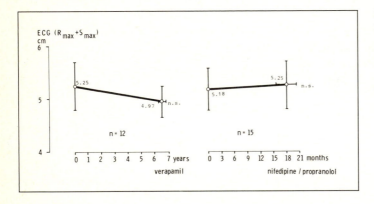

Fig. 2. Changes of the So-kolow-index in the subgroup of 12 patients pretreated with verapamil and during nifedipine-propranolol therapy in all 15 patients. n.s: not significant.

X-ray findings

No significant changes during verapamil and nifedipine-propranolol treatment could be found using conventional chest X-rays in the standing position. There was no occurrence of and no increase in pulmonary congestion.

The heart size, assessed by the help of heart volume determinations in the sitting position with elevated legs, showed no significant changes during the total observation period: during pretreatment with verapamil in 12 patients, mean heart volume had decreased from 934 ± 233 to 877 ± 198 ml/1.73 m^2 body surface (not significant). During nifedipine-propranolol treatment, heart volume increased in 11 patients and decreased in four. The total group of 15 patients showed a mean significant increase from 877 ± 214 to 947 ± 246 ml/1.73 m^2 body surface area ($p < 0.05$) (Fig. 3).

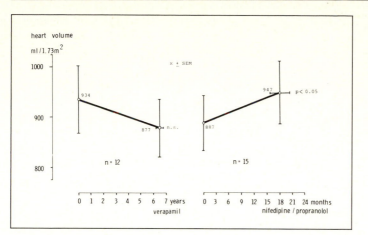

Fig. 3. Heart volume determinations in the patient group pretreated with verapamil in the group during combined nifedipine-propranolol therapy.

Echocardiography

The changes during the two treatment periods assessed by echocardiography were minor. During verapamil pre-treatment in 12 patients, left atrial diameter decreased from 40.2 ± 10 to 38.2 ± 8 mm ($p < 0.05$). The diameter of the interventricular septum was 22.5 ± 4 vs. 21.0 ± 4 mm and of the posterior wall 13.2 ± 3 before and 12.7 ± 3 mm during verapamil (n.s.).

During nifedipine-propranolol treatment, there was a significant increase in the mean left atrial diameter of all 15 patients from 40.0 ± 9 to 42.0 ± 9 mm ($p < 0.05$). Left ventricular wall thickness showed no clear change. The initial mean interventricular septal thickness was 20.5 ± 3 mm, and during combination therapy 21.5 ± 3 mm (n.s.). At the same time, the measurements of the posterior wall were 13.1 ± 2 and 13.6 ± 2 mm (n.s.) (Fig. 4).

Comparison between clinical and hemodynamic findings

The present study, comparising 15 patients, showed no relationship between treatment results and the initial left ventricular filling pressure or the left ventricular pressure gradients, at rest or following provocation, measured during cardiac catheterization. Although the four patients who developed dizziness or syncope had resting or latent obstruction, they did not belong to those with the highest gradients (Tables 1 and 3).

Discussion

The present study was based on the hypothesis that the hemodynamic effects of propranolol on supernormal left ventricular systolic function at rest, and of nifedipine on impaired diastolic function would lead to a clinically quantifiable improvement in cardiac function. The high contractility at rest and the left ventricular outflow tract gradient, as typical features of obstructive cardiomyopathy, show great variability, since they depend on sympathetic tone. Consequently, beta-blockers were employed as soon as available in the treatment of hypertrophic cardiomyopathy (8, 10, 25). Clinical investigations showed only minor effects on the ventricular systolic function at rest. An increase in the

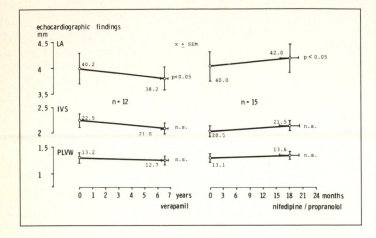

Fig. 4. Echocardiographic measurements during verapamil pretreatment in the subgroup and during nifedipine-propranolol therapy in the total patient group.

ventricular pressure gradient following provocation, however, could be prevented (14, 17, 25). In contrast, chronic reduction of outflow tract obstruction was proven in only some of these patients (3, 15, 36). There is some controversy regarding the effects of beta-blockers on diastolic ventricular function. Some patients showed a decrease in filling pressure following acute administration (55). This might have been due to the individual dosage and the mode of administration (12, 14, 25). An even greater variability with respect to filling pressure during long-term treatment (3, 39, 55) occurred, where a further increase or reviving increase was usually observed (36). Concurrent to hemodynamic findings, the clinical course of the disease varied with beta-blocker treatment. As well as deterioration, clinical improvement has been reported with strict high-dose and long-term treatment (3, 4, 10, 15, 16, 55). However, in most patients there was no correlation between hemodynamic and clinical findings (39, 55). Often, only an initial clinical improvement in a low percentage of patients was reported (34, 39, 55). Significant differences with untreated control patients could not be established (8, 36). Rather, a decrease in stress tolerance with reduced cardiac output and increased pulmonary circulation pressure occurred (39). Thus, the results of beta-blocker treatment in general are disappointing, particularly because prognosis cannot be improved (22, 34, 36, 39).

As a result, there has been some discussion as to whether the combination of beta-blockers and calcium antagonists might be a beneficial therapeutic approach (11, 16, 35). This drug combination has resulted from conclusions drawn shortly after the first report on the clinically quantifiable efficacy of calcium antagonists (28, 32). It was indicated that left ventricular filling can be improved. Nifedipine has a marked effect on ventricular diastolic function (4, 33, 35, 37, 38, 48, 49); verapamil and diltiazem, however, also show systolic effects (2, 23, 29, 30, 45, 47). In some patients, calcium antagonists caused an increase in intraventricular obstruction due to marked peripheral vasodilatation (4, 33, 48, 49). Intravenous, and especially over-rapid administration, causes a sudden drop in afterload. We did not see these effects following slow verapamil injection (29, 30).

For the combined therapy, we chose propranolol as the betablocker, because this agent shows no intrinsic sympathomimetic activity which could have produced an attenuation

Table 3. Results of verapamil and nifedipine-propranolol treatment.

Pat.	Findings under verapamil-therapy				Findings under nifedipine-propranolol-therapy						
	Sok.-index (mV)		heart volume (ml/1.73 m²)		Sok.-index (mV)		heart volume		subjective		
No.	before	during	before	during	before	during	before	during	better	equal	worse
1	–	–	–	–	3.8	3.2	760	720		×	
2	6.2	4.7	755	722	4.6	4.5	670	833		×	
3	–	–	–	–	8.0	8.0	760	775		×	
4	4.9	4.9	815	840	5.5	5.0	915	853		×	
5	3.5	4.4	685	700	4.4	5.1	905	820	×		
6	3.5	3.5	905	765	3.5	3.4	755	778			×
7	5.1	5.1	900	750	4.4	5.1	740	921		×	
8	9.0	6.1	1265	930	6.4	5.9	930	990			×
9	6.7	6.8	880	835	7.4	8.0	780	827	×		
10	4.5	3.0	1470	1390	3.1	3.4	1515	1638			×
11	4.1	4.5	900	1050	4.6	5.5	1095	1230			×
12	5.6	5.3	930	1000	5.8	6.4	1050	1168			×
13	–	–	–	–	2.7	2.9	950	1072			×
14	4.3	5.6	660	695	6.6	7.4	730	723			×
15	5.6	5.8	1045	850	6.9	4.9	750	861			×

Sokolow-index was calculated as the sum of the greatest S- and R-waves in the precordial leads (in mV); normal radiological heart volume determinations were < 790 and < 720 ml/1.73 m² in men and women, respectively.

of the desired effects. In addition, long-term treatment results have, to date, only been obtained for high-dose propranolol treatment (15, 16). We chose nifedipine as the calcium antagonist to avoid as far as possible an additional negative chronotropic and dromotropic effect at a correspondingly high oral dosage — which might be more possible with verapamil and diltiazem — and to produce the pronounced effects on left ventricular diastolic dynamics which are described. In addition, data has shown beneficial acute effects on ventricular dynamics by nifedipine being further improved by propranolol and vice versa (20). On the basis of several studies it might be expected that the decrease in cardiac output due to beta-blockade (39) could be compensated by an increased brought about by concomitant calcium antagonistic medication (20, 48). Accordingly, an increase in left ventricular obstruction, due to an afterload reduction caused by nifedipine, might therefore be counterbalanced. The effects of beta-blockade with a reduction in ventricular outflow tract obstruction per se, with unaltered or reduced filling pressure as a result of nifedipine, might lead to improved well-being and objective improvement, for example in ECG or echocardiography, comparable to treatment with verapamil alone.

Since no impressive beneficial effects during the 18-month treatment period with nifedipine-propranolol occurred, the first question was whether this was due to patient selection. Most of the patients had been pretreated with verapamil and although they did not show a pronounced improvement when compared with the total patient group, there was nevertheless a slight subjective and objective improvement. During the following nifedipine-propranolol treatment, most patients experienced deterioration, as did those patients who had hitherto received no treatment. Thus, it is unlikely that patients had been selected whose chronic disease was not responsive to any medication, since their condition improved following calcium antagonistic therapy alone.

The nifedipine-propranolol dosages could not be increased due to side effects. Intolerable side effects necessitated withdrawal of medication in five patients. The other ten patients exhibited side effects which were, however, tolerable.

If the combination of nifedipine and propranolol was actually superior to verapamil treatment alone, this therapy should have led to subjective and objective improvment. Since this was not the case, initial data were reexamined in order to establish whether an improvement occurred in certain well-defined cases. Treatment results, however, seemed to depend neither on left ventricular filling pressure, nor on the degree intraventricular obstruction. In addition, the results of primary treatment with verapamil did not allow conclusions about the effectiveness of subsequent nifedipine-propranolol treatment.

Thus, it is possible that the hemodynamic effects of nifedipine and propranolol may have cancelled each other out. Since a reduction (48) or no change (4) in obstruction has been reported for nifedipine (48), the advantageous effect on left ventricular systolic function due to beta-blockers should be enhanced rather than neutralized (35). Beta-blockers lead to an increase in filling pressure, particularly during exercise (39), which might possibly neutralize the countercurrent beneficial effect of nifedipine (33, 37, 38). In the past, some patients have reported immediate improvement in dyspnea paralleling a decrease in left ventricular filling pressure, following intravenous or intracoronary administration of verapamil. Correspondingly, in other patients with marked pulmonary congestion, the sublingual administration of nifedipine in acute cases brought about an impressive improvement in dyspnea. At the moment we have no hemodynamic measurements related to acute administration of combined therapy, but on the other hand no clinical improvement in dyspnea has been achieved following acute or longterm administration.

In conclusion, it seems likely that the combination of nifedipine and propranolol has an additional effect on ventricular systolic function, but the effects cancel each other out with respect to ventricular diastolic function. If no clinical improvement in patients with hypertrophic cardiomyopathy treated with nifedipine — propranolol occurs, then overall improvement (symptoms, clinical findings and prognosis) can only be expected if the therapy improves ventricular diastolic function. To date, such improvement has only been shown during high-dose monotherapy with calcium antagonists, as well as after surgery with myotomy-myectomy.

Summary: Fifteen (14 male and one female) patients with hypertrophic cardiomyopathy, ranging from 22 to 67 (mean: 45.5) years of age were treated with oral nifedipine and propranolol for 6 to 24 (mean: 18) months. Twelve of the patients had been pretreated with a mean oral dose of 560 mg verapamil for 60 up to 93 (mean: 78.5) months, showing slight subjective and objective improvement. Treatment with nifedipine-propranolol was terminated in five cases due to deterioration or side effects after 6 and 12 months, respectively. During combined therapy, two patients reported subjective improvement, but in five cases there was no change and eight patients reported deterioration. The mean Sokolow-index showed no change. The radiologically determined heart volume increased in 11/15 patients and significantly in the mean of all patients from 887 ± 239 to 947 ± 246 ml/m^2. In addition, echocardiographic measurements showed a significant increase in left atrial diameter from 40.0 ± 9 to 42.1 ± 9 mm, whereas ventricular wall thickness remained unchanged. Thus, high dose verapamil therapy seems superior to nifedipine-propranolol therapy in most patients with hypertrophic cardiomyopathy.

References

1. Adelmann AG, Wigle ED, Ranganathan N, Webb GB, Kidd BSL, Bigelow WG, Silver MD (1972) The clinical course in muscular subaortic stenosis. A retrospective and prospective study of 60 hemodynamically proved cases. Ann Intern Med 77: 515—525
2. Anderson DM, Raff GL, Ports TA, Brundage BH, Parmley, WW, Chatterjee K (1984) Hypertrophic obstructive cardiomyopathy — Effects of acute and chronic verapamil treatment on left ventricular systolic and diastolic function. Br Heart J 51: 523—529
3. Assmann H, Assmann, I, Fiehring, H, Dittrich P, Eger H (1975) Verlaufsbeobachtungen bei der idiopathischen hypertrophischen subaortalen Stenose unter Propranololbehandlung. Dtsch Gesundhwes 30: 918—920
4. Betocchi S, Cannon III RO, Watson RM, Bonow RO, Ostrow HG, Epstein SE, Rosing DR (1985) Effects of sublingual nifedipine on hemodynamics and systolic and diastolic function in patients with hypertrophic cardiomyopathy. Circulation 72: 1001—1007
5. Bonow RO, Rosing DR, Bacharach SL, Grenn MV, Kent KM, Lipson LC, Maron BJ, Leon MB, Epstein SE (1981) Effects of Verapamil on Left Ventricular Systolic Function and Diastolic Filling in Patients with Hypertrophic Cardiomyopathy. Circulation 64: 787—796
6. Bonow RO, Frederick TM, Bacharach SL, Green MV, Goose PW, Maron BJ, Rosing DR (1983) Atrial systole and left ventricular filling in hypertrophic cardiomypathy: effect of verapamil. Am J Cardiol 51: 1386—1391

7. Braunwald E, Lambrew CT, Rockhoff SD, Ross J, Morrow AG (1967) Idiopathic hypertrophic subaortic stenosis. 1. A description of the disease based upon an analysis of 64 patients. Circulation 30 suppl IV: IV-3-IV-217

8. Cherian G, Brockington, IF, Shah PM, Oakley CM, Goodwin JF (1966) Beta-adrenergic blokade in hypertrophic obstructive cardiomyopathy. Br Med J 1: 895

9. Circo E, Maron BJ, Bonow RO, Cannon RO, Epstein SE (1984) Relation Between Marked Changes in Left Ventricular Outflow Tract Gradient and Disease Progression in Hypertrophic Cardiomyopathy. Am J Cardiol 53: 1103—1109

10. Cohen LS, Braunwald E (1967) Amelioration of angina pectoris in idiopathic hypertrophic subaortic stenosis with beta adrenergic blockade. Circulation 35: 847—851

11. Cserhalmi L, Aßmann I, Glavanow M, Rev J, Kelecserneyi Z (1984) Langzeittherapie der hypertrophischen obstruktiven und nichtobstruktiven Kardiomyopathie mit Nifedipin im Vergleich zu Propranolol. Zschr ges inn Med 39: 330—335

12. Edwards RHT, Kristinsson A, Warrell DA, Goodwin JF (1970) Effects of propranolol on response to exercise in hypertrophic obstructive cardiomyopathy. Br Heart J 32: 219—225

13. Ensslen R, Schwarz F, Thormann J, Schlepper M (1977) Auswurffraktion und Reserve des linken Ventrikels bei hypertrophischer obstruktiver Kardiomyopathie. Z Kardiol 66: 663—640

14. Flamm MD, Harrison DC, Hancock EW (1968) Muscular subaortic stenosis. Prevention of outflow obstruction with propranolol. Circulation 38: 846—858

15. Frank MJ, Abdulla AM, Canedo MI, Saylors RE (1978) Long-term medical management of hypertrophic obstructive cardiomyopathy. Am J Cardiol 42: 993—1001

16. Frank MJ, Watkins LO, Abdulla AM (1985) Management with Beta-Adrenergic Blocking Drugs. In: ten Cate FJ (ed) Hypertorphic Cardiomyopathy. Clinical Recognition and Management. M Dekker, New—York—Basel, pp 155—172

17. Goodwin JF, Shah PM, Oakley CM, Cohen J, Yipintsoi T, Pocock W (1964) The clinical pharmacology of hypertrophic obstructive cardiomyopathy. In: Wolstenholme GEW, O'Connor M (eds) Ciba-Foundation-Symposium: Cardiomyopathies. Churchill Ltd, London, pp 189—213

18. Goodwin JF, Oakley CM (1972) The cardiomyopathies. Br Heart J 34: 545—552

19. Goodwin JF (1982) The frontiers of cardiomyopathy. Br Heart J 48: 1—18

20. Gotsman MS, Lewis BS (1974) Left ventricular volumes and compliance in hypertrophic cardiomyopathy. Chest 66: 489

21. Grant C, Raphael MJ, Steiner RE, Goodwin JF (1968) Left Ventricular Volume and Hypertrophy in Outflow Obstruction. Cardiovasc Res 4: 346

22. Haberer, Hess OM, Jenni R, Krayenbühl HP (1983) Hypertrophe obstruktive Kardiomyopathie: Spontanverlauf im Vergleich zur Langzeittherapie mit Propranolol und Verapamil. Z Kardiol 72: 487—493

23. Hanrath P, Mathey DG, Kremer P, Sonntag F, Bleifeld W (1980) Effect of verapamil on left ventricular isovolumic relaxation time and regional left ventriuclar filling in hypertrophic cardiomyopathy. Am J Cardiol 45: 1258—1264

24. Hanrath P, Mathey DG, Siegert R, Bleifeld W (1980) Left Ventricular Relaxation and Filling Pattern in Different Forms of Left Ventricular Hypertrophy: An Echocardiographic Study. Am J Cardiol 45: 15—23

25. Harrison DC, Braunwald E, Glick G, Mason DT, Chitsey CA, Ross Jr S (1964) Effects of beta-adrenergic blockade on the circulation, with particular reference to observations in patients with hypertrophic subaortic stenosis. Circulation 29: 84—98

26. Hess OM, Goebel NH, Luescher H, Schneider J, Angehrn W, Krayenbühl HP (1979) Left ventricular function in patients with hypertrophic nonobstructive cardiomyopathy. Eur J Cardiol 9/2: 129

27. Hess OM, Grimm J, Krayenbühl HP (1983) Diastolic function in hypertrophic cardiomyopathy: effects of propranolol and verapamil on diastolic stiffness. Eur Heart J 4 (Suppl): 47

28. Hopf R, Keller M, Kaltenbach M (1976) Die Behandlung der hypertrophen obstruktiven Kardiomyopathie mit Verapamil. Verh dtsch Ges Inn Med 82, Bd. II, 1054

29. Hopf R, Kaltenbach M (1984) Einfluß hoher Dosen von Verapamil auf die linksventrikuläre Hämodynamik. In: F Gross (Hrsgb): Die Bedeutung der Kalziumantagonisten für die Hochdrucktherapie. MMW Medizin Verlag München, S 41—57

30. Hopf R, Rodrian S, Kaltenbach M (1986) Behandlung der hypertrophen Kardiomyopathie mit Kalziumantagonisten — Eine Zehnjahresbilanz. Therapiewoche 36: 1433—1454
31. Jenni R, Ruffmann K, Vieli A, Anliker M, Krayenbühl HP (1985) Dynamics of aortic flow in hypertrophic cardiomyopathy. Eur Heart J 6: 391—398
32. Kaltenbach M, Hopf R, Keller M (1976) Calciumantagonistische Therapie bei hypertroph obstruktiver Kardiomyopathie. Dtsch Med Wschr 101: 1284—1287
33. Krayenbühl HP, Hess OM, Senn M, Ritter M (1984) Effects of Calcium Antagonists on Left Ventricular Diastolic Funtion in Hypertrophic Cardiomyopathy. In: Althaus U, Burckhardt D, Vogt E (eds), Calcium-Antagonismus. Universimed-Verlag, Frankfurt, pp 250—258
34. Kuhn H, Loogen F (1978) Die Anwendung von Beta-Rezeptorenblockern bei hypertrophischer obstruktiver Kardiomyopathie (HOCM). Internist 19: 527—531
35. Landmark K, Sire S, Thanlow E, Amlie JP, Nitter-Hange S (1982) Haemodynamic effects of nifedipine and propranolol in patients with hypertrophic obstructive cardiomyopathy. Br Heart J 48: 19—26
36. Loogen F, Kuhn H, Krelhans W (1978) Natural history of hypertrophic obstructive cardiomyopathy and the effect of therapy. In: Kaltenbach M, Loogen F, Olsen EGJ (eds) Cardiomyopathy and Myocardial Biopsy. Springer-Verlag, Heidelberg—New York, p 286—299
37. Lorell BH, Paulus WJ, Grossman W, Wynne J, Cohn PF, Braunwald E (1980) Improved diastolic function and systolic performance in hypertrophic cardiomyopathy after nifedipine. New Engl J Med 303: 801—803
38. Lorell BH, Paulus WJ, Grossman W, Wynne J, Cohn PF (1982) Modification of abnormal left ventricular diastolic properties by nifedipine in patients with hypertrophic cardiomyopathy. Circulation 65: 500—507
39. Lösse B, Kuhn H, Krönert H, Rafflenbeul D, Kirscher P, Schulte HD, Loogen F (1980) Hämodynamische Auswirkungen konservativer und operativer Therapie bei hypertrophischer obstruktiver Kardiomyopathie. Z Kardiol 69: 470—477
40. Lösse B, Kuhn H, Loogen F (1982) Klinische und hämodynamische Effekte von Verapamil bei hypertrophischer obstruktiver Kardiomyopathie. Z Kardiol 71: 813—819
41. Maron BJ, Kenry WL, Clark CE, Redwood DR, Roberts WC, Epstein SE (1976) Asymetric septal hypertrophy in childhood. Circulation 53: 9—19
42. Masini V, Ceci V, Malinconico U, Milazzotto (1981) Therapeutic evaluation of pindolol and verapamil in hypertrophic obstructive cardiomyopathy. G Ital Cardiol 11: 1729—1737
43. McKenna W, Deanfield J, Faruqi A, England D, Oakley C, Goodwin J (1981) Prognosis in hypertrophic and hemodynamic features. Am J Cardiol 47: 532—538
44. Murgo JP (1982) Does outflow obstruction exist in hypertrophic cardiomyopathy? New Engl J Med 307: 1008—1009
45. Nagao M, Omote S, Takizawa A, Yasue H (1983) Effect of diltiazem on left ventricular isovolumic relaxation time in patients with hypertrophic cardiomyopathy. Jpn Circulation J 47: 54—58
46. Oakley CM, Goodwin JF (1973) Spontaneous loss of left ventricular outflow tract obstruction in hypertrophic cardiomyopathy. Recent Adv Stud Cardiac Struct Metab 2: 669—675
47. Rosing DR, Kent KM, Borer JS, Seides SF, Maron BJ, Epstein SE (1979) Verapamil therapy: a new appraoch to the pharmacologic treatment of hypertrophic cardiomyopathy. I Hemodynamic effects. Circulation 60: 1201—1207
48. Schanzenbächer P, Schick KD, Kochsiek K (1982) Nifedipin bei hypertrophisch obstruktiver Kardiomyopatie. Dtsch med Wschr 107: 1842—1846
49. Senn M, Hess OM, Krayenbühl HP (1982) Nifedipin in der Behandlung der hypertrophen, nichtobstruktiven Kardiomyopathie. Schweiz. med Wschr 38: 1312—1317
50. Speiser K, Krayenbühl HP (1979) Dynamik der linksventrikulären Füllung nach akuter Betablockade bei der hypertrophen obstruktiven Kardiomyopathie. Z Kardiol 68: 271
51. Stenson RE, Flamm Jr MD, Harrison DC, Hancock EW (1973) Hypertrophic Subaortic Stenosis: Clinical and Hemodynamic Effects of Long-Term Propranolol Therapy. Am J Cardiol 31: 763—773
52. Suwa M, Hirota Y, Kawamura K (1984) Improvement in left ventricular diastolic function during intravenous and oral diltiazem therapy in patients with hypertrophic cardiomyopathy: an echocardiographic study. Am J Cardiol 54: 1047—1053

53. Swanton EH, Brooskby IAB, Jenkins BS, Webb-Peploe MW (1977) Hemodynamic studies of beta-blockade in hypertrophic obstructive cardiomyopathy. Eur J Cardiol 5/4: 327—341

54. Shah PM, Adelman AG, Wigle ED, Gobel FL, Burchell HB, Hardarson T, Curiel R, Calzada CS, Oakley CM, Goodwin JF (1973) The natural (and unnatural) history of hypertrophic obstructive cardiomyopathy. A multicenter study. Circ Res 34, suppl II: 179—195

55. Sowton E (1976) Betarezeptorenblocker bei hypertropher Kardiomyopathie. In: Schweizer W (Hrsg): Die Betablocker. Gegenwart und Zukunft. Verlag Huber H, Bern—Stuttgart—Wien, pp 239—258

56. Spiller P, Brenner C, Karsch KR, Loogen F, Neuhaus KL (1977) Systolische und diastolische Funktion des linken Ventrikels bei hyertrophischer obstruktiver Kardiomyopathie. Z Kardiol 66: 483—490

57. Wigle ED, Hembecker RD, Guyton RW (1962) Idiopathic ventricular septal hypertrophy causing muscular subaortic stenosis. Circulation 26: 325—340

Authors' address:
Priv.-Doz. Dr. R. Hopf, Abteilung für Kardiologie, Zentrum der Inneren Medizin, Klinikum der Johann Wolfgang-Goethe Universität, Theodor Stern Kai Nr. 7, D-6000 Frankfurt/Main 70, F.R.G.

Long-term treatment of hypertrophic cardiomyopathy with verapamil or propranolol in matched pairs of patients: Results of a multicenter study

G. Kober[1], R. Hopf[1], G. Biamino[2], P. Bubenheimer[3], K. Förster[4], K. H. Kuck[5], P. Hanrath[5], K.-E. v. Olshausen[6], M. Schlepper[4], and M. Kaltenbach[1]

[1] Zentrum der Inneren Medizin, Abteilung für Kardiologie, Universitäts-klinikum Frankfurt
[2] Universitätsklinikum Steglitz, Berlin
[3] Benedikt Kreutz-Rehabilitationszentrum Bad Krozingen
[4] Kerckhoff-Klinik Bad Nauheim
[5] II. Medizinische Universitätsklinik, Kardiologische Abteilung, Hamburg
[6] Medizinische Klinik, Abteilung Innere Medizin III, Universität Heidelberg

Introduction

According to definition, hypertrophic cardiomyopathy (HCM) is a myocardial disease of unknown origin. Initially, types with and without obstruction of the left or right ventricle were separated as different diseases.

Today most investigators consider hypertrophic obstructive (HOCM) and non-obstructive (HNCM) cardiomyopathy simply as differing pictures of the same etiologically unknown disease. This concept is in agreement with the fact that the asymmetric hypertrophic process is not uniformly distributed over both ventricles, rather it is predominantly located in one of the ventricles or in different parts of the interventricular septum or the ventricular free wall itself.

As in other diseases of unknown origin, therapy of HCM is basically an empiric one, based on theoretical concepts. Medical treatment mainly consists of beta-blockers, especially propranolol (1—3) or calcium antagonists (4, 5). So far, no studies are available comparing the long-term effects of both compounds in similar patient groups. The purpose of this study is to compare the effect of treatment with either verapamil or propranolol on two groups of patients similar in symptoms and objective findings.

Method

Six centers from Bad Krozingen, Bad Nauheim, Berlin, Frankfurt, Hamburg, Heidelberg participated in the joint-study. These centers reported to the organizers in Frankfurt a total of 137 newly diagnosed patients with HCM with and without left ventricular obstruction. None had previously been treated with verapamil or propranolol.

Diagnosis was based on clinical findings, ECG, carotid pulse tracing, echocardiogram as well as right and left heart catheterization including attempts to provoke an intra-ventricular gradient. In the majority of patients a left ventricular biopsy was also performed.

At the organizational headquarters, the patients were allocated to one of two different regimes of therapy, to form matched pairs. One patient from each pair received an initial dosage of 3 × 40 mg propranolol, the other 3 × 80 mg verapamil. Dosage was increased, according to the tolerance of the individual patient, to a daily dosage of 3 × 80 mg to 3 × 160 mg propranolol, or 3 × 160 to 3 × 240 mg verapamil (Table 1).

The matched pairs were formed on the basis of the same sex, age difference of not more than 5 years, subjective symptoms, auscultatory findings, signs of hypertrophy in the ECG and left ventricular gradient at rest ($\pm$ 20 mm Hg) and following provocation ($\pm$ 40 mm Hg).

Therapy was continued for a period of 2 years. Follow-up studies began 4 weeks after the start of therapy, and repeated every 3 months. All non-invasive data were checked after 1 year and after 2 years. Two years after start of therapy, a repeat catheterization was scheduled which was performed in 69 patients.

Of 137 patients entering the study, 37 pairs completed the 2-year follow-up. 20 pairs of patients had an invasive follow-up investigation. 16 patients finished the 2-year follow-

Table 1. Multicenter treatment of HCM (daily doses).

Verapamil (mg)	Propranolol (mg)
3 × 80 (240)	3 × 40 (120)
3 × 120 (360)	3 × 80 (240)
3 × 160 (480)	3 × 120 (360)
3 × 240 (720)	3 × 160 (480)

Table 2. Follow-up of patient numbers in the study.

Patients who	entered the study	137	100%
Completed follow-up			
	37 pairs	74 }	
	without partner	16 }	66%
Dropped out,	therapy-related	11	8%
	loss follow-up	26	19%
	no drug intake	4	
	pretreated	3	
	false diagnosis	1	
	sudden death	1	
	(on verapamil)		
	pregnancy	1	

up without a matching partner. The study was discontinued in 11 patients due to side effects, 26 patients due to incomplete follow-up and ten due to various other reasons (Table 2). One patient died suddenly during verapamil treatment.

Therapy-related reasons for termination of allocated therapy were: inefficacy in three propranolol patients and in one verapamil patient, congestive heart failure and bronchial asthma in two propranolol patients, gastrointestinal difficulties (two in each group) and dizziness in one verapamil patient (Table 3).

The data from the beginning of therapy are compiled in Table 4. Among all data there was only a minor, but statistically significant, difference between both groups in the Sokolow-indices. There was no difference with respect to age, sex, symptoms, clinical and echocardiographic findings, aortic and left ventricular pressures, including the pressure gradient at rest and following provocation. The mean final dosage of verapamil was 493 mg/day and 340 mg/day of propranolol.

Results

Figure 1 shows the change in clinical symptoms, heart rate, Sokolow index and maximum left ventricular gradient in both groups.

Symptoms according to the NYHA-classification improved significantly ($p < 0.005$) in the verapamil group, but remained unchanged after propranolol. Heart rate decreased in both groups. The Sokolow index decreased significantly after verapamil, whereas no change could be observed following propranolol. The maximum left ventricular gradient during provocation maneuvers decreased in both groups, reaching statistical significance only after propranolol.

When the mean changes of the parameters between entrance into the study and at 2 years' follow-up were compared (Fig. 2) the reduction in NYHA classification and in Sokolow index after verapamil was statistically significant from propranolol. The more pronounced decrease in heart rate and in maximum gradient following propranolol could not be confirmed statistically in comparison to verapamil.

The systolic murmur and the echocardiographic parameters (Table 5) as well as left ventricular systolic and enddiastolic pressures and the gradient at rest (Table 6) did not change significantly and showed no difference in either group.

In Table 7, responders and non-responders to the individual therapy were separated in the form of improved, unchanged or deteriorated data. Symptoms improved in one

Table 3. Therapy-related reasons for terminating therapy.

	Propranolol	Verapamil
Ineffective	3	1
Congestive heart failure	1	—
Asthma bronchiale	1	—
Gastrointestinal complaints	2	2
Dizziness	—	1
	7	4

Table 4. Mean data in two groups (37 patients each) of patients before treatment with verapamil or propranolol.

	Verapamil	Propranolol
Age (years)	45±12	45±12
Sex (♂ : ♀)	28 : 9	28 : 9
NYHA	2.3±0.7	2.1±0.6
Angina pectoris (*n*)	22	27
Syncope (*n*)	5	5
Palpitations (*n*)	20	15
Dyspnea (*n*)	22	25
Heart rate (b/min)	71±13	72±13
Systolic murmur		
Grade 1 + 2 (*n*)	10	11
3 + 4 (*n*)	26	23
Sokolow index (mV)	4.5±1.3	3.9±1.4 $p<0.05$
Septum diameter (mm)	19.9±5.8	20.9±4.4
Posterior wall (mm)	13.4±3.4	13.8±3.0
Sept: post. wall	1.5±0.4	1.6±0.4
LVEDP (mm Hg)	14± 8	15± 8
LVSP-apex (mm Hg)	168±33	158±42
AoSP	132±24	137±28
AoDP	76±14	80±19
LV-Grad. (rest)	36±32	24±38
LV-Grad. (post ES)	75±72	75±59
LV-Grad. (orciprenalin)	98±71	91±64
LV-Grad. (max. provoc)	122±69	111±61
Med. (mg/day)	493±136	340±135

third of the patients in either group, but deteriorated in one quarter of the propranolol and in only one of the verapamil patients. The Sokolow index improved twice as often after verapamil. Echocardiographic diameters and left ventricular gradients improved more frequently and deteriorated in less patients following verapamil.

In Table 8, objective data are compared for patients who clinically improved, remained unchanged or deteriorated. Improvement or unchanged clinical class was independent of changes in the Sokolow index. In both subgroups, no change was seen after propranolol but a reduction following verapamil. Heart rate decrease was similar in all three propranolol subgroups with the lowest 2-year value in the improved patients. The improved verapamil patients showed some decrease in heart rate during treatment, but markedly higher values compared to the propranolol group.

Discussion

The aim of medical treatment in HCM is to improve symptoms, to reduce hypertrophy or at least to slow down further progression and to improve prognosis.

Beta-blockers are aimed at reducing the increased contractility and protecting the heart from nervous and humoral sympathetic stimuli. Calcium antagonists are expected to

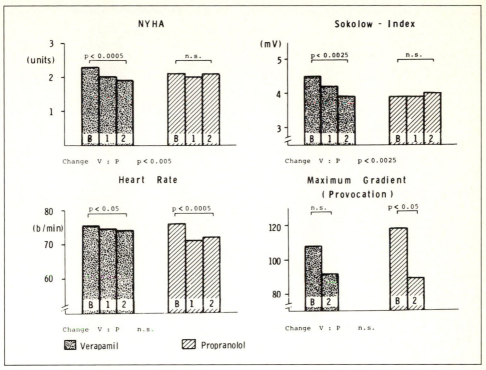

Fig. 1. Course of NYHA classification, Sokolow index, heart rate and maximum LV-gradient before (B), and 1 (1) and 2 (2) years following verapamil or propranolol treatment.

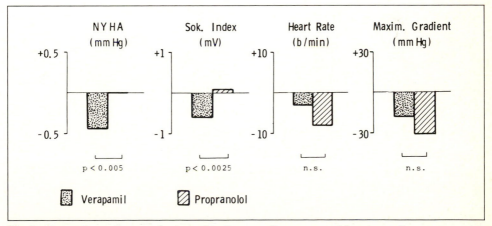

Fig. 2. Comparison of mean changes after 2 years of treatment with verapamil or propranolol. Verapamil significantly improved symptomatology (NYHA classification) and reduced left ventricular hypertrophy, according to the Sokolow index; propranolol did not. No significant differences were found between the respective therapy groups with regard to reduction in resting heart rate and maximum left ventricular gradient.

Table 5. Echocardiographic parameters before (B), 1 year (1Y) and 2 years (2Y) following verapamil or propranolol treatment.

		Verapamil		Propranolol		V : P
Septal diameter (mm)	B	19.9±5.8		20.9		N.S.
	1Y	20.7±4.4	N.S.	21.3	N.S.	N.S.
	2Y	21.0±3.8		21.6		N.S.
	B : 2Y	+ 1.1		+ 0.7		N.S.
Posterior wall diameter (mm)	B	13.4		13.8		N.S.
	1Y	13.5	N.S.	13,1	N.S.	N.S.
	2Y	13.9		14,1		N.S.
	B : 2Y	+ 0.5		+ 0.6		N.S.
Sept:Post. wall	B	1.45		1.57		N.S.
	1Y	1.54	N.S.	1.60	N.S.	N.S.
	2Y	1.51		1.54		N.S.
	B : 2Y	+ 0.06		−0.03		N.S.

Table 6. Hemodynamic parameters before and 2 years (2 Yrs) following verapamil or propranolol treatment.

		Verapamil	Propranolol	
LVEDP	before	14± 8	15± 8	
(mm Hg)	2 Yrs	15± 6	18± 8	
	change	+ 1	+ 3	N.S.
LVSPapex	before	168±33	158±42	
(mm Hg)	2 Yrs	156±37	151±35	
	change	−12	−7	N.S.
LVSPbase	before	132±24	137±28	
(mm Hg)	2 Yrs	135±30	137±22	
	change	+ 3	0	N.S.
AoDP	before	76±14	80±19	
(mm Hg)	2 Yrs	78±11	79± 9	
	change	+ 2	−1	N.S.
LVGrad-rest	before	36	21	
(mm Hg)	2 Yrs	21	14	
	change	−15	−7	N.S.

reduce the influence of calcium ions at the contractile proteins in the cardiac muscle. It is assumed that an excess or an increased sensitivity towards calcium ions stimulates the hypertrophic process and may cause structural damage.

A great number of studies confirm the beneficial hemodynamic effects of acutely administered beta-blockers (9—11), predominantly propranolol, or calcium antagonists (9, 10, 12—17), predominantly verapamil.

There are only few studies on the long-term results of chronic treatment with either substance.

Table 7. Percentage of patients who improved, remained unchanged or deteriorated, from symptoms and objective data during 2 years of verapamil (V) or propranolol (P) treatment.

	% improved		% unchanged		% deteriorated	
	P	V	P	V	P	V
NYHA-class. (border ± 0.5 classes)	32	37	44	60	24	3
Sokolow index (border ± 0.5 mV)	23	55	57	31	20	14
Septal diameter (± 5%)	24	34	30	25	45	41
Relation Septum: Posterior wall	36	50	15	13	49	37
LV-Gradient, rest (Δ ± 5 mm Hg)	12	33	44	53	44	14
LV-Gradient (max. prov.) (Δ ± 20 mm Hg)	38	56	38	22	25	22

Table 8. Relation between changes in symptomatology and objective parameters.

		New York Heart Association Classification (NYHA)					
		improved (≥ 0.5 classes)		unchanged (< ± 0.5 classes)		deteriorated (≥ 0.5 classes)	
		P	V	P	V	P	V*
Sokolow index (mV)	before	3.6	4.2	4.2	4.6	4.3	3.1
	2 yrs	3.6	3.4	4.2	4.1	4.5	3.8
Heart rate (beats/min)	before	68	78	74	69	72	65
	2 yrs	61	70	65	66	66	72
Septal diam. (mm)	before	21.7	21.1	19.7	19.6	21.8	28
	2 yrs	21.5	20.3	20.5	21.1	24.3	29
Dosage (mg)		336	502	304	477	430	480

* one patient

Reports are rare of good or sufficient long-term results with propranolol (19, 20) but frequent of a high number of treatment failures (11, 21—23) or significant side effects with a predominantly high-dose therapy. On the other hand, there are a considerable number of follow-up observations with chronic verapamil therapy showing mainly favourable results (16, 24—28).

It is even more difficult to compare the efficacy of the two forms of therapy during long-term treatment as, to date, there are only comparisons of acute hemodynamic measurements or comparisons of different patient groups, treated at different times.

In general, an objective assessment of the results of chronic oral treatment of HCM is difficult. Thus, in most acute and chronic studies in the literature, changes in symptomatology or physical capacitance are the focus of follow-up investigations. For many reasons it is even more difficult to obtain objective changes in a multi-center trial, compared to a single center-trial. Results reaching statistical significance in patients treated in one center are often significant at a lower level, or not significant at all in pooled data from different centers.

To detect the advantages of either therapeutic approach in this study, a comparison of two patient groups was performed who were, as far as possible, homogenous with respect to the initial findings and who were consequently treated as identically as possible within the different groups, according to their individual tolerances. Comparison between the matched pairs was designed in order to prevent different treatments of possibly different stages and forms or etiologies of the disease.

Analysis of the initial findings from the patients showed that this aim, to compare homogenous groups, had been achieved to a great extent. A small but significant difference between both groups existed only with respect to the Sokolow index.

Both therapeutic approaches were performed at high dosages. Propranolol at a mean dosage of 340 mg/day corresponds to the dose described as effective by Frank et al. (19, 20). With this dosage, blockade of more than 90% of the beta-receptors can be anticipated (29, 39, 31) which, in our example, resulted in a significant decrease in heart rate. After 2 years of propranolol treatment, the heart rate decreased from 74 to 64 beats/min, with values in the subgroups of between 61 and 66 beats/min (Table 8). The decrease in heart rate was markedly less pronounced with verapamil (mean 71 to 68 beats/min). This different reduction in heart rate, however, could not be statistically confirmed.

Evaluating the course of the hypertrophic parameters, there is a significant decrease in the Sokolow index with verapamil, but not with propranolol. This confirms the findings of other investigators and of our earlier studies. The echocardiographic findings showed no changes in either group. The maximum left ventricular gradient, mostly measured following provocation, decreased in both regimens but reached statistical significance only with propranolol. Comparing the changes in the two groups, no different behaviour was noticed.

The interpretation of the reduction in the Sokolow index, despite unchanged echocardiographic wall dimensions, is difficult. Since no change in the excitation and conduction of the heart was seen in the electrocardiogram and no change in the diameters of the left ventricular chamber was found, an electrical artifact comparable to e.g., the Brody effect (32) does not seem responsible. It seems to be more likely that the sensitivity of the electrocardiogram to detect changes in muscle cell hypertrophy is higher than the echocardiographic dimensions which cannot differentiate, e.g., between muscle and scar tissue.

In general, verapamil led to subjective improvement of the described symptoms and stress tolerance; however, propranolol did not. As shown in Table 7 from individual data this can be explained by a higher rate of responders to verapamil treatment, but more so by a higher rate of patients whose symptoms deteriorated during propranolol treatment.

On the whole, side effects were rare. Termination of specific therapy was necessary slightly more often in patients treated with propranolol. Only one patient in the study (treated with verapamil) died.

This multi-center study principally confirms the results of several single-center studies in which one of the medical concepts was followed or in which historical comparisons were tried (6, 28). As could be shown, verapamil is advantageous to propranolol in relieving symptoms and reducing the increased Sokolow index. Reduction in heart rate and left ventricular gradients is rather more pronounced with propranolol, but differences between both drugs are not significant. Thus, a decrease in heart rate and intraventricular gradient is not the prerequisite for an improvement in symptoms. In addition, side effects requiring termination of therapy are less pronounced in patients treated with verapamil when compared to propranolol.

Summary: The effects of a 2-year treatment with high-dose propranolol (mean, 340 ± 135 mg/day) and verapamil (mean, 493 ± 136 mg/day) were compared in two groups of patients with hypertrophic cardiomyopathy. Both groups were broadly identical at the beginning of the trial and were formed of matched pairs. Out of 137 patients entering the study, 37 pairs completed the 2 year follow-up. The mean group symptomatology (NYHA-classification) improved significantly only following verapamil treatment. Individual improvement was seen more often following verapamil (V), but deterioration was almost exclusively seen during propranolol (P) treatment. Reduction of the Sokolow-index was significant in the V group only. Reduction in the resting heart rate and maximum gradient was more pronounced following P. No correlation could be found between the change in clinical symptoms and electrocardiographic, echocardiographic or hemodynamic data, nor to the dosage of V or P administered.

From clinical and echocardiographic findings and in respect of side effects, V is advantageous over P in the treatment of hypertrophic cardiomyopathy, although a considerable number of patients improve after P. Objective data do not allow one to anticipate responders or non-responders to either treatment.

References

1. Harrison D, Braunwald E, Glich G, Mason DT, Chidsey CA, Ross J Jr (1964) Effects of β-adrenergic blockade on the circulation with particular reference to observations in patients with hypertrophic subaortic stenosis. Circulation 29: 84
2. Lösse B, Kuhn H, Loogen F (1982) Functional results in medically and surgically treated patients with hypertrophic obstructive cardiomyopathy. In: Kaltenbach M, Epstein SE (eds), Hypertrophic Cardiomyopathy. Springer Berlin—Heidelberg—New York, pp, 251—260
3. Kuhn H, Loogen F (1978) Die Anwendung von Beta-Rezeptorenblockern bei hypertrophischer Kardiomyopathy (HOCM). Internist 19: 527—531
4. Kober G, Schmidt-Moritz A, Hopf R, Kaltenbach M (1983) Long-term treatment of hypertrophic obstructive cardiomyopathy — usefulness of verapamil. Eur Heart J 4: 165—174
5. Hopf R, Rodrian S, Kaltenbach M (1986) Behandlung der hypertrophen Kardiomyopathy mit Kalziumantagonisten. Therapiewoche 36: 1433—1454
6. Lösse B, Kuhn H, Loogen F (1982) Klinische und hämodynamische Effekte von Verapamil bei hypertrophischer obstruktiver Kardiomyopathie. Z Kardiol 71: 813—819
7. Maron BJ, Merill, WH, Freier PA, Kent KM, Epstein SE, Morrow AG (1978) Long-term clinical course and symptomatic status of patients after operation for hypertrophic subaortic stenosis. Circulation 57: 1205—1213
8. Agnew TM, Barratt-Boyes BG, Brandt PWT, Roche AHG, Lowe JB, O'Brien KP (1977) Surgical resection in idiopathic hypertrophic subaortic stenosis with a combined approach through aorta and left ventricle: a long-term follow-up study in 49 patients. J Thor Cardiovasc Surg 74: 307—316

9. Bonow RO, Rosing DR, Bacharach SL, Green MV, Kent KM, Lipson LC, Maron BJ, Leon MB, Epstein SE (1981) Effects of verapamil on left ventricular systolic function and diastolic filling in patients with hypertrophic cardiomyopathy. Circulation 64: 787—796

10. Landmark K, Sire S, Thaulow E, Amlie JP, Nitter-Hauge S (1982) Hemodynamic effects of nifedipine and propranolol in patients with hypertrophic obstructive cardiomyopathy. Br Heart J 48: 19—26

11. Stenson RE, Flamm MD Jr, Harrison DC, Hancock EW (1973) Hypertrophic subaortic stenosis. Clinical and hemodynamic effects of long-term propranolol therapy. Am J Cardiol 31: 763—773

12. Schmid P, Pavek P, Klein W (1979) Echokardiographische und hämodynamische Untersuchungen zur Beeinflussung der hypertrophischen obstruktiven Kardiomyopathie durch Verapamil. Z Kardiol 68: 89—92

13. Vincenzi M, Morlino T, Allegri P, Barbierei E, Cappelletti F, de Lio U, Ometto R, Maiolino P (1981) Changes in cardiovascular function induced by verapamil in healthy subjects and in patients with ischemic heart disease. Clin Cardiol 4: 15—21

14. Spicer RL, Rocchini AP, Crowley DC, Vasiliades J, Rosenthal A (1983) Hemodynamic effects of verapamil in children and adolescents with hypertrophic cardiomyopathy. Circulation 67: 413—420

15. Rosing DR, Kent KM, Borer JS, Seides SF, Maron BJ, Epstein SE (1979) Verapamil therapy: a new approach to the pharmacologic treatment of hypertrophic cardiomyopathy. I. Hemodynamic effects. Circulation 60: 1201—1207

16. Rosing DR, Kent KM, Maron BJ, Epstein SE (1979) Verapamil therapy: a new approach to the pharmacologic treatment of hypertrophic cardiomyopathy. II. Effects on exercise capacity and symptomatic status. Circulation 60: 1208—1213

17. Senn M, Hess OM, Krayenbühl HP (1982) Nifedipin in der Behandlung der hypertrophen, nichtobstruktiven Kardiomyopathie. Schweiz Med Wschr 112: 1312—1317

18. Hanrath P, Mathey DG, Kremer P, Sonntag F, Bleifeld W (1980) Effect of verapamil on left ventricular isovolumic relaxation time and regional left ventricular filling in hypertrophic cardiomyopathy. Am J Cardiol 45: 1258—1264

19. Frank MJ, Abdulla AM, Canedo MI, Saylors RE (1978) Long-term medical management of hypertrophic obstructive cardiomyopathy. Am J Cardiol 42: 993—1001

20. Canedo MI, Frank MJ (1981) Therapy of hypertrophic cardiomyopathy: medical or surgical? Clinical and pathophysiologic considerations. Am J Cardiol 48: 383—388

21. Wigle ED, Adelman AG, Felderhof CH (1974) Medical and surgical treatment of the cardiomyopathies. Circ Res 34, 35 Suppl II: II—196—II—223

22. Goodwin JF (1974) Prospects and predictions for the cardiomyopathies. Circulation 50: 210—219

23. Loogen F, Krelhaus W, Kuhn H (1976) Verlaufsbeobachtungen der hypertrophischen obstruktiven Kardiomyopathie (HOCM). Z Kardiol 65: 511—521

24. Kaltenbach M, Hopf R (1982) Konservative medikamentöse Behandlung der hypertrophen Myokardiopathie. Z Kardiol 71: 795—805

25. Kaltenbach M, Hopf R, Kober G, Bussmann WD, Keller M, Petersen Y (1979) Treatment of hypertrophic obstructive cardiomyopathy with verapamil. Br Heart J 42: 35—42

26. Kaltenbach M, Hopf R, Keller M (1976) Calciumantagonistische Therapie bei hypertroph obstructiver Kardiomyopathie. Dtsch Med Wschr 101: 1284—1287

27. Masini V, Ceci V, Malinconico U, Milazotto F (1981) Therapeutic evaluation of pindolol and verapamil in hypertrophic obstructive cardiomyopathy. G Ital Cardiol II: 1729—1737

28. Haberer T, Hess OM, Jenni R, Krayenbühl HP (1983) Hypertrophe obstruktive Kardiomyopathie: Spontanverlauf im Vergleich zu Langzeittherapie mit Propranolol und Verapamil. Z Kardiol 72: 487—493

29. Shand DG (1975) Drug therapy: propranolol. N Engl J Med 293: 280—285

30. Chidsey C, Pine M, Favrot L, Smith S, Leonetti G, Morselli P, Zanchetti A (1976) The use of drug concentration measurements in studies of the therapeutic responses to propranolol. Postgr Med J 52 (S4): 26—32

31. Vucovich RA, Foley JE, Brown B, Willard DA, Buckley MO, Kelly D, Fitzgerald D, Torney W, Darragh A (1979) Effect of β-blockers on exercise double product (systolic blood pressure X heart rate). Br J Clin Pharmacol 7 (Suppl 2): 167—172
32. Brody DA (1956) Theoretical analysis of intracavitory blood mass influence on the heart-lead relationship. Circ Res 4: 731

Authors' address:
Prof. Dr. med. G. Kober, Abteilung für Kardiologie, Zentrum der Inneren Medizin, Klinikum der Universität, Theodor-Stern-Kai 7, D-6000 Frankfurt am Main, F.R.G.

Hemodynamic long-term results after medical and surgical therapy of hypertrophic cardiomyopathies

B. Lösse, F. Loogen, and H. D. Schulte*

Dept. of Cardiology, Pneumology and Angiology and * Dept. of Thoracic and Cardiovascular Surgery, University of Düsseldorf, F.R.G.

Introduction

Nearly 30 years after the first modern descriptions of hypertrophic cardiomyopathy (10, 50), the ideal form of therapy, which should be low-risk and effective in all patients with this disease, has not yet been found. Most information was gathered in chronological order on surgical therapy and the application of beta-adrenergic blocking and calcium-antagonistic drugs. None of these therapy forms is causal. The primary effort is, therefore, directed at ameliorating the patient's disabling symptoms, increasing their reduced exercise capacity, and prolonging life. Functional limitation is primarily caused by hemodynamic impairment and rhythm disturbances. Hemodynamic measurements, particularly when performed during exercise, are therefore a suitable method for comparing and quantifying the effectiveness of different forms of therapy.

There are numerous reports on the long-term effects of these therapeutic procedures on clinical symptoms and resting hemodynamics (1, 3, 5, 11—15, 17, 20—22, 25—34, 38, 42, 45—47, 49, 51, 52). However, only a few published data are available concerning the longterm hemodynamic effects during exercise (9, 11, 17, 29—33, 38, 47). Moreover, these studies are usually limited to follow-up periods of only several weeks or months.

In this study, we present results of hemodynamic measurements during exercise in a large number of patients with hypertrophic cardiomyopathy before and during medical treatment, as well as after surgery, with observation periods of up to 90 months. The study is focused on the following four objectives: (1) to compare the clinical and hemodynamic efficacy of propranolol, verapamil and surgery after mean follow-up periods of 3 to 9 months; (2) to compare the hemodynamic efficacy of verapamil with regard to the site of intraventricular obstruction, i.e. in typical subvalvular or atypical midventricular obstructive as well as in non-obstructive hypertrophic cardiomyopathy; (3) to compare the verapamil-induced clinical and hemodynamic effects observed during the first year of treatment with those after a mean of more than 3 years; (4) to compare the effects of surgical treatment recorded during the first postoperative year with those after a mean of 4.5 years.

Methods

Study population

The study is based on hemodynamic measurements during exercise in 112 patients, 34 females and 78 males, aged from 16 to 72 years at the initial measurement. 100 patients suffered from hypertrophic obstructive cardiomyopathy (HOCM), 12 from hypertrophic non-obstructive cardiomyopathy (HNCM). The diagnosis had been confirmed in all patients by heart catheterization, including pressure measurements and left (in most cases also right) ventricular angiography. All patients with HOCM had basal and/or provocable pressure gradients of 30 mm Hg or more within the left ventricle, with the obstruction being located either typically, in the subvalvular region, or atypically, in the midventricular portion of the left ventricle. Additionally, 33 patients also exhibited right ventricular outflow gradients of 5 to 55 mm Hg at rest. Patients with HNCM were characterized by the absence of outflow obstruction at rest or on provocation.

Of the 100 patients with HOCM, 13 patients underwent exercise hemodynamic investigations before and during treatment with propranolol, 68 patients before and during treatment with verapamil, and 31 patients before and after surgical treatment (Table 1). All 12 patients with HNCM were treated with verapamil. The addition of these patient numbers exceeds that of the total study population, because 12 patients with HOCM were subsequently examined on two therapeutic regimens (four patients propranolol and verapamil, four patients propranolol and surgery). 23 of the 68 HOCM patients treated with verapamil and 10 of the 31 operated patients underwent a further investigative procedure after several years (Table 1).

Inclusion into the study was not through a special selection but was determined by the informed consent of the patients, by the capacity of our hemodynamic laboratory and by the traditional therapeutic regimen in our institution. This consisted of an initial medical treatment with propranolol which, from 1978, was progressively replaced by verapamil. If medical treatment failed to control symptoms, surgery was advised. Surgical treatment consisted in all cases of transaortal subvalvular septal myectomy often combined with additional myotomy (44).

In view of their clinical symptoms and their initial heart catheterization data (Table 2), patients admitted to surgery were on an average in a more advanced stage of the disease than the medically treated patients. This is reflected by higher left ventricular enddiastolic pressures and higher intraventricular pressure gradients. There was no significant difference between the groups of different medical treatment. It has to be men-

Table 1. Hemodynamic effects of medical and surgical therapy in HCM.

	Therapy	No. of patients	Observation period (months)		Dose (mg)
HOCM	propranolol	13	3.0±0.6		198±20
HOCM	verapamil	68	5.5±0.3		432±11
HOCM	myectomy	31	9.1±1.3		
HNCM	verapamil	12	4.8±0.5		393±32
HOCM	verapamil	23	5.2±0.5	38.3±3.9	448±16
HOCM	myectomy	10	12.2±3.1	52.4±6.3	

Table 2. Hemodynamic characteristics at heart catheterization and maximal exercise capacity of patients with hypertrophic obstructive (HOCM) and nonobstructive (HNCM) cardiomyopathy.

	HOCM			HNCM verapamil
	propranolol	verapamil	myectomy	
No. of patients	13	68	31	12
Sex (male:female)	7:6	46:22	25:6	9:3
Age (years)	41.1± 2.4	43.1±1.6	43.9±2.2	47.5±3.5
EDP_{LV} (mm Hg)	16.3± 2.0	14.3±0.8	19.1±1.2	15.3±1.4
$P_{LV,}$ basal (mm Hg)	40.8±11.6	28.7±4.5	60.3±6.8	0
$P_{LV,}$ provoked (mm Hg)	129.2±12.9	115.1±7.0	139.1±7.6	0
$P_{RV,}$ basal (mm Hg)	17.5± 5.2	18.7±3.4	20.6±4.2	0
	($n = 4$)	($n = 22$)	($n = 13$)	
Exercise capacity (W)	75.0± 7.4	83.5±3.5	66.9±3.7	93.8±6.3

Abbreviations: EDP_{LV} = left ventricular enddiastolic pressure; P_{LV} = left ventricular outflow tract gradient; P_{RV} = right ventricular outflow tract gradient.

tioned, however, that four patients of the propranolol group and nine patients of the verapamil group later had to be admitted for surgery.

Hemodynamic investigations

The methods of exercise testing and hemodynamic monitoring were not changed throughout the years of follow-up. Exercise tests were performed with all patients in the supine position on a bicycle ergometer. Work load was increased in steps of 25 W to a maximum, terminated by angina, dyspnea or exhaustion. Heart rate, pulmonary artery pressure (Swan-Ganz catheter), systemic artery pressure (cannulated radial or brachial artery) and total body oxygen consumption (paramagnetic method, Oxycon, Mijnhardt) were continuously measured. Pulmonary arterial wedge pressure and oxygen content in pulmonary and systemic arteries (Lex-O_2-Con, Lexington Instruments) were discontinuously measured at rest and at each exercise level after reaching a steady-state of constant heart rate and oxygen consumption. For this reason, each exercise level was maintained for 5—7 min. Cardiac output was calculated from total body oxygen consumption and arterio-venous oxygen content difference, and stroke volume from cardiac output and heart rate. In a very few cases, cardiac output measurements both before and after therapeutic intervention were performed using the thermodilution method.

Initial pretreatment measurements were performed immediately before initiation of medical therapy or, in the case of operated patients, 3 days to 28 months (mean 6.1 ± 1.8 months) before surgery. The therapeutic effects were assessed by a second measurement after a mean of 3 to 9 months and, in subgroups of verapamil-treated and operated patients, by a third measurement after a mean of 38 or 52 months, respectively (Table 1).

Drug dosage

The daily dose of propranolol was 120 to 360 (mean 198 ± 20) mg. It was adjusted to achieve a resting heart rate of between 50 and 60 beats per minute. In the case of verapamil treatment, a daily dose of 480 mg was attempted but not reached in all patients due to side effects (dizziness, obstipation, edema). Thus, the mean daily dose was 432 ± 11 mg in HOCM patients and 393 ± 32 mg in HNCM patients. In the subgroup of 23 HOCM patients investigated repeatedly on verapamil, the daily dosage was 448 ± 16 mg. All surgically treated patients had been pretreated with propranolol and/or verapamil without satisfactory benefit. Pre- and post-operative measurements were performed in 24 of the 31 patients without medical therapy (medication discontinued for at least 3 days) or on identical medical therapy. Of the remaining seven patients, one received 160 mg propranolol only at the preoperative test, whereas four patients were on 30 to 120 mg propranolol and two patients on 240 mg verapamil only at the postoperative test, because of tachyarrhythmias observed in the early postoperative period.

Statistical analysis

All results are expressed as the mean ± standard error of the mean. Data were compared using Student's two-tailed t-test for paired data.

Results

Follow-up below 1 year

The changes in the degree of functional limitation (according to the classification of the New York Heart Association), observed during the first year of medical treatment or

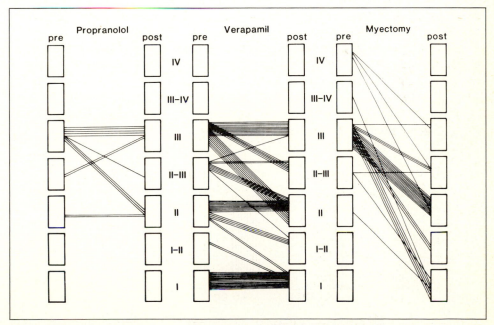

Fig. 1. Changes in functional class after propranolol (3.0 ± 0.6 months, 13 patients), verapamil (5.5 ± 0.3 months, 68 patients) and surgical therapy (9.1 ± 1.3 months, 31 patients).

Table 3. Changes in clinical symptoms after different forms of therapy for HOCM. Figures in parentheses represent patient proportions considering only initially symptomatic patients of worse than NYHA class II.

Dose (mg)	Follow-up (months)	No. of patients	Symptoms		
			improved	unchanged	worsened
Propranolol	198±20	3.0±0.6	13	31%	54%	15%
Verapamil	432±11	5.5±0.3	68	41%	58%	1%
			(52)	(54%)	(44%)	(2%)
Myectomy		9.1±1.3	31	94%	6%	0%

after surgery, are illustrated in Fig. 1 and summarized in Table 3. In the propranolol group, four patients improved, but two patients deteriorated, whereas the remaining seven patients remained unchanged. In the verapamil group, only one patient deteriorated. On the other hand, 28 patients improved, and the remaining 39 patients remained unchanged. It should be pointed out, however, that 16 of these patients already were in class I before initiation of therapy and, thus, could not improve further. The best results regarding clinical symptoms were observed after surgical therapy. All but two unchanging patients improved. Of even greater importance is the fact that, in contrast to the medically treated patients, a considerable number of patients (about one third) improved by more than one NYHA class.

The different response to therapy is also reflected by the changes in exercise tolerance (Fig. 2). There was, on average, no change in the propranolol-treated patients, whereas the verapamil-treated patients and especially the operated patients showed significant increases in tolerated work load.

Figure 3 illustrates the hemodynamic changes which were observed in each individual patient at the highest common exercise level in the pre- and post-intervention exercise

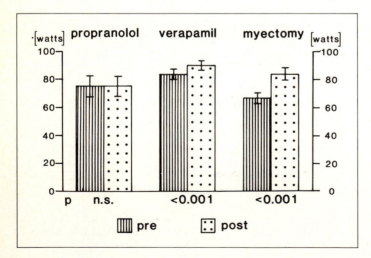

Fig. 2. Changes in exercise tolerance (mean ± standard error of the mean) after therapy of HOCM with propranolol, verapamil or myectomy. Same patients as in Fig. 1.

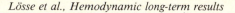

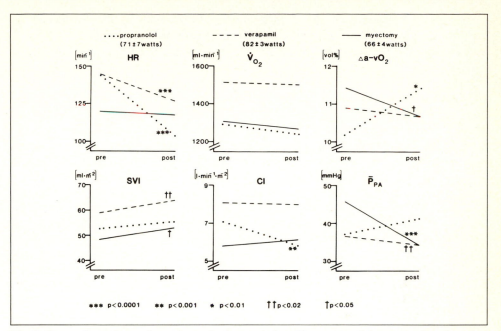

Fig. 3. Comparison of mean hemodynamic changes induced by propranolol, verapamil and surgical therapy. Same patients and duration of therapy as in Fig. 1. Comparisons were made individually for each patient at the highest common exercise level reached before and after therapeutic intervention. Mean maximal work loads were different in the three patient groups and are indicated at the top. Upper row (from the left): heart rate, total body oxygen consumption, arterio-venous oxygen difference. Lower row: stroke volume index, cardiac index, mean pulmonary artery pressure.

test. The differences in the initial control values reflect the different degrees of severity of disease in the three patient groups and, thus, the different mean workloads. Furthermore, it should be mentioned that individual responses to treatment were quite heterogeneous. On average, however, propranolol induced a marked fall in heart rate which could not be compensated for by the slight increase in stroke volume. As a consequence, cardiac output fell significantly with a concomitant increase in arterio-venous oxygen difference. Mean pulmonary artery pressure, already pathologically increased, showed a tendency towards a further rise.

Verapamil induced a smaller fall in heart rate which was, in contrast to propranolol, compensated for by a significant increase in stroke volume. Hence, cardiac output remained constant. Also in contrast to propranolol, mean pulmonary artery pressure fell significantly.

Surgical therapy induced no change in heart rate. Since stroke volume increased significantly, there was also a slight but not significant increase in cardiac output, accompanied by a significant fall in arterio-venous oxygen difference. Of utmost importance for the patients' symptoms, in contrast to the propranolol-treated patients, and much more pronounced than in the verapamil-treated patients, a substantial fall in the originally highly elevated pulmonary artery pressure could be observed.

As already mentioned, 16 out of the 68 verapamil-treated patients were already in NYHA class I before initiation of therapy and were thus not able to experience further symptomatic improvement. We therefore tested the question of whether the amount of verapamil-induced hemodynamic changes was dependent on the initial functional classification. For this reason, patients were subdivided into three subgroups: (1) better than NYHA class II (18 patients), (2) NYHA class II (16 patients), (3) worse than NYHA class II (34 patients). As can be seen in Fig. 4, the hemodynamic changes in the subgroups paralleled those observed in the whole group. In general, there were no significant differences between the subgroups, except the fall in mean pulmonary artery pressure, which was most prominent and significant only in the most initially impaired subgroup of patients worse than NYHA class II.

In order to test whether the existence and the site of an intraventricular obstruction had an influence on the hemodynamic response to verapamil, subgroups of HOCM patients with typical subvalvular obstruction ($n = 42$) and with atypical midventricular obstruction ($n = 13$) were compared and opposed to the group of patients with HNCM ($n = 12$). As demonstrated in Fig. 5, the verapamil-induced changes in hemodynamic parameters were of the same kind in both forms of obstructive hypertrophic cardiomyopathy, with a significant fall in exercise heart rate and pulmonary artery pressure. In contrast, in patients with HNCM there was a tendency towards a rise in exercise pul-

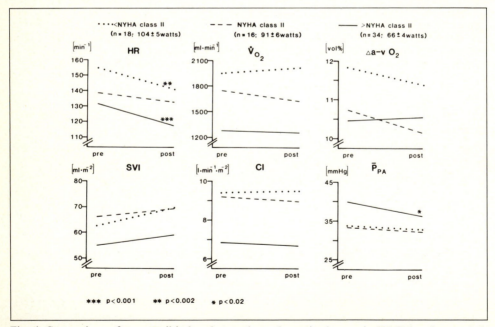

Fig. 4. Comparison of verapamil-induced mean hemodynamic changes in HOCM patients subdivided according to their different functional limitation. Same patients as in the previous figures. Comparisons were made individually for each patient at the highest common exercise level reached before and after therapy. Mean maximal work loads were different in the three patient groups and are indicated at the top. Arrangement of hemodynamic parameters and abbreviations as in Fig. 3.

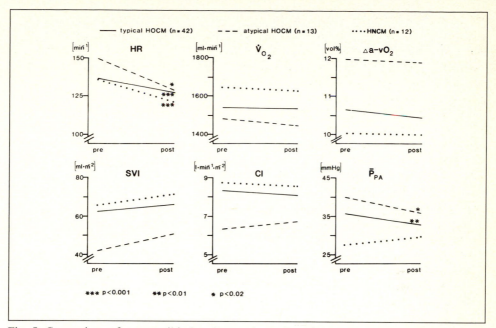

Fig. 5. Comparison of verapamil-induced mean hemodynamic changes in patients with typical HOCM (subvalvular obstruction), atypical HOCM (midventricular obstruction) and HNCM. Comparisons were made individually for each patient at the highest common exercise level reached before and after therapy of 5.5 ± 0.3 months duration in HOCM patients and 4.75 ± 0.5 months in HNCM patients. Mean maximal work loads were different in the three patient groups: 84.5 ± 4.5 watts in typical HOCM, 73.1 ± 7.2 watts in atypical HOCM, 89.6 ± 5.7 watts in HNCM. Arrangement of hemodynamic parameters and abbreviations as in Fig. 3.

monary artery pressure on verapamil, whereas the changes in the other hemodynamic parameters were similar to those observed in the obstructive forms of the disease. The changes in pulmonary artery pressure were not, however, significant. In addition, the initial values before therapy were lower than in the patients with HOCM which may have influenced behavior under therapy.

Follow-up of more than 3 years

To answer the clinically important question of how long the early therapeutic benefits persist, repeat studies were performed after several years in a group of the patients treated with verapamil or surgery. In the case of verapamil, the second study under therapy was undertaken in 23 patients, an average of 38.3 ± 3.9 months (range: 17 to 82 months) after the beginning of therapy. The drug dosage was not changed significantly throughout the observation period. It was 450.4 ± 11.3 mg at the first year study and 445.2 ± 22.3 mg at the late study. In the case of ten surgically treated patients, the second postoperative study was performed a mean of 52.4 ± 6.3 months (range 24 to 90 months) after surgery. Postoperative medication, introduced in some patients in the early postoperative period

Table 4. Additiional medical therapy in surgically treated patients with HOCM.

Patient No.	preop.	1. postop.	2. postop.
1	—	—	—
2	—	—	—
3	—	—	—
4	—	—	—
5	—	β—bl	—
6	—	d	d, v
7	(β—bl)	—	—
8	(β—bl)	β—bl	β—bl
9	((β—bl))	β—bl	—
10	((β—bl))	v	v

β—bl = beta-adrenergic blocking agents, v = verapamil, d = digitalis; ( ) = discontinued 48 h before the study, (( )) = discontinued 72 h before the study.

to control tachyarrhythmias, was changed during the follow-up period in three patients (Table 4).

The changes in functional limitation are illustrated in Fig. 6. It can be seen that the beneficial effects observed during the first year of verapamil treatment in 14 of the 23 patients did not persist in all cases. There were only two patients who experienced increasing benefit during long-term therapy. On the other hand, in seven of the 14 initially improved patients, symptoms deteriorated to the pre-treatment level, and one of the initially unchanged patients was even more symptomatic in the late study. In the surgically treated patients, in contrast, re-deteriorations in symptomatology were counterba-

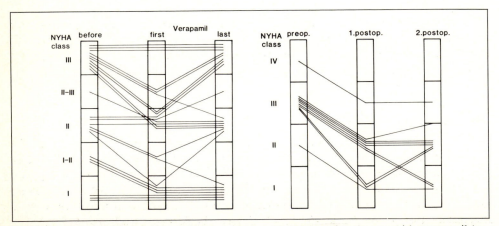

Fig. 6. Serial changes in functional class in patients with HOCM after therapy with verapamil (n = 23; first study, an average of 5.2 ± 0.5 months, last study 38.3 ± 3.9 months, after beginning of therapy) or surgery (n = 10; first postop. study, a mean of 12.2 ± 3.1 months, second postop. study 52.4 ± 6.3 months, after surgery).

lanced by further improvements. Furthermore, if symptoms deteriorated during the interval between the first and the late postoperative study, they never reached the preoperative level.

As a consequence of the different long-term responses of functional limitation, there were also differences in exercise capacity (Fig. 7). The small increase in exercise tolerance observed during the first year of verapamil treatment was not maintained as far as the late study. In strong contrast to these findings, surgically treated patients experienced a substantial increase in exercise capacity during the first postoperative year and further increase up to the late study. As a result, operated patients reached higher exercise levels in the late study than the verapamil-treated patients, although they had been more restricted before the beginning of therapy.

The different long-term response of clinical symptoms and exercise capacity to verapamil and surgical therapy is explained by the different behaviour of hemodynamic parameters. It should be pointed out once more that the individual hemodynamic changes were quite heterogeneous. On average, the initial beneficial effects observed during the first year of verapamil treatment — i.e., a fall in heart rate and pulmonary artery pressure, increase in cardiac output and stroke volume during exercise — were diminished or even abolished at the late study. Only the fall in heart rate persisted (Fig. 8). In contrast to these disappointing results, the beneficial hemodynamic changes observed during the first year after surgical therapy — i.e., a fall in exercise heart rate and pulmonary artery pressure, increase in cardiac output and stroke volume — not only per-

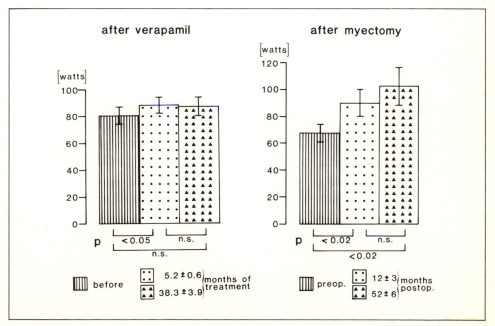

Fig. 7. Serial changes in exercise tolerance (mean ± standard error of the mean) of HOCM with verapamil or surgery. Same patients as in Fig. 6.

sisted but were even more pronounced in the late postoperative study (Fig. 9). It seems unlikely that the minor changes in additional medical treatment (Table 4) were responsible for this progressive improvement.

Discussion

General considerations

This study was not designed as a randomized study but summarizes our therapeutic experiences over the past 11 years of dealing with this disease. Hemodynamic exercise measurements were initiated at a time when propranolol was the drug of choice for medical treatment. Shortly thereafter the first encouraging results of verapamil therapy were published (21). Due to the disappointing results of propranolol therapy, which we had observed thus far and which were confirmed by the findings included in this study, we changed our therapeutic concept in favor of verapamil, which progressively became the drug of choice after 1978. During the whole study period, surgery was advised when medical treatment failed to improve severely symptomatic patients or when severe symptoms recurred in patients who had initially responded to medical treatment.

We are aware that the lack of randomization may be a major point of criticism. Nevertheless we do believe that the data presented in this study are valuable in comparing the effects of different forms of therapy. Resting hemodynamic characteristics at heart catheterization (Table 2) and pre-treatment heart rates and exercise pulmonary artery pressure (Fig. 3) demonstrate no significant differences between the groups of HOCM

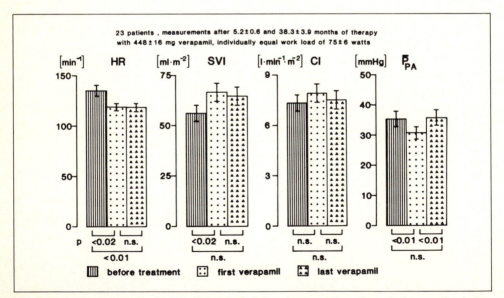

Fig. 8. Serial hemodynamic changes (from the left: heart rate, stroke volume index, cardiac index, mean pulmonary artery pressure) during therapy with verapamil in 23 patients with HOCM. Registrations were made in each individual at the highest common exercise level reached in all three studies (average for all studies 75 ± 6 W). Mean values ± standard error of the mean.

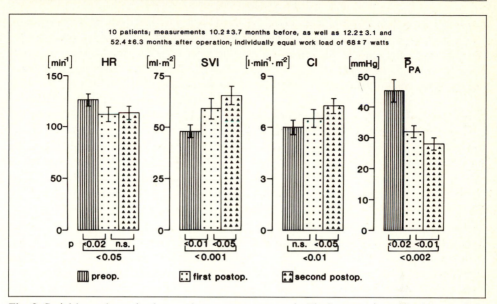

Fig. 9. Serial hemodynamic changes (same parameters as in Fig 9, mean ± standard error of the mean) after surgical therapy in 10 patients with HOCM. Registrations were made in each individual at the highest common exercise level reached in all three studies (average for all studies: 68 ±7 W).

patients undergoing different medical therapy, although there is a trend toward a slightly higher degree of impairment (especially regarding intraventricular gradients and left ventricular enddiastolic pressures) in the propranolol group. Clearly, the surgically treated patients represent a selection of more severely restricted patients, as compared to the medically treated patients, because surgery was advised only in highly symptomatic patients after an unsuccessful trial of medical therapy. It is for this reason that four patients of the propranolol group and nine of the verapamil group later had to be admitted for surgery and, thus, contribute essentially to the surgical group. For these reasons, the comparably more beneficial clinical and hemodynamic effects of surgical therapy gain further emphasis.

Strict randomization may be considered for short-term studies but for ethical reasons it is unsuitable at least for the long-term treatment of HOCM. In view of the marked differences in hemodynamic and symptomatic response to medical and surgical therapy presented in this study and also reported by other institutions (3, 26, 34, 42, 52), randomization should not cause exclusion of symptomatic patients, unresponsive to a trial of medical therapy, from the more substantial benefits of surgery, merely for experimental reasons. It should therefore only be considered for asymptomatic or mildly symptomatic patients.

Medical therapy

The mode of action of the employed pharmacological agents propranolol and verapamil is as yet not fully understood. The administration of propranolol is based on its negative inotropic effects and on the demonstration of reduced left ventricular outflow tract gradients at rest and during mild exercise (12, 13, 18, 47), whereas there are controversial opinions as to whether left ventricular relaxation and diastolic distensibility are also favourably affected (7, 19, 48). Verapamil has also been shown to reduce left ventricular outflow tract gradients (20, 21, 40, 43), and its beneficial effects on left ventricular diastolic relaxation and distensibility are well established (2, 4, 6—8, 16, 19, 43).

Our data demonstrate that verapamil, given for several months, is on average superior to propranolol in the treatment of HOCM with regard to clinical symptoms, exercise tolerance and beneficial hemodynamic response. A comparison over longer treatment periods is not possible because we have not sufficient exercise hemodynamic data available for longer periods of therapy with propranolol. Therefore, the objection of Frank et al. (13, 14), that a mean interval of two years of high-dose beta-adrenergic blocking therapy is required for attainment of maximum functional improvement, cannot be completely refuted. The value of Frank's study seems, however, to be limited by a large number of patients who were lost to follow-up or had poor compliance. Furthermore, a considerable number of patients additionally required diuretics, antiarrhythmics or pacemaker therapy so that the proper effects of propranolol were possibly blurred. As other investigators (1, 52) have found, in our experience patients did not usually tolerate the high doses of propranolol recommended by Frank, but reacted with side effects when attempts to further increased dosage were made.

The hemodynamic exercise measurements presented in this study demonstrate marked differences in the response to propranolol and verapamil. With regard to clinical symptoms and exercise capacity, the contrasting influence of both pharmacologic agents on cardiac output and pulmonary artery pressure appears to be of greatest importance. Whereas propranolol induced a marked reduction in cardiac output and a slight further increase in elevated exercise pulmonary artery pressures, verapamil exerted no depression of cardiac output and reduced pulmonary artery pressures significantly. This is probably the reason why exercise tolerance significantly improved after verapamil but did not change after propranolol. The negative effect of propranolol seems to be mainly caused by the marked depression in heart rate which could not be adequately compensated for by the small increase in stroke volume during exercise. In contrast, the fall in heart rate induced by verapamil was smaller and fully compensated for by a greater increase in stroke volume.

The differences in exercise hemodynamics explain the differences in exercise tolerance and the different rate of symptomatic improvement. Symptomatic benefit in 31 % of the patients after propranolol and in 41 % of the patients (54 %, if only initially symptomatic patients of worse than NYHA class I are considered) after verapamil agrees favourably with the majority of previous studies from our own department (24, 27, 31) and those of other investigators (5, 37, 39, 41, 45). There are, however, reports of higher rates of clinical improvement after extremely high doses of propranolol (13, 14) as well as after verapamil (20—22). Whereas these propranolol studies may be biased, at least in part, by special selection of patients and additional drug therapy, the reasons for the reported high success rates after verapamil are not completely clear. One reason could be the administration of higher verapamil doses of an average 520 to 530 mg, as compared to a mean of 432 mg in our study. Our patients did not usually tolerate higher doses, however. Therefore, a difference in the patient populations has to be discussed as a further factor. As the data presented in this study suggest, less seriously impaired patients with HOCM, as well as patients with HNCM, seem to experience, on average less symptomatic and hemodynamic (especially in terms of exercise pulmonary artery pressure) benefit from verapamil than the initially more severely impaired patients. Another reason for higher success rates with verapamil could be the longer duration of treatment as compared to our study. This explanation appears, unlikely, however, in view of our long-term observations which more often showed recurrence of symptoms than progressive improvement.

Recurrence of symptoms and hemodynamic impairment, in spite of continuous therapy, is a problem that has also been observed by other authors during treatment with verapamil (8, 39, 42), propranolol (1, 42, 45) or, more recently, disopyramide (52). In our long-term study, half of the initially improved patients returned to the pre-treatment level of functional impairment and four of them had to be operated upon. Simultaneously, the initial hemodynamic improvements were alleviated or abolished. It is difficult to ascertain whether these events have to be attributed to loss of drug efficacy or to progression of the underlying disease. Withdrawal experiments after long-term therapy (8), which we have also performed in a very few patients, indicate a persistent effect of verapamil and thus favour the second possibility.

Surgical therapy

Surgical therapy in the form of septal myectomy is usually thought to exert its beneficial effects by reducing or abolishing the subaortic obstruction (5, 28, 34, 38, 42, 49, 52). Whether and to what extent an improvement in diastolic function contributes to symptomatic benefits, is still under discussion (38, 42, 52).

In view of the reported postoperative reduction of the preoperatively mostly supernormal left ventricular ejection fraction (9, 32), our measurements of a postoperative increase in stroke volume by an average of 10 % (Fig. 3) are indicative of an increase in left ventricular enddiastolic volume. Whereas the average increase in stroke volume was as high as after verapamil treatment, surgery induced a far greater reduction in exercise pulmonary artery pressure. Since heart rate was not depressed, as it was after medical therapy, postoperative increase in stroke volume was also accompanied by a significant increase in cardiac output. These substantial hemodynamic benefits are probably the reason why surgical therapy improved clinical symptoms and exercise tolerance far more often and more substantially than both forms of medical treatment. Our findings of symptomatic improvement in 94 % of the patients agree favourably with reports by other investigators (5, 26, 34) and confirm the opinion of Wigle et al. (52) that the symptomatic relief afforded by surgery far exceeds that achieved with any form of drug therapy. Furthermore, they confirm the practice of other institutions with surgical experience, that report substantial symptomatic benefit from surgery in patients unresponsive to medical treatment (3, 5, 26, 34, 42, 52).

Since there is no evidence that surgery alters the basic disease process, scepticism has been expressed with regard to the late outcome in operated patients (36). This seemed to be supported by reports on recurrence of symptoms in 3 % to 36 % of initially improved patients during long-term postoperative follow-up for mean periods of 4.6 to 13.4

years (3, 23, 34, 42, 49). The reasons for this re-deterioration are not clear. Serial post-operative catheterizations, performed 1 to 15 years after operation, gave no evidence of postoperative recurrence of left ventricular outflow gradient (3, 28, 34). Although this does not exclude increasing left ventricular hypertrophy or occasionally observed progressive left ventricular dilatation (3, 34, 35, 51) as causes of symptomatic impairment, other causes not related to HOCM may be, at least in part, responsible for the late recurrence of symptomatic limitation, e.g., serious concomitant disease (coronary artery disease, chronic obstructive pulmonary disease, hypertension) or physiologic reduction in physical capacity due to increasing age. Bearing in mind that surgical therapy, as well as medical therapy, does not correct the underlying heart muscle disease, one would expect a certain rate of recurring symptoms in the postoperative course. A comparison with reported rates of clinical deterioration in untreated or medically treated patients (1, 5, 23, 27, 37, 45, 47) is, however, in favour of surgery, as the rate of recurring symptoms is smaller.

The results of our long-term studies in patients treated with verapamil or surgery demonstrate striking differences in favour of surgery: (1) The incidence of early symptomatic and hemodynamic benefit is higher in surgically treated patients; (2) The recurrence rate of symptoms during long-term follow-up is smaller in the surgical group; (3) If symptoms recur, they do not usually reach the preoperative level of severity in surgically treated patients as they do in medically treated patients; (4) In contrast to the findings in medically treated patients, beneficial effects on exercise hemodynamics and exercise capacity less often alleviate but rather persist and intensify during long-term follow-up in surgically treated patients. In summary, despite the limited number of patients, in agreement with other authors (3, 34, 52) these findings suggest that surgery alters the course of HOCM more dramatically than medical treatment.

Clinical implications

Although the symptomatic and hemodynamic response to medical therapy with propranolol or verapamil may individually vary in patients with hypertrophic cardiomyopathy, verapamil appears on average to be superior to propranolol (and should therefore be preferred) with respect to changes in clinical symptoms and exercise capacity as well as in stroke volume, cardiac output, mean pulmonary artery pressure and arterio-venous oxygen difference during exercise. The beneficial effects of verapamil are independent of the site of intraventricular obstruction (subvalvular or midventricular), but seem to be better in both forms of HOCM than in HNCM. The most impressive improvements in HOCM with respect to symptoms and hemodynamics, however, are achieved with surgery. As far as long-term results are concerned, surgically treated patients experience more frequent, more substantial and, of utmost importance, more long-lasting benefits from therapy than do medically treated patients.

Summary: The therapeutic effectiveness of propranolol, verapamil and surgery (trans-aortal subvalvular myectomy) in hypertrophic cardiomyopathy was assessed in 100 patients with hypertrophic obstructive cardiomyopathy (HOCM) and 12 patients with hypertrophic non-obstructive cardiomyopathy (HNCM) by means of exercise tests with hemodynamic measurements. The effects of propranolol were assessed in 13 HOCM patients, of verapamil in 68 HOCM patients and 12 HNCM patients, and of surgery in 31 HOCM patients after a mean of 3 to 9 months. Of the 68 verapamil-treated patients, 23 were reexamined once more after a mean of 38 months. Ten of the 31 surgically treated patients were reexamined after a mean of 52 months.

In the studies performed within the first year of medical treatment or after surgery, verapamil was clinically and hemodynamically superior to propranolol, but not as effective as surgical treatment. Functional limitation according to the NYHA classification improved after propranolol in 31 % of the patients, after verapamil in 41 %, and after surgery in 94 % of the cases. Improvements by more than one NYHA class were observed exclusively after surgical treatment. Maximal exercise capacity was, on average, not changed after propranolol, but increased after verapamil and, more substantially, after surgery. These different responses to treatment could be attributed to hemodynamic changes, especially concerning heart rate, stroke volume, cardiac output, arterio-venous oxygen difference and pulmonary artery presssure. In the case of verapamil, the beneficial hemodynamic effects occured independently of the site of intraventricular obstruction in HOCM (subvalvular or midventricular), but seemed to be superior in HOCM as compared to HNCM.

The late reexaminations, an average of 38 months after beginning verapamil treatment and 52 months after surgery, demonstrated that the initial salutary clinical and hemodynamic effects of verapamil were not maintained during long-term follow-up in the majority of patients, whereas they persisted or even intensified during long-term observation after surgery.

References

1. Adelman AG, Wigle ED, Ranganathan N, Webb GD, Kidd BSL, Bigelow WG, Silver MD (1972) The clinical course in muscular subaortic stenosis: a retrospective and prospective study of 60 hemodynamically proved cases. Ann Intern Med 77: 515—524
2. Anderson DM, Raff GL, Ports TA, Brundage BH, Parmley WW, Chatterjee K (1984) Hypertrophic obstructive cardiomyopathy. Effects of acute and chronic verapamil treatment on left ventricular systolic and diastolic function. Br Heart J 51: 523—529
3. Beahrs MM, Tajik AJ, Seward JB, Giuliani ER, McGoon DC (1983) Hypertrophic obstructive cardiomyopathy: Ten- to 21-year follow-up after partial septal myectomy. Am J Cardiol 51: 1160—1166
4. Betocchi S, Bonow RO, Bacharach SL, Rosing DR, Maron BJ, Green MV (1986) Isovolumic relaxation period in hypertrophic cardiomyopathy: Assessment by radionuclide angiography. J Am Coll Cardiol 7: 74—81
5. Bigelow W, Trimble AS, Wigle ED, Adelman AG, Felderhof C (1974) The treatment of muscular subaortic stenosis. J Thorac Cardiovasc Surg 68: 384—391
6. Bonow RO (1985) Effects of calcium-channel blocking agents on left ventricular diastolic function in hypertrophic cardiomyopathy and in coronary artery disease. Am J Cardiol 55: 172B—178B
7. Bonow RO, Rosing DR, Bacharach SL, Green MV, Kent KM, Lipson LC, Maron BJ, Leon MB, Epstein SE (1981) Effects of verapamil on left ventricular systolic function and diastolic filling in patients with hypertrophic cardiomyopathy. Circulation 64: 787—796
8. Bonow RO, Rosing DR, Epstein SE (1983) The acute and chronic effects of verapamil on left ventricular function in patients with hypertrophic cardiomyopathy. Eur Heart J 4, Suppl F: 57—65

9. Borer JS, Bacharach SL, Green MV, Kent KM, Rosing DR, Seides SF, Morrow AG, Epstein SE (1979) Effect of septal myotomy and myectomy on left ventricular systolic function at rest and during exercise in patients with IHSS. Circulation 60, Suppl I: 82—87

10. Brock RC (1957) Functional obstruction of the left ventricle, Guys Hosp Rep 106: 221—238

11. Edwards RHT, Kristinsson A, Warrell DA, Goodwin JF (1970) Effects of propranolol on response to exercise in hypertrophic obstructive cardiomyopathy. Br Heart J 32: 219—225

12. Flamm MD, Harrison DC, Hancock EW (1968) Muscular subaortic stenosis. Prevention of outflow obstruction with propranolol. Circulation 38: 846—858

13. Frank MJ, Abdulla AM, Canedo MI, Saylors RE (1978) Long-term medical management of hypertrophic obstructive cardiomyopathy. Am J Cardiol 42: 993—1001

14. Frank MJ, Abdulla AM, Watkins LO, Prisant L, Stefadouros MA (1983) Long-term medical management of hypertrophic cardiomyopathy: usefulness of propranolol. Eur Heart J 4, Suppl F: 155—164

15. Haberer T, Hess OM, Jenni R, Krayenbühl HP (1983) Hypertrophe obstruktive Kardiomyopathie: Spontanverlauf im Vergleich zur Langzeittherapie mit Propranolol and Verapamil. Z Kardiol 72: 487—493

16. Hanrath P, Mathey DG, Kremer P, Sonntag F, Bleifeld W (1980) Effect of verapamil on left ventricular isovolumic relaxation time and regional left ventricular filling in hypertrophic cardiomyopathy. Am J Cardiol 45: 1258—1264

17. Hanrath P, Schlüter M, Sonntag F, Diemert J, Bleifeld W (1983) Influence of verapamil therapy on left ventricular performance at rest and during exercise in hypertrophic cardiomyopathy. Am J Cardiol 52: 544—548

18. Harrison DC, Braunwald E, Glick G, Mason DT, Chidsey CA, Ross J Jr (1964) Effects of beta adrenergic blockade on the circulation, with particular reference to observation in patients with hypertrophic subaortic stenosis. Circulation 29: 84—98

19. Hess OM, Grimm J, Krayenbuehl HP (1983) Diastolic function in hypertrophic cardiomyopathy: effects of propranolol and verapamil on diastolic stiffness. Eur Heart J 4, Suppl F: 47—56

20. Kaltenbach M, Hopf R (1985) Treatment of hypertrophic cardiomyopathy: relation to pathological mechanisms. J Mol Cell Cardiol 17: 59—68

21. Kaltenbach M, Hopf R, Kober G, Bussmann WD, Keller M, Petersen Y (1979) Treatment of hypertrophic obstructive cardiomyopathy with verapamil. Br Heart J 42: 35—42

22. Kober G, Schmidt-Moritz A, Hopf R, Kaltenbach M (1983) Long-term treatment of hypertrophic obstructive cardiomyopathy — usefulness of verapamil. Eur Heart J 4, Suppl F: 165—174

23. Kuhn H, Gietzen F, Mercier J, Lösse B, Köhler E, Schulte HD, Bircks W, Loogen F (1983) Untersuchungen zur Klinik, zum Verlauf und zur Prognose der hypertrophischen Kardiomyopathie. Z Kardiol 72: 83—98

24. Kuhn H, Loogen F (1978) Die Anwendung von Beta-Rezeptorenblockern bei hypertrophischer obstruktiver Kardiomyopathie (HOCM). Internist 19: 527—531

25. Kuhn H, Thelen U, Leuner C, Köhler E, Bluschke V (1980) Langzeitbehandlung der hypertrophischen nicht obstruktiven Kardiomyopathie (HNCM) mit Verapamil. Z Kardiol 69: 669—675

26. von der Lohe E, Müller-Haake C, von Essen R, Effert S, Messmer BJ (1984) Septumresektion bei hypertropher obstruktiver Kardiomyopathie: Langzeitergebnisse bei 33 Patienten. Dtsch med Wschr 109: 1749—1753

27. Loogen F, Kuhn H, Gietzen F, Lösse B, Schulte HD, Bircks W (1983) Clinical course and prognosis of patients with typical and atypical hypertrophic obstructive and with hypertrophic non-obstructive cardiomyopathy. Eur Heart J 4, Suppl F: 145—153

28. Loogen F, Kuhn H, Krelhaus W (1978) Natural history of hypertrophic obstructive cardiomyopathy. In: Kaltenbach M, Loogen F, Olsen EGJ (eds) Cardiomyopathy and Myocardial Biopsy. Springer-Verlag, Berlin-Heidelberg—New York, pp 286—299

29. Lösse B, Kuhn H, Krönert H, Rafflenbeul D, Kirschner P, Schulte HD, Loogen F (1980) Hämodynamische Auswirkungen konservativer und operativer Therapie bei hypertrophischer obstruktiver Kardiomyopathie. Z Kardiol 69: 470—477

30. Lösse B, Kuhn H, Loogen F (1982) Results of exercise testing in medically and surgically treated patients with hypertrophic cardiomyopathy. In: Kaltenbach M, Epstein SE (eds) Hypertrophic Cardiomyopathy; Springer-Verlag, Berlin—Heidelberg—New York, pp 251—260

31. Lösse B, Kuhn H, Loogen F (1982) Klinische und hämodynamische Effekte von Verapamil bei hypertrophischer obstruktiver Kardiomyopathie. Z Kardiol 71: 813—819
32. Lösse B, Kuhn H, Loogen F, Schulte HD (1983) Exercise performance in hypertrophic cardio-myopathies. Eur Heart J 4, Suppl F: 197—208
33. Lösse B, Loogen F, Schulte HD (1984) Frühe und späte hämodynamische Veränderungen nach operativer Therapie der hypertrophischen obstruktiven Kardiomyopathie. Z Kardiol 73: 654—662
34. Maron BJ, Merrill WH, Freier PA, Kent KM, Epstein SE, Morrow AG (1978) Long-term clinical course and symptomatic status of patients after operation for hypertrophic subaortic stenosis. Circulation 57: 1205—1213
35. Oakley CM (1971) Hypertrophic obstructive cardiomyopathy — patterns of progression. In: Wolstenholme GEW, O'Connor M (eds) Hypertrophic Obstructive Cardiomyopathy. Ciba Foundation Symposium; Churchill, London, pp 9—29
36. Oakley CM (1975) Surgical correction of ASH. Circulation 51: 951—952
37. Powell WJ Jr, Whiting RB, Dinsmore RE, Sanders CA (1973) Symptomatic prognosis in patients with hypertrophic subaortic stenosis (IHSS). Am J Med 55: 15—24
38. Redwood DR, Goldstein RE, Hirshfeld J, Borer JS, Morganroth J, Morrow AG, Epstein SE (1979) Exercise performance after septal myotomy and myectomy in patients with obstructive hypertrophic cardiomyopathy. Am J Cardiol 44: 215—220
39. Rosing DR, Condit JR, Maron BJ, Kent KM, Leon MB, Bonow RO, Lipson LC, Epstein SE (1981) Verapamil therapy: a new approach to the pharmacologic treatment of hypertrophic cardiomyopathy: III: Effects of long-term administration. Am J Cardiol 48: 545—553
40. Rosing DR, Kent KM, Borer JS, Seides SF, Maron BJ, Epstein SE (1979) Verapamil therapy: a new approach to the pharmacologic treatment of hypertrophic cardiomyopathy. I. Hemodynamic effects. Circulation 60: 1201—1207
41. Rosing DR, Kent KM, Maron BJ, Epstein SE (1979) Verapamil therapy: a new approach to the pharmacologic treatment of hypertrophic cardiomyopathy. II. Effects on exercise capacity and symptomatic status. Circulation 60: 1208—1213
42. Rothlin ME, Gobet D, Haberer T, Krayenbühl HP (1983) Surgical treatment versus medical treatment in hypertrophic obstructive cardiomyopathy. Eur Heart J 4, Suppl F: 215—223
43. Schmid P, Pavek P, Klein W (1979) Echokardiographische und hämodynamische Untersuchungen zur Beeinflussung der hypertrophischen obstruktiven Kardiomyopathie durch Verapamil. Z Kardiol 68: 89—92
44. Schulte HD, Bircks W, Körfer R, Kuhn H (1981) Surgical aspects of typical subaortic and atypical midventricular hypertrophic obstructive cardiomyopathy (HOCM). Thorac Cardiovasc Surg 29: 375—380
45. Shah PM, Adelman AG, Wigle ED, Gobel FL, Burchell HB, Hardarson T, Curiel R, De la Calzada C, Oakley CM, Goodwin JF (1974) The natural (and unnatural) history of hypertrophic obstructive cardiomyopathy. Circ Res 34/35, Suppl II: 179—195
46. Spicer RL, Rocchini AP, Crowley DC, Rosenthal A (1984) Chronic verapamil therapy in pediatric and young adult patients with hypertrophic cardiomyopathy. Am J Cardiol 53: 1614—1619
47. Stenson RE, Flamm MD Jr, Harrison DC, Hancock EW (1973) Hypertrophic subaortic stenosis: clinical and hemodynamic effects of long-term propranolol therapy. Am J Cardiol 31: 763—773
48. Swanton RH, Brooksby IAB, Jenkins BS, Webb-Peploe MM (1977) Hemodynamic studies of β blockade in hypertrophic obstructive cardiomyopathy. Eur J Cardiol 5/4: 327—341
49. Tajik AJ, Giuliani GR, Weidman WH, Brandenburg RD, McGoon DC (1974) Idiopathic hypertrophic subaortic stenosis. Long-term surgical follow-up. Am J Cardiol 34: 815—822
50. Teare RD (1958) Asymmetrical hypertrophy of the heart in young adults. BR Heart J 20: 1—8
51. Turina J, Jenni R, Krayenbuehl HP, Turina M, Rothlin M (1986) Echocardiographic findings late after myectomy in hypertrophic obstructive cadiomyopathy. Eur Heart J 7: 685—692
52. Wigle ED, Sasson Z, Handerson MA, Ruddy TD, Fulop J, Rakowski H, Williams WG (1985) Hypertrophic cardiomyopathy. The importance of the site and the extent of hypertrophy. A review. Progr Cardiovasc Dis 28: 1—8

Authors' address:
Prof. Dr. med. Benno Lösse, Medizinische Klinik und Poliklinik der Universität, Abteilung für Kardiologie, Pneumologie und Angiologie, Moorenstr. 5, D-4000 Düsseldorf, F.R.G.

Programmed electrical stimulation in patients with hypertrophic cardiomyopathy

K.-H. Kuck, K.-P. Kunze, M. Geiger, A. Costard, and M. Schlüter

Department of Cardiology, University Hospital Eppendorf, Hamburg, F.R.G.

Introduction

Sudden death is a well known complication of hypertrophic cardiomyopathy with or without obstruction (10, 12, 20). Nonsustained ventricular tachycardia detected by ambulatory electrocardiography has been associated with subsequent sudden death or cardiac arrest (21, 23, 25, 26), but it is a nonspecific finding in the disease.

Nonsustained ventricular tachycardia is often slow and asymptomatic and its presence does not provide a causal relationship between ventricular arrhythmias and symptomatic episodes. However, treatment to prevent sudden death is primarily based on findings of ambulatory monitoring. Programmed electrical stimulation has been used in the diagnosis and therapy of patients at risk for syncope or sudden death and a variety of underlying cardiac disorders (9, 22, 28). The use of this technique in patients with hypertrophic cardiomyopathy has been limited to a few reports on selected patients (2, 14, 29). Therefore, we initiated a prospective study in consecutive patients with hypertrophic cardiomyopathy who had either a history of cardiac arrest or syncope, or no history of documented or suspected symptomatic ventricular arrhythmias. All patients underwent programmed electrical stimulation. This report presents the stimulation results of all patients at the time of inclusion into the study.

Methods

The study group consisted of 54 consecutive patients with hypertrophic cardiomyopathy; three patients had a history of cardiac arrest (group A), eight patients had a history of syncope (group B), and 43 patients had no history of either documented or suspected ventricular arrhythmias (group C). In group A, two patients had ventricular fibrillation documented on the electrocardiogram, obtained at the time of cardiac arrest. In one patient cardiac arrest occurred during school sports; in the other patient, at rest. The remaining patient had documented rapid ventricular tachycardia (rate 300 bpm) at the time of cardiac arrest. In group B, syncopal attacks ranged from one to five episodes per patient. In none of these was the cause of syncope known. An electrocardiographic registration at the time of syncope was not available in any patient. In three patients syncope was exercise-related; in the other patients syncopal attacks occurred at rest as well as during exercise. In group C, all patients complained of dyspnea, angina or occasional episodes of palpitations.

All patients were off any medication for at least seven half-lives before inclusion into the study. M-mode and two-dimensional echocardiographic data were obtained in all but nine patients, in whom the ultrasonic imaging quality was inadequate. The criterion used for the echocardiographic diagnosis of hypertrophic cardiomyopathy was the demonstration of a non-dilated hypertrophic left ventricle in the absence of any other cardiac or systemic disease that itself was capable of producing left ventricular hypertrophy (8, 18). The distribution pattern of left ventricular hypertrophy was determined according to Maron et al. (19).

All patients underwent a standard hemodynamic study including right and left heart catheterization and coronary angiography. Only patients with normal coronary arteries were included in this study. After informed consent had been obtained, a complete electrophysiologic study was performed 1 to 4 days after the hemodynamic investigation. 6-F catheters were passed through both femoral veins and/or through the left brachial or subclavian vein and through the right femoral artery using the Seldinger technique, and were positioned in the heart under fluoroscopic guidance. Quadripolar catheters were placed high in the right atrium, coronary sinus, and right and left ventricles. A bipolar catheter or a hexapolar closely spaced electrode catheter (Mansfield Scientific Inc.) was placed across the tricuspid valve to record the His bundle electrogram. A Siemens 16-channel electrocardiographer was used for continuous display and recording of the endocardial electrograms and of three to six surface electrocardiograms. A stimulator (ERA-HIS, Biotronik GmbH, FRG) was used to deliver rectangular pulses of 1 ms in duration and a constant current of twice diastolic threshold.

Detailed information on the stimulation protocol used in our laboratory has been given previously (17). Atrial stimulation included right and left atrial stimulation (the latter via the coronary sinus) at three different cycle lengths (640, 510, 440 ms) with the single extrastimulus technique. Right atrium and coronary sinus were then paced at increasing rates up to the Wenckebach cycle length. Ventricular pacing was performed first from the right and then from the left ventricle, using the extrastimulus technique. A maximum of two extrastimuli were delivered during sinus rhythm and at the same basic cycle lenghts as during atrial stimulation. Finally, right ventricular stimulation was performed at increasing rates up to a minimal cycle length of 300 ms.

Definitions

Induced ventricular arrhythmias — Repetitive ventricular response: three to five consecutive ventricular beats; nonsustained ventricular tachycardia: more than five ventricular responses, terminating spontaneously in less than 30 s. Sustained ventricular tachycardia: that with a duration of more than 30 s, unless termination is forced earlier because of hemodynamic deterioration. Ventricular fibrillation: ventricular rhythm without identifiable QRS complexes in the surface leads. Ventricular tachycardias with a continuously changing QRS configuration were termed polymorphic; those with a uniform QRS complex were termed monomorphic. The endpoint of the study was either the initiation of a sustained ventricular tachycardia or ventricular fibrillation or the completion of the stimulation protocol.

Table 1. Clinical, electrocardiographic, echocardiographic and hemodynamic data of patients with hypertrophic cardiomyopathy.

Characteristics		Group A (n = 3)	Group B (n = 8)	Group C (n = 43)
Age		43±20 yrs	45±15 yrs	48±13 yrs
Sex male		1 pt	5 pts	26 pts
female		2 pts	3 pts	17 pts
Family history of SD		–	3 pts	12 pts
Electrocardiography				
rhythm	sinus	2 pts	8 pts	41 pts
	AFib	1 pt	–	2 pts
QRS morphology	normal	3 pts	2 pts	12 pts
	LVH	–	6 pts	27 pts
	LBBB	–	–	2 pts
	RBBB	–	–	–
	unspecific BBB	–	–	1 pt
	preexcitation	–	–	1 pt
QRS width		100±20 ms	95±12 ms	101±18 ms
Echocardiography				
VS thickness		26±2 mm	26±7	24±5 mm
VS/PW		3.1±1.3	2.1±0.8	2.0±0.6
		⌐— $p<0.005$ —⌐	⌐— NS —⌐	
		⌐———————— $p<0.005$ ————————⌐		
Distribution of LVH				
	I	–	1 pt	2 pts
	II	1 pt	1 pt	11 pts
Maron class	III	2 pts	5 pts	21 pts
	IV	–	–	1 pt
Hemodynamics				
LV no gradient		3 pts	3 pts	17 pts
gradient	rest	–	73±25 mmHg	82±39 mmHg
	provocable	–	108±49 mmHg	121±60 mmHg
RV no gradient		–	–	34 pts
gradient	rest	–	–	16±11 mmHg
Enddiast. pressure LV		14±2 mmHg	14±8 mmHg	15± 9 mmHg
	RV	4±2 mmHg	5±3 mmHg	4± 2 mmHg

AFib = atrial fibrillation; BBB = bundle branch block; LBBB = left bundle branch block; LVH = left ventricular hypertrophy; PW = posterior wall; RBBB = right bundle branch block; SD = sudden death; VS = ventricular septum; pt = patient

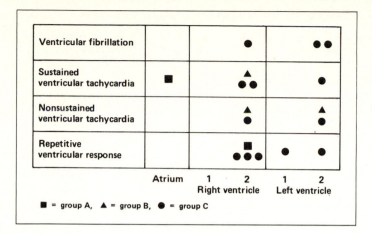

Fig. 1. Incidence of induced ventricular arrhythmias as a function of the stimulation mode in patients with hypertrophic cardiomyopathy. 1,2 = number of extrastimuli.

Statistical analysis

Data are expressed as means ± 1 standard deviation. Comparisons of sets of data were made using Student's *t*-test. Differences between distributions were analyzed by the chi-square test. A probability value of $p < 0.05$ was considered statistically significant.

Results

Clinical, electrocardiographic, echocardiographic and hemodynamic data of patient groups are summarized in Table 1. There were no statistically significant differences among patients of groups A, B and C, except for the echocardiographic ventricular septum/posterior free wall ratio, which was significantly greater in group A than in groups B and C.

Ventricular arrhythmias were induced in two patients from group A, in three from group B and in 13 from group C. The type and incidence of induced ventricular arrhythmias did not differ significantly between patients of groups A, B and C (Fig. 1).

The modes of initiation of ventricular tachycardia and fibrillation are shown in Table 2. Atrial stimulation induced a ventricular arrhythmia in only one group A patient, who had exercise-induced cardiac arrest. In this patient, right atrial stimulation at a cycle length of 250 ms led to induction of a rapid ventricular tachycardia (cycle length 180 ms), deteriorating into ventricular fibrillation. This patient's Wenckebach cycle length of 250 ms represented the lower limit of all recorded Wenckebach cycle lengths which ranged up to 450 ms. Mean Wenckebach cycle length was 275 ± 35 ms for group A, 333 ± 33 ms for group B and 320 ± 61 ms for group C. Because of the limited number of patients in group A, no statistical comparison with group B and C Wenckebach cycle lengths was made.

Inducibility of ventricular arrhythmia increased significantly by adding a second extrastimulus during right ventricular pacing and by left ventricular stimulation with two extrastimuli (Fig. 1). The coupling interval of the extrastimulus inducing ventricular arrhythmia was 206 ± 35 ms. This coupling interval was not statistically different from

Table 2. Mode of initiation of ventricular tachycardia and fibrillation and characteristics of ventricular tachycardia.

	pt.	Stimulation			Ventricular tachycardia		
		site	mode		CL	morphology	duration
Group A							
sus VT	H.A.	RA	At CL 250 ms during pacing at increasing rates		180	LBBB	VF after 8 s
Group							
n sus VT	B.G.	RV	BCL 510	S_2S_3 270/260	230	polymorphic	6 beats
	M.J.	LV	BCL 510	S_2S_3 230/190	250	polymorphic	10 beats
sus VT	S.B.	RV	BCL 510	S_2S_3 240/160	180	RBBB	VF after 4 s
Group C							
n sus VT	H.P.	LV	BCL 440	S_2S_3 260/230	220	BBB	9 beats
	J.L.	RV	BCL 510	S_2S_3 290/240	350	polymorphic	6 beats
sus VT	H.S.	LV	BCL 640	S_2S_3 260/180	180	polymorphic	VF after 8 s
	K.K.	RV	BCL 440	S_2S_3 220/190	220	polymorphic	VF after 12 s
	S.H.	RV	BCL 440	S_2S_3 250/220	210	polymorphic	VF after 6 s
VF	H.R.	RV	SR	S_1S_2 200/250			
	B.H.	LV	SR	S_1S_2 250/180			
	H.G.	LV	BCL 510	S_2S_3 250/170			

CL = cycle length; LBBB = left bundle branch block; LV = left ventricle; n sus VT = nonsustained ventricular tachycardia; RA = right atrium; RBBB = right bundle branch block; RV = right ventricle; sus VT = sustained ventricular tachycardia; VF = ventricular fibrillation.

the effective refractory periods during right and left ventricular pacing in patients without induced ventricular arrhythmias (Table 3).

Induced sustained ventricular arrhythmias were ventricular tachycardia in five patients and ventricular fibrillation in three. Sustained ventricular tachycardia was always rapid, with a mean cycles length of 194 ± 20 ms. Ventricular tachycardia always deteriorated into ventricular fibrillation after 8 ± 3 s and required DC countershock for termination.

Patients of group A, B and C in whom sustained ventricular arrhythmias were induced did not differ in electrocardiographic, echocardiographic or hemodynamic data from patients without induced ventricular arrhythmias.

Discussion

Several mechanisms may be responsible for sudden death in patients with hypertrophic cardiomyopathy. Sudden increase of the intraventricular pressure gradient in patients with left ventricular outflow obstruction, supraventricular arrhythmias with or without accessory atrioventricular pathways (3, 15, 29), bradyarrhythmias (13) and complete

Table 3. Right and left ventricular effective refractory periods (ms).

Site	BCL	No. of ES	Group A (n = 3)	Group B (n = 8)	Group C (n = 43)
Right ventricle	640	1	260±15	250±34	264±27
	510	1	247±18	248±39	246±25
	440	1	236±15	225±24	230±22
	640	2	225±40	196±34	210±26
	510	2	210±19	183±31	193±26
	440	2	205±25	178±30	187±25
Left ventricle	640	1	240±13	263±17	263±21
	510	1	230±12	238±31	246±19
	440	1	220±12	234±34	236±25
	640	2	192±14	240±28	209±29
	510	2	195±14	207±66	199±29
	440	2	190±12	210±57	193±28

BCL = basic cycle length; ES = extrastimuli

heart block (7) have been reported. A prominent factor possibly related to sudden death is the occurrence of ventricular tachyarrhythmias which, in a high number of patients, are detected during long-term electrocardiographic monitoring (23, 25, 26). Some authors have been able to show a close relationship between the occurrence of more than two consecutive premature beats during Holter monitoring and subsequent sudden death (21, 25). However, nonsustained ventricular tachycardia on Holter monitoring is almost always slow and asymptomatic, and therefore the presence of these nonsustained arrhythmias does not establish a causal relationship between arrhythmias and symptomatic episodes. More likely they seem to be only a marker for subsequent fatal events. Other variables, in addition to nonsustained slow ventricular tachycardia, or other arrhythmias, may be responsible for the induction of a terminal event (24).

The inducibility of ventricular tachyarrhythmias by programmed electrical stimulation has been suggested to predict potential sudden death in patients after acute myocardial infarction without previously documented ventricular arrhythmias (11, 27). Few studies on the use of the technique in selected patients with hypertrophic cardiomyopathy have been reported (2, 14, 29). Following reports on the fatal outcome of electrophysiologic studies in patients with hypertrophic cardiomyopathy (15, 30), we were well aware of the potential hazard of this approach, but, because of the limited specificity of ambulatory ECG monitoring and the lack of any other technique to identify patients at risk of sudden cardiac death, we felt that there was the need for such an investigation.

Anderson et al. (2) have reported programmed electrical stimulation of the right ventricle in patients with obstructive hypertrophic cardiomyopathy undergoing myotomy or myectomy, who were studied in the operating room under general anesthesia and under their chronic medication. The stimulation protocol included right ventricular pacing with a maximum of three extrastimuli. Under these conditions, ventricular arrhythmias could be induced in all 17 patients, with ventricular fibrillation in five patients, sustained ventricular tachycardia in nine patients, nonsustained ventricular tachycardia in one patient, and repetitive ventricular response in two patients. In three of the 14 patients with ventricular fibrillation or sustained ventricular tachycardia, the arrhythmias were induced by two extrastimuli, while three extrastimuli had to be applied in the remaining 11 patients. However, the prognostic value to the inducibility of ventricular arrhythmias by three ventricular extrastimuli is not definitely known, and it has been shown that severe ventricular arrhythmias can be induced by more than two extrastimuli, even in normal patients without previously documented ventricular arrhythmias (5).

The same limitations hold for a recent study in seven symptomatic patients, with cardiac arrest in three patients, syncope in one and presyncope in two (14). Induced arrhythmias were ventricular fibrillation in one patient, ventricular tachycardia in three and supraventricular tachycardia in two. Follow-up of these patients was uneventful under a medical therapy guided by electrophysiologic testing. The authors suggested that electrophysiologic investigation may be useful to identify the cause of symptoms in patients with hypertrophic cardiomyopathy and to select prophylactic therapy. However, since no "asymptomatic" patients with hypertrophic cardiomyopathy were included, the specificity of their findings is unknown — particularly with a stimulation protocol which included a maximum of three extrastimuli.

In our investigation, 54 consecutive patients with both obstructive and non-obstructive hypertrophic cardiomyopathy were studied. No patient was under therapy, and the stimulation protocol was limited to two ventricular extrastimuli. The study population included three different groups of patients. Firstly, patients with a history of cardiac arrest due to ventricular arrhythmias; secondly, patients with a history of syncope without documented arrhythmias at the time of syncope and, thirdly, patients without documented or suspectd sustained ventricular arrhythmias. The incidence and type of induced ventricular arrhythmias did not differ among those patients.

Interestingly, sustained ventricular arrhythmia always consisted of a rapid ventricular tachycardia or ventricular fibrillation. A slow ventricular tachycardia was never induced.

Induction of a rapid ventricular tachycardia with ventricular fibrillation has been shown to be nonspecific in patients with coronary artery disease and myocardial infarction (16). The fact that these types of arrhythmia were induced in "asymptomatic" and "symptomatic" patients with hypertrophic cardiomyopathy may also indicate the nonspecificity of the induction of these arrhythmias by programmed stimulation. In one patient, cardiac arrest, caused by exercise-induced ventricular fibrillation, was the first documented sign of hypertrophic cardiomyopathy. It is well known that syncope or cardiac arrest may be the first manifestation of the disease (20). Rapid ventricular tachycardia deteriorating into ventricular fibrillation had been induced in this patient by pacing the right atrium at increasing rates. The inducibility of rapid ventricular tachycardia or ventricular fibrillation by atrial pacing is a very rare finding in patients without an accessory pathway. It has been described in another two patients with hypertrophic cardiomyopathy (29, 31), and this finding is possibly specific to patients with hypertrophic cardiomyopathy.

Repetitive ventricular response or nonsustained ventricular tachycardia was induced in ten patients. The prognostic value of the inducibility of these types of arrhythmia in normal patients without documented ventricular arrhythmias is low (1, 5), they may be predictive of the spontaneous occurrence of severe ventricular arrhythmias in patients with coronary artery disease (4). The significance of their occurrence in the setting of hypertrophic cardiomyopathy is uncertain.

The vulnerability of patients with cardiac arrest or of patients with non-documented ventricular tachycardia to the induction of ventricular arrhythmias from the left ventricle is not known. In patients with coronary artery disease, it has been shown that the sensitivity to inducing ventricular arrhythmias is higher for a protocol including left ventricular stimulation than for one restricted to right ventricular stimulation (6). In our study, all patients, symptomatic or asymptomatic, underwent left ventricular stimulation when no sustained arrhythmias were induced from the right ventricle. Left ventricular stimulation was deliberately included into our protocol on purpose, because hypertrophic cardiomyopathy is primarily a disease of the left ventricle. However, the sensitivity and specificity of left ventricular stimulation in this setting must be assessed in long-term follow-up studies.

We conclude that programmed electrical stimulation with a maximum of two ventricular extrastimuli in patients with hypertrophic cardiomyopathy cannot distinguish between patients with cardiac arrest or syncope and "asymptomatic" patients. The induction of a rapid ventricular tachycardia by atrial stimulation in the absence of an accessory atrioventricular connection may be a specific finding to identify patients at risk of exercise-induced ventricular fibrillation.

Summary: Programmed electrical stimulation was performed in 54 consecutive patients with hypertrophic cardiomyopathy. Three patients had a history of cardiac arrest due to ventricular tachyarrhythmias (group A), eight patients had a history of syncope of unknown origin (group B), and 43 patients were „asymptomatic", i.e. they had no documented or suspected symptomatic ventricular arrhythmias (group C). There were no differences among the groups with respect to electrocardiographic, echocardiographic or hemodynamic data. Ventricular arrhythmias were induced by atrial and right and left ventricular stimulation with a maximum of two extrastimuli in 18 patients. Induced arrhythmias were repetitive ventricular response in six patients, nonsustained ventricular tachycardia in four, sustained ventricular tachycardia in five, and ventricular fibrillation in three patients. Ventricular tachycardia was always rapid with a mean cycle length of 194 ± 20 ms. In one group A patient, rapid ventricular tachycardia was induced during atrial stimulation. The type and incidence of induced ventricular arrhythmias did not differ among the three groups. It is concluded that programmed stimulation with a maximum of two ventricular extrastimuli cannot distinguish between patients with hypertrophic cardiomyopathy who had either cardiac arrest or syncope or were "asymptomatic".

References

1. Akhtar M (1981) The clinical significance of the repetitive ventricular response. Circulation 63: 773—775
2. Anderson KP, Stinson EB, Derby GC, Oyer PE, Mason JW (1983) Vulnerability of patients with obstructive hypertrophic cardiomyopathy to ventricular arrhythmia induction in the operating room. Am J Cardiol 51: 811—816

3. Bonhour JB, Bory M, Bourmayan C, Chiffoleau S, Favereau X, Foussard C, Komajda M, Lassabe G, Morand Ph, Neiman JL (1974) Tachycardie supraventriculaires au cours des myocardiopathies obstructives. Arch Mal Coeur 74: 993—999
4. Breithardt G, Seipel L, Meyer T, Abendroth RR (1982) Prognostic significance of repetitive ventricular response during programmed ventricular stimulation. Am J Cardiol 49: 693—698
5. Brugada P, Abdollah H, Heddle B, Wellens HJJ (1983) Results of a ventricular stimulation protocol using a maximum of 4 premature stimuli in patients without documented or suspected ventricular arrhythmias. Am J Cardiol 52: 1214—1218
6. Buxton AE, Waxman HL, Marchlinski FE, Unterecker WJ, Waspe LE, Josephson ME (1984) Study of patients with documented sustained ventricular tachyarrhythmias. Circulation 69: 532—540
7. Chmielewski CA, Riley RS, Mahendran A, Most AS (1977) Complete heart block as a cause of syncope in asymmetric septal hypertrophy. Am Heart J 93: 91—93
8. DeMaria A, Bommer W, Lee G, Mason DT (1980) Value and limitations of 2-dimensional echocardiography in assessment of cardiomyopathy. Am J Cardiol 46: 1224—1231
9. DiMarco JP, Garan H, Harthorne JW, Ruskin JW (1981) Intracardiac electrophysiologic techniques in recurrent syncope of unknown cause. Ann Intern Med 95: 542—548
10. Frank S, Braunwald E (1968) Idiopathic hypertrophic subaortic stenosis. Clinical analysis of 126 patients with emphasis of the natural history. Circulation 37: 759—788
11. Hamer A, Vohra J, Hunt D, Sloman G (1982) Prediction of sudden death by electrophysiologic studies in high risk patients surviving acute myocardial infarction. Am J Cardiol 50: 223—229
12. Hardarson T, de la Calzada CS, Curiel R, Goodwin JF (1973) Prognosis and mortality of hypertrophic obstructive cardiomyopathy. Lancet 2: 1462—1467
13. Joseph S, Balcon R, McDonald L (1972) Syncope in hypertrophic obstructive cardiomyopathy due to asystole. Br Heart J 34: 974—976
14. Kowey PR, Eisenberg R, Engel TR (1984) Sustained arrhythmias in hypertrophic obstructive cardiomyopathy. N Engl J Med 310: 1566—1569
15. Krikler DM, Davies MJ, Fowland E, Goodwin JF, Evans RC, Shaw DB (1980) Sudden death in hypertrophic cardiomyopathy: associated accessory atrioventricular pathways. Br Heart J 43: 245—251
16. Kuck KH, Costard A, Schlüter M, Kunze KP (1986) Significance of timing programmed electrical stimulation after acute myocardial infarction. J Am Coll Cardiol 8: 1279—1288
17. Kunze KP, Kuck KH, Schlüter M, Kuch B, Bleifeld W (1984) Electrophysiologic and clinical effects of intravenous and oral encainide in accessory atrioventricular pathway. Am J Cardiol 54: 323—329
18. Maron BJ, Epstein SE (1979) Hypertrophic cardiomyopathy: a discussion of nomenclature. Am J Cardiol 43: 1242—1244
19. Maron BJ, Gottdiener JS, Epstein SE (1981) Patterns and significance of distribution of left ventricular hypertrophy in hypertrophic cardiomyopathy. Am J Cardiol 48: 418—428
20. Maron BJ, Roberts WC, Edwards JE, McAllister HA, Foley DD, Epstein SE (1978) Sudden death in patients with hypertrophic cardiomyopathy; characterization of 26 patients without functional limitation. Am J Cardiol 41: 803—810
21. Maron BJ, Savage DD, Wolfgang JK, Epstein SE (1981) The prognostic significance of 24 hour ambulatory electrocardiographic monitoring in patients with hypertrophic cardiomyopathy: a prospective study. Am J Cardiol 48: 252—257
22. Mason JW, Winkle RA (1980) Accuracy of the ventricular tachycardia induction study for predicting long-term efficacy and inefficacy of antiarrhythmic drugs. N Engl J Med 303: 1073—1077
23. Mc Kenna WJ, Chetty S, Oakley CM, Goodwin JF (1980) Arrhythmia in hypertrophic cardiomyopathy: exercise and 48 hour ambulatory electrocardiographic assessment with and without adrenergic blocking therapy. Am J Cardiol 45: 1—5
24. Mc Kenna WJ, Goodwin JF (1981) The natural history of hypertrophic cardiomyopathy. Curr Prog Cardiol 6: 1—25
25. Mc Kenna WJ, England D, Doi YL, Deanfield JE, Oakley C, Goodwin JF (1981) Arrhythmia in hypertrophic cardiomyopathy. I. Influence on prognosis. Br Heart J 46: 168—172

26. Mc Kenna WJ, England D, Oakley C, Goodwin J (1980) Detection of arrhythmia in hypertrophic cardiomyopathy: prospective study. Circulation 62 (Suppl III): 187 (Abstract)
27. Richards DA, Cody DV, Denniss AR, Russel AP, Young AA, Uther JE (1983) Ventricular electrical instability: a predictor of death after myocardial infarction. Am J Cardiol 51: 75—80
28. Ruskin JN, DiMarco JP, Garan H (1980) Out of hospital cardiac arrest: electrophysiologic observations and selection of long-term antiarrhythmia therapy. N Engl J Med 303: 607—613
29. Stafford WJ, Trohman RG, Bilsker M, Zaman J, Castellanos A, Myerburg RJ (1986) Cardiac arrest in an adolescent with atrial fibrillation and hypertrophic cardiomyopathy. J Am Coll Cardiol 7: 701—704
30. Wellens JHH, Bär FW, Vanagt EJ (1980) Death after ajmaline administration. Am J Cardiol 45: 905 (Letter)
31. Wellens HJJ, Bär FWHM, Vanagt EJDM, Brugada P (1982) Medical treatment of ventricular tachycardia: considerations in the selection of patients for surgical treatment. Am J Cardiol 49: 186—193

Authors' address:
Karl-Heinz Kuck, M.D., Department of Cardiology, University Hospital Eppendorf, Martinistr. 52, 2000 Hamburg 20, F.R.G.

10-year results and survival of patients with hypertrophic cardiomyopathy treated with calcium antagonists

R. Hopf and M. Kaltenbach

Zentrum der Inneren Medizin, Klinikum der J.-W. Goethe-Universität, Frankfurt/Main, F.R.G.

Introduction

To date, the etiology of hypertrophic cardiomyopathy remains unclear. In consequence, no causal therapy is available. The only approach is treatment of symptoms, aiming to reduce or relieve complaints, minimizing disease progression, thereby reducing the high annual mortality rate of about 3.5%. The hemodynamic characteristics of the disease offer the possibility of a therapeutic approach.

The longest known features of hypertrophic cardiomyopathy are most often normal or even super-normal contractility at rest with concomitant reduced contractility reserve and an intraventricular pressure gradient in the obstructive form of the disease. Regarding the specific features of systolic ventricular function, it is logical to introduce beta-blocker treatment with sympathicolytic activity. Following acute administration, impressive changes in systolic ventricular dynamics can be confirmed. However, longterm results have been disappointing (2, 4, 6, 7, 15, 20, 31, 33). The most important feature of hypertrophic cardiomyopathy is the impaired diastolic ventricular filling behavior due to the hypertrophic and thus "stiffer" myocardium (3, 7, 9, 18, 22).

In 1976 we reported preliminarily favourable results achieved through calcium antagonist treatment in patients suffering from hypertrophic cardiomyopathy (10, 13). These encouraging findings have been confirmed by numerous other authors (15, 25, 26, 27, 30). An improvement in diastolic ventricular filling behavior was postulated as the reason for the positive therapeutic results obtained by calcium antagonists (1, 3, 9, 18, 26, 29, 30).

This report deals with long-term calcium antagonist treatment in patients with hypertrophic cardiomyopathy. Some patients have been followed up for more than 10 years.

Patients and methods

Patients

The results presented here are based on the course of the disease in 84 patients treated with oral doses of calcium antagonists following confirmation of the diagnosis by echocardiogram and heart catheterization. The patient group consisted of 20 women and 64 men, aged from 12 to 64 years at the onset of therapy.

23 patients displayed hypertrophic, non-obstructive cardiomyopathy with left ventricular outflow tract gradients not exceeding 30 mm Hg. The other 61 patients displayed the obstructive form. In 22 of them, there was no gradient at rest; in the others, gradients ranged between 12 and 125 mm Hg (mean: 57 mm Hg). Following provocation, the highest left ventricular pressure gradients in patients with obstructive cardiomyopathy ranged from 32 to 290 mm Hg (mean, 100 mm Hg). Additionally, 18 patients exhibited right ventricular pressure gradients of at least 14 mm Hg, ranging from 10 to 27 mm Hg. Left ventricular filling pressure for all patients was between 5 and 48 mm Hg (mean, 20 mm Hg).

Therapy

None of the 84 patients was excluded from the therapy-study because of disease severity. Premedication (most often beta-blockers) was discontinued in all patients for at least 2 weeks prior to treatment with calcium antagonists. Fifty-six patients were treated with a daily dose of 320 to 640 mg orally administered verapamil. The mean dose was 515 mg. 27 patients, 15 of whom had also received verapamil previously, were treated with a daily oral dose of 75 to 250 mg (mean 158 mg) gallopamil. One female patient received nifedipine, 30 mg daily. The duration of treatment for the total patient group was 40 to 133 months (mean 52 months). Thus, these results are based on a total of 362 patient treatment years. Of the total of 84 patients, 35 were treated with calcium antagonists for more than 5 years.

Additional treatment

Due to edema or persistent pulmonary congestion, it was necessary to initiate a concomitant saluretic therapy in 12 cases. In 8 patients, antiarrhythmic medications were prescribed due to confirmed rhythm disturbances. Because of anamnestically established thromboembolism or intermittent atrial fibrillation, four patients were treated with salicylates or anticoagulants. One patient, suffering from tachyarrhythmia, received digitalis medication after not responding to other therapy.

Follow-up investigations

After the onset of calcium antagonistic treatment, the patients underwent follow-up investigations at regular intervals — if possible — during the first 3 months, then at 6- to 12-month intervals. The follow-up investigations included an ECG, carotid pulse tracing, echocardiogram, chest X-ray and radiologic assessment of the heart volume.

31 patients underwent follow-up angiography after 8 to 55 months of treatment (mean 31 months). Of these patients, 25 demonstrated obstructive and six nonobstructive hypertrophic cardiomyopathy. The aim was to check the hemodynamic effects of long-term treatment.

One patient was scheduled for surgery, another died while on the waiting list.

One female patient died during verapamil therapy before follow-up data could be obtained. For assessment of prognosis during treatment with calcium antagonists, however, this patient is included when considering causes of death.

Documentation

The same instrument was used for all ECG monitoring in each patient. It was calibrated exactly and no filter was used. The Sokolow-index was calculated from the maximal R and S amplitudes in the precordial Wilson leads and used to evaluate the course of the disease.

The heart size was calculated from two heart volume X-ray determinations in the supine or sitting position with the legs positioned at the same height as the atria (15). For better comparison the heart size was calculated for the mean body surface area of 1.73 m² (relative heart volume). Heart volume assessment was performed additionally to the conventional chest X-ray in the standing position.

Echocardiographic follow-up investigations were only performed in a subgroup of patients, since the technique was introduced in 1976. Before 1976, one patient group had already been treated 1 or 2 years. In addition, echocardiographic measurements could not be obtained for all patients, due to technical or anatomic difficulties. The patients underwent m-mode as well as 2-dimensional echocardiography. Interventricular septum and posterior wall measurements were assessed in the area of pronounced width and evaluated by an observer, who was unaware of treatment status.

To reduce variability caused by technical and individual factors (range for repeated investigations in the same patient within 1 week: for echo-measurements 2 mm, for ECG 0.4 mV and for heart volume about 7%), individual findings were assessed as follows: for each patient the mean values for all data acquired during calcium antagonist therapy (ECG, heart volume, echocardiograms) were calculated and compared with individual initial values. The mean values for each of the initial findings and the data following therapy were also assessed. Student's t-test for paired data was employed for statistical evaluation. The statistical borderline for significance was set at $2\,p < 0.05$.

Results

Subjective complaints

Prior to therapy with calcium antagonists, the patients complained of typical symptoms, particularly dyspnea and angina pectoris. Only ten patients were symptom-free. Sixty-two out of 74 previously symptomatic patients reported improvement or complete relief of symptoms during therapy; i.e. a subjective improvement in 84%. In 19 patients there was no change. This group, however, comprised nine of those ten patients with previously unimpaired physical stress tolerance. In one initially asymptomatic patient, physical stress tolerance slightly decreased, and syncope was suffered for the first time. In another patient symptoms and stress tolerance deteriorated.

The improvement of pre-existing exertional dyspnea or angina pectoris was most impressive when compared with the other symptoms. Most patients, previously complaining of signs of collapse or syncope reported that symptoms improved or even disappeared with therapy (Table 1). According to the New York Heart Association (NYHA) classification an improvement of functional class from a mean of 2.6 to 1.9 was achieved, taking the 84 patients into account (Fig. 1). No patient showed initial improvement but renewed deterioration during longterm treatment.

Table 1. Symptoms in 84 patients with hypertrophic cardiomyopathy prior to calcium antagonist therapy and changes of symptoms during treatment.

before	n =	during therapy with calciumantagonists				
		disappeared	improved	unchanged	worsened	new appeared
dyspnea	48	3	25	18	2	
angina pectoris	46	3	28	12	3	
syncope/collapse arrhythmias	14	9	3	2		2
palpitations	19	7	4	5	3	2
vertigo	10	1	7	1	1	
weakness	11	3	5	3	1	
diaphoresis	7	1	3	2		
edema	7			7	1	5
no complaints	10			9	1	
embolism	3					
mitral stenosis	1					
myocardial infarction	1					

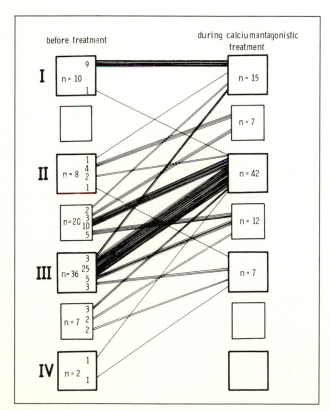

Fig. 1. Clinical course of 84 patients with hypertrophic cardiomyopathy during treatment with calcium antagonists according to NYHA classification (one patient died prior to the 1st follow-up investigation).

Electrocardiography

Repeat electrocardiograms were available for 61 patients prior to the onset of therapy with calcium antagonists. The observation-period ranged from 3 to 33 months (mean: 24 months). The majority of these patients had been receiving high dose beta-blockers. The Sokolow-index was 4.78 before and 4.85 mV (N.S.) during therapy, and despite it. The course during calcium antagonist treatment was electrocardiographically documented in 82 patients. 42 patients showed a decrease in the Sokolow-index, 27 showed no change (less than 5%) and nine showed an increase. The mean Sokolow-index significantly decreased from 5.0 to 4.5 mV in the total patient population ($2p < 0.001$). In patients showing improvement, the reduction in the Sokolow-index could generally be observed during the first 2 years of treatment. This was evident when comparing the initial findings for each patient with the data recorded in a subgroup of 69 patients during the 18th to 24th month of treatment. During this period, the therapeutic effect occurred. Further treatment showed no renewed increase in the Sokolow-index in these patients, as results from 56 patients treated for a longer period show (Fig. 2). Repolarization-disturbances were not quantitatively evaluated, but generally receded parallel to the reduction in QRS amplitude. In some cases the ECG tracing returned to normal values, when evaluated according to the Sokolow-index and repolarization disturbances.

Conventional chest X-ray findings and radiologic heart volume determination

The cardiac configuration as well as cardiac size, evaluated by conventional chest X-rays in the standing position, remained unchanged during calcium antagonist treatment. There was no case of newly developed pulmonary congestion and no increase in pre-existing pulmonary congestion in any patient.

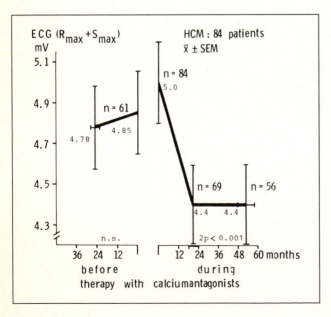

Fig. 2. Changes in Sokolow-index (calculated from the largest R and S amplitudes in the precordial leads).

Heart size was carefully documented using repeated heart volume measurements. The course of the disease prior to the onset of therapy with calcium antagonists was documented in 40 patients. The mean observation period was 24 months, and the mean heart volume of these patients increased significantly during this period (from a mean of 904 to 980 ml/1.73 m² body surface area) even though the patients were treated with highly dosed beta-blockers ($2p < 0.001$). During the course of calcium antagonist treatment, complete radiologic findings were available for 82 patients. Heart volume decreased in 39 cases, remained unchanged in 34 patients (change of less than 5%) and increased in nine patients. The mean heart volume of the total group of 82 patients significantly decreased from 947 to 895 ml/1.73 m² body surface area ($2p < 0.001$). Analogous to the ECG findings, improvement was seen within the first 2 years of treatment (Fig. 3). In 66 patients who underwent follow-up investigations 18 to 24 months after the start of therapy, the heart volume decreased from 947 to 871 ml/1.73 m² body surface area. The initial decrease in heart size was not followed by a renewed increase in any patient.

The comparison between left ventricular enddiastolic pressure and changes in heart volume — as observed under therapy — clearly showed that heart volume decreased independent of the level of filling pressure (Fig. 4).

Echocardiographic findings

Typical for hypertrophic cardiomyopathy, the patients exhibited normal or small left ventricular diameters. There was neither a clear systolic nor diastolic increase in left ventricular diameter during treatment with calcium antagonists. The left atrial diameter was increased in 80% of the patients.

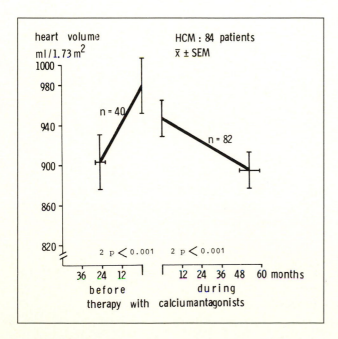

Fig. 3. Changes of X-ray-assessed heart volume.

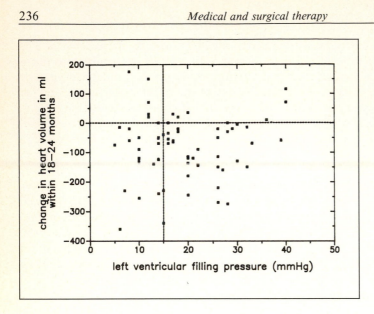

Fig. 4. Changes in X-ray-assessed heart volume during therapy with calcium antagonists. Patients with high left ventricular enddiastolic pressure usually showed the same amount of decrease in heart size.

Prior to the onset of calcium antagonist therapy, follow-up investigations (mean duration 40 months) could be documented in a subgroup of 15 patients. During that time these patients had been exclusively treated with beta-blockers and showed a tendency towards an increase in the left atrial diameter from 4.23 to 4.42 cm during the observation period as well as a non-significant increase of septal thickness from 2.39 to 2.53 cm and of the posteroir wall from 1.5 to 1.53 cm (N.S.). During therapy with calcium

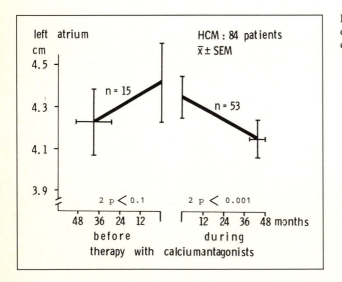

Fig. 5. Changes in echocardiographically-assessed left atrial diameter.

antagonists the mean left atrial diameter decreased significantly from 4.35 to 4.15 ($2p < 0.001$) in a total of 53 patients. Again, the decrease was established, predominantly within the first 18 to 24 months. No definite repeat increase in diameter was noticed during the following course of treatment (Fig. 5). Left ventricular wall thickness remained nearly unchanged: intraventricular septal thickness 2.4 vs. 2.24 and the posterior wall 1.43 vs. 1.35 cm, changes not being significant (Fig. 6).

Results of follow-up heart catheterization

In 32 patients a second heart catheterization was performed after a mean treatment period of 31 months, to evaluate whether hemodynamic parameters had been influenced by the calcium antagonist treatment. Clinical improvement was seen in 15 patients, in another there was no therapeutic effect and two patients presented with clinical worsening. The mean pressure gradient at rest decreased nonsignificantly in 25 patients with the obstructive form of hypertrophic cardiomyopathy, from 40 to 29 mm Hg and the maximum gradient following provocation from 109 to 76 mm Hg ($2p < 0.005$).

The mean of all 32 patients showed an unchanged enddiastolic left ventricular pressure (19.6 vs. 19.1 mm Hg).

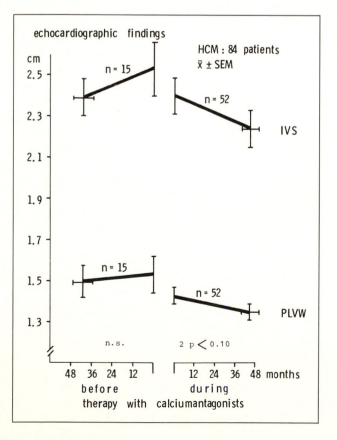

Fig. 6. Changes in echocardiographically-assessed wall thickness of the left ventricle (IVS: interventricular septal wall; PLVW: left ventricular posterior wall).

Side effects

Only one patient treated with 480 mg verapamil per day exhibited a first degree AV-block (PR-interval 0.30 s). A reduction of the dosage to 320 mg led to normalization of the atrioventricular conduction. Seven patients had pre-existing edema of the legs and five patients developed edema during calcium antagonistic therapy. In these 12 cases, additional therapy with diuretics was initiated. Heart failure did not occur in any of the 84 patients. Three patients presented with pre-existing episodes of acute pulmonary congestion, which subsided during therapy. In these cases, 10 mg of sublingual nifedipine was effective within a few minutes, and the efficacy was intensified when oral furosemide was given additionally. Several patients exhibited radiological signs of pre-existing pulmonary congestion, but no new incidence arose during therapy. Some patients complained of diaphoresis, headaches and dizziness following therapy. Typically for this treatment, after several weeks or months of continued therapy these symptoms disappeared. Patients frequently complained of obstipation. In some, it became necessary to prescribe laxatives.

Deaths

Nine patients died during the 4 to 133 months of calcium antagonist therapy. Eight of them had been treated with verapamil, one was the only patient treated with nifedipine. Six deaths were caused by hypertrophic myocardial disease. In four cases, typical sudden death occurred, following 16, 22, 53, and 55 months of therapy. In another patient, treated with verapamil for 113 months, sudden death could not be confirmed with certainty, but is likely. One patient, suffering from hypertrophic non-obstructive cardiomyopathy, died after 47 months of therapy with protracted cardiogenic shock. The histologic investigation in this case showed extensive disseminated fibrosis of the myocardium. Three other patients died from other causes: one patient of a cerebral vascular process (duration of therapy: 24 months). A further patient died of cardiac forward failure due to a concomitant high-grade mitral stenosis for which she did not agree to cardiac surgery, she had received therapy for 54 months; and one patient died several weeks after a traffic accident due to a shock lung. It cannot be ruled out that despite 37 months of therapy with verapamil a syncope had led to this accident.

Thus the mean annual mortality rate, based on 362 patient-treatment-years, for all patients, was 2.5% and 1.7% for those patients who died definitely due to hypertrophic cardiomyopathy. Calculating the survival probability (test of Kaplan and Meier), any given patient with hypertrophic cardiomyopathy at the onset of verapamil treatment, gives an individual 10-year survival probability greater than 82% (Fig. 7).

Discussion

The clinical picture and course of the disease in the patient with hypertrophic cardiomyopathy are unpredictable. Symptom-free patients with unimpaired stress tolerance may have a normal life expectance or die of sudden cardiac death. On the other hand, the disease is not necessarily continuously progressive in symptomatic patients. Standstills of longer duration are not unusual. Therefore, the decision to initiate therapy must

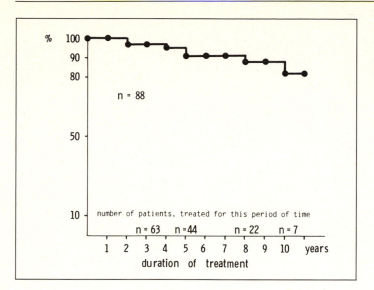

Fig. 7. 10-year survival probability of patients with hypertrophic cardiomyopathy treated with calcium antagonists, calculated by the Kaplan and Meier test.

take into consideration the symptomatic aspect, as well as a possible improvement in prognosis.

Regarding these demands, beta-blockers did not fulfill expectations. Initial improvement of findings in many patients could not be confirmed by long-term studies (13, 16). Potentially life threatening rhythm disturbances still occurred (6), despite subjective improvement in symptoms under high doses of beta-blockers. Thus, it is not surprising that the annual mortality rate of about 3.5% could not be reduced by beta-blocker therapy (8, 13).

Beta-blockers exert an impressive effect on the sympathicotonically modulated systolic ventricular function (32, 33) which is altered in HCM patients due to dynamic obstruction (12, 20). However, an acute drop (33) in filling pressure or a reduction after long-term oral treatment (2, 33) can only be observed in some patients. The impaired systolic ventricular dynamics seem to be of minor importance, since the emptying of the ventricles is completed earlier than in healthy individuals (22). This hypothesis, however, is still under discussion (12). Impaired diastolic relaxation and filling may be the more important hemodynamic characteristics in hypertrophic cardiomyopathy and thus are discussed with regard to the incidence of sudden death (22). According to our experience, calcium antagonists, especially verapamil-like substances influence the systolic ventricular function and produce a decrease in pressure gradient and contractility (11). This is supported by the literature (61, 25, 26, 30). Calcium antagonists, however, particularly improve the diastolic ventricular function (1, 3, 9, 17, 25). The latter effect has also been proven for nifedipine (18, 19, 28, 29) and diltiazem (23, 31). The filling pressure is decreased not only at rest, but during exercise. After intravenous administration of 10 mg verapamil, patients suffering from HCM showed a non-significant decrease in filling pressure at rest from 20.3 to 16.7 mm Hg. During exercise tests a decrease in pressure rise from 36.3 to 27.5 ($2p < 0.005$) (11) occurred, thus supporting the data of other investigators (16). This may explain the improved stress tolerance of patients treated with calcium antagonists, compared to those treated with beta-blockers (4, 8, 17, 20, 26). The decrease in filling pressure cannot be confirmed as only acute effect since the effectiveness of chronic treatment is even more pronounced. Calcium antagonists bring about long-term improvement in subjective symptoms and clinical findings. Apart from the dosage, the length of the treatment period is important.

Calcium antagonists induce a marked improvement in clinical severity, but the question of improved prognosis must be discussed. Our findings confirm earlier studies (11) showing that the annual mortality rate could be reduced to less than 2% with consequent high-dose verapamil or gallopamil treatment. We are now able to draw conclusions from a representative number of patients and a sufficiently long follow-up period and our results agree with those of other investigators (8). The antiarrhythmic effectiveness of verapamil may play a certain role in this process; this effect has been shown to be superior when compared to pindolol (20). On the other hand, there is no possibility of treating ventricular tachycardias with verapamil as is possible with classical antiarrhythmic medications or amiodarone in particular (7, 21). Therefore, the improvement in systolic and especially diastolic ventricular dynamics possibly has a beneficial effect on ectopia development, thus reducing the risk of sudden death (22). However, it seems prudent to decide on an individual basis, whether calcium antagonist treatment should be complemented by antiarrhythmics. Our positive results are possibly due to this therapeutic approach.

The literature reports a case of sudden death due to asystole following verapamil medication (24). In this case, previous therapy with digitalis had been discontinued some days beforehand. The documented conduction block, therefore, may have been caused by the additional effect of verapamil and digoxin on the conduction system. Non-fatal electrophysiologic and hemodynamic complications have been reported (5). Thus, the dosage should be adjusted according to individual conditions. Prior to the start of chronic therapy at high dosage, an ECG following a single administration of oral test doses of 160 mg verapamil or 50 mg gallapomil was performed. No complications due to calcium antagonist treatment occurred after testing and individual dosage adjustment. There were also no undesired hemodynamic effects in patients with high filling pressure. These patients sometimes showed impressive longterm improvements. Additional treatment with saluretics should be initiated, if necessary.

Calcium antagonists have proven successful for the treatment of hypertrophic cardiomyopathy and may be considered superior when compared to beta-blockers. Thus, they represent an alternative as well as an additional treatment to surgery. On the basis of our experience, the use of substances like verapamil may be considered superior to others, due to their beneficial effect on systolic and diastolic ventricular function and their — hypothetically — direct as well as indirect antiarrhythmic effects. On the whole, these qualities improve prognosis in patients with hypertrophic cardiomyopathy.

Summary: Hypertrophic cardiomyopathy is characterized by progredient myocardial hypertrophy causing ventricular systolic and diastolic dysfunction. Long-term results of beta-blocker therapy have been disappointing. Neither the impaired ventricular filling or the prognosis are improved. In contrast, calcium antagonists mainly influence diastolic ventricular dynamics, but also have beneficial effects on systolic function. The results of long-term therapy with calcium antagonists, including patients treated for more than 10 years, are presented here. A total of 84 consecutive patients (mean age 43 years; 20 female and 64 male) with confirmed hypertrophic cardiomyopathy were treated with high doses of calcium antagonists (mean doses of 515 mg verapamil or 158 mg gallopamil per day). In the course of therapy with a mean duration of 52 months, heart size — assessed by X-ray technique — and Sokolow-index in the ECG decreased significantly (heart volume: from 947 to 885 ml/1.73 m² body surface; Sokolow-index: from 5.0 to 4.5 mV). The echocardiogram showed a significant decrease in left atrial diameter, whereas wall thickness only tended to decrease. Hemodynamic control investigations confirmed an improvement in systolic as well as in diastolic ventricular function (mean follow-up period was 31 months). According to these findings the condition and stress tolerance improved in 84% of the patients. Therapy with calcium antagonists also improved prognosis: without treatment or following treatment with beta-blocking agents, annual mortality is approximately 3.5%, whereas in the described patient population mortality dropped to less than 2%. Thus, a calcium antagonist is the medication of first choice for patients with hypertrophic cardiomyopathy.

References

1. Anderson DM, Raff GL, Ports TA, Brundage BH, Parmley, WW, Chatterjee K (1984) Hypertrophic obstructive cardiomyopathy — Effects of acute and chronic verapamil treatment on left ventricular systolic and diastolic function. Br Heart J 51: 523—529
2. Assmann H, Assmann I, Fiehring H, Dittrich P, Eger H (1975) Verlaufsbeobahctungen bei der idiopathischen hypertrophischen subaortalen Stenose unter Propranololbehandlung. Dtsch Gesundhwes 30: 918—920
3. Bonow R, Frederick TM, Bacharach SL, Green MV, Goose PW, Maron BJ, Rosing DR (1983) Atrial systole and left ventricular filling in hypertrophic cardiomyopathy: effect of verapamil. Am J Cardiol 51: 1386—1391
4. Cserhalmi L, Aßmann I, Glavanov M, Rev J, Kelecseneyi Z (1984) Langzeittherapie der hypertrophischen obstruktiven und nichtobstruktiven Kardiomyopathie mit Nifedipin im Vergleich zu Propranolol. Z Ges Inn Med 39: 330—335
5. Epstein SE, Rosing DR (1981) Verapamil: its potential for causing serious complications in patients with hypertrophic cardiomyopathy. Circulation 64: 437—441
6. Frank MJ, Abdulla AM, Canedo MI, Saylors RE (1978) Longterm medical management of hypertrophic obstructive cardiomyopathy. Am J Cardiol 42: 993—1001
7. Goodwin JF (1982) The frontiers of cardiomyopathy. Br Heart J 48: 1—18
8. Haberer T, Hess OM, Jenni R, Krayenbühl HP (1983) Hypertrophe obstruktive Kardiomyopathie: Spontanverlauf im Vergleich zur Langzeittherapie mit Propranolol und Verapamil. Z Kardiol 72: 487—493
9. Hanrath P, Mathey DG, Kremer P, Sonntag F, Bleifeld W (1980) Effect of verapamil on left ventricular isovolumic relaxation time and regional left ventricular filling in hypertrophic cardiomyopathy. Am J Cardiol 45: 1258—1264
10. Hopf R, Keller M, Kaltenbach M (1976) Die Behandlung der hypertrophen obstruktiven Kardiomyopathie mit Verapamil. Verh Dtsch Ges Inn Med 82, Bd II: 1054
11. Hopf R, Kaltenbach M (1982) Die Hypertrophe Kardiomypathie. Möglichkeiten der Kalziumantagonistischen Behandlung. Thieme, Suttgart—New York
12. Jenni R, Ruffmann K, Vieli A, Anliker M, Krayenbühl HP (1985) Dynamics of aortic flow in hypertrophic cardiomyopathy. Eur Heart J 6: 391—398
13. Kaltenbach M, Hopf R, Keller M (1976) Calciumantagonistische Therapie bei hypertroph obstruktiver Kardiomyopathie. Dtsch med Wschr 101: 1284—1287

14. Kaltenbach M, Hopf R, Müller M, Riemann HE (1983) Vergleich verschiedener Methoden zur röntgenologischen Herzvolumenbestimmung. In: Kaltenbach M, Klepzig H (Hrsgb.): Röntgenologische Herzvolumenbestimmung. Springer-Verlag Berlin—Heidelberg—New York, pp 18—25
15. Kuhn H, Loogen F (1978) Die Anwendung von Beta-Rezeptorenblockern bei hypertrophischer obstruktiver Kardiomyopathie (HOCM). Internist 19: 527—531
16. Kuhn H, Thelen U, Leuner C, Köhler E, Bluschke V (1980) Langzeitbehandlung der hypertrophischen nicht obstruktiven Kardiomyopathie (HNCM) mit Verapamil. Z Kardiol 69: 669—675
17. Lösse B, Kuhn H, Loogen F (1982) Klinische und hämodynamische Effekte von Verapamil bei hypertrophischer obstruktiver Kardiomypathie. Z Kardiol 71: 813—819
18. Lorell BH, Paulus WJ, Grossmann W, Wynne J, Cohn PF, Braunwald E (1980) Improved diastolic function and systolic performance in hypertrophic cardiomyopathy after nifedipine. N Engl J Med 303: 801—803
19. Lorell BH, Paulus WJ, Grossmann W, Wynne J, Cohn PF (1982) Modification of abnormal left ventricular diastolic properties by nifedipine in patients with hypertrophic cardiomyopathy. Circulation 67: 500—507
20. Masini V, Ceci V, Malinoconico U, Milazzotto F (1981) Therapeutic evaluation of pindolol and verapamil in hypertrophic obstructive cardiomyopathy. G Ital Cardiol 11: 1729—1737
21. McKenna EJ, Harris L, Perez G, Krikler DM, Oakley C, Goodwin JF (1981) Arrhythmia in hypertrophic cardiomyocapthy. VII: Comparison of amiodarone and verapamil in treatment. Br Heart J 46: 173—178
22. Murgo JP (1982) Does outflow obstruction exist in hypertrophic cardiomyopathy? N Engl J Med 307: 1008—1009
23. Nagao M, Omote S, Takizawa A, Yasue H (1983) Effect of diltiazem on left ventricular isovolumic relaxation time in patients with hypertrophic cardiomyopathy. Jpn Circ J 47: 54—58
24. Perrot B, Danchin N, Terrier de la Chaise A (1984) Verapamil: a cause of sudden death in a patient with hypertrophic cardiomyopathy. Br Heart J 51: 352—354
25. Rosing DR, Kent KM, Borer JS, Seides SF, Maron BJ, Epstein SE (1979) Verapamil therapy: a new approach to the pharmacologic treatment of hypertrophic cardiomyopathy. I Hemodynamic effects. Circulation 60: 1201—1207
26. Rosing DR, Kent KM, Maron BJ, Epstein SE (1979) Verapamil treatment of hypertrophic cardiomyopathy. II Effects on exercise capacity and symptomatic status. Circulation 60: 1208—1213
27. Rosing DR, Condit J, Maron BJ, Kent KM, Leon MB, Bonow RO, Lipson LC, Epstein SE (1981) Verapamil therapy: a new approach to the pharmacologic treatment of hypertrophic cardiomyopathy. III Effects of long-term administration. Am J Cardiol 48: 545—553
28. Schanzenbächer P, Schick KD, Kochsiek K (1982) Nifedipin bei hypertrophisch obstruktiver Kardiomyopathie. Dtsch med Wschr 107: 1842—1846
29. Senn M, Hess OM, Krayenbühl HP (1982) Nifedipin in der Behandlung der hypertrophen, nicht-obstruktiven Kardiomyopathie. Schweiz med Wschr 38: 1312—1317
30. Spicer RL, Rocchini AP, Crowley DC, Rosenthal A (1984) Chronic verapamil therapy in pediatric and young adult patients with hypertrophic cardiomyopathy. Am J Cardiol 53: 1614—1619
31. Suwa M, Hirota Y, Kawamura K (1984) Improvement in left ventricular diastolic function during intravenous and oral diltiazem therapy in patients with hypertrophic cardiomyopathy: an echocardiographic study. Am J Cardiol 54: 1047—1053
32. Swanton EH, Brooksby IAB, Jenkins BS, Webb-Peploe MM (1977) Hemodynamic studies of beta-blockade in hypertrophic obstructive cardiomyopathy. Eur J Cardiol 5/4: 327—341
33. Stenson RE, Flamm Jr MD, Harrison DC, Hancock EW (1973) Hypertrophic subaortic stenosis. Clinical and hemodynamic effects of long-term propranolol therapy. Am J Cardiol 32: 763—773

Authors' address:
Priv.-Doz. Dr. R. Hopf, Abteilung für Kardiologie, Zentrum der Inneren Medizin, Klinikum der Johann-Wolfgang Goethe-Universität, Theodor Stern Kai Nr. 7, D-6000 Frankfurt/Main 70, F.R.G.

Techniques and complications of transaortic subvalvular myectomy in patients with hypertrophic obstructive cardiomyopathy (HOCM)

H. D. Schulte, W. Bircks, B. Lösse

Department of Thoracic and Cardiovascular Surgery and Department of Cardiology, Pulmonology, and Angiology University of Düsseldorf, F.R.G.

Introduction

Studies on the natural history of patients with hypertrophic obstructive cardiomyopathy (HOCM) demonstrate a slowly continuing deterioration, characterized additionally by development of mitral insufficiency, atrial fibrillation, congestive heart failure, and sudden death (10, 25, 27, 35, 38, 41). This development can be partly interrupted with different medical therapeutic regimens for HOCM using β-blocking agents and/or calcium antagonists, as demonstrated by recent clinical investigations (7, 15, 20). However, there are some patients who do not respond adequately on a long-term basis to conservative treatment, or they deteriorate again after an initially impressive clinical improvement. These patients may become candidates for surgical treatment.

Several surgical techniques have been employed. We have followed a modified Morrow technique (transaortic subvalvular myectomy [29, 34, 36]).

The basis of this contribution is our own surgical experience with 212 patients who were operated upon by only two surgeons from 1963 to May 31, 1986. This group of patients included 18 patients with a so-called atypical (midventricular) obstruction which, in all our cases, was accompanied by a typical subvalvular muscular obstruction.

Patients and Methods

Most of our surgical patients were investigated, pretreated, and followed by members of our own cardiological department, who have documented their interest in all types of cardiomyopathies for many years. In addition, however, a considerable number of patients were sent for surgery after failing medical therapy by other cardiological groups in Germany, Austria, and Denmark.

Indications for surgical treatment

Our list of surgical indications (Table 1) clearly demonstrates that all patients have to be pretreated medically for at least several months before surgery (7, 26, 33, 34). With the exception of 12 patients in clinical class IV, all patients belonged to clinical class III

Table 1. Indications for surgical treatment.

Inadequate response to medical therapy (β-blocking agents, calcium-antagonists) Clinical class III or IV (NYHA) Considerable systolic gradient (LV-ascending aorta, intraventricular) at rest or after provocation (> 50 mm Hg) Paradoxical pressure behaviour

(NYHA). Most of our patients had a systolic gradient between the ascending aorta and the left ventricle of distinctly more than 50 mm Hg at invasive investigations: Some patients had less or no obviously measurable gradient at rest; however, they demonstrated a substantially effective gradient after provocation (post-extrasystolic beat, Valsalva maneuver, isoprenaline, physical exertion).

Present surgical procedure

For technical facilitation of the surgical procedure, the use of a headlight for the surgeon, complete relaxation of the myocardium by means of cold crystalloid, high volume cardioplegia (Bretschneider), tilting of the operation-table to the left, and pushing the relaxed lateral LV-wall towards the LV-outflow tract have proven extremely useful. In addition, we have developed special instruments for precise in situ preparation, in order to avoid complications and injuries of the aortic and mitral valves, as well as to the intraseptal conduction system, and for better and deeper retraction to allow a precise and sufficient myectomy deep into the left ventricle.

The original Morrow procedure (29) was modified because our intra-operative simultaneous pressure tracings (LV, ascending aorta with and without provocation) after myectomy in many cases indicated an insufficient relief of the systolic gradient and/or a continuing paradoxical pressure behaviour (Brockenbrough phenomenon).

Therefore, the subvalvular myectomy was extended to the left into the commissure of the left and right coronary cusps. This incision for myotomy had been earlier recommended by Bigelow and coworkers (5). The more extended myectomy was continued into the LV in the direction of the apex between the bases of the anterior and posterior papillary muscles. If necessary, the bulging hypertrophic parts of the lateral LV wall, especially in cases with visible deviation of the posterior papillary muscle and/or chordae towards the hypertrophied ventricular septum, would also be removed. Additionally, the resection of the thickened fibrotic endocardial layer within the LV outflow tract was performed, as earlier recommended, also by Morrow (18).

Our own surgical experience

From 1963 to May 31, 1986, a total of 212 patients were operated on, 194 of whom belonged to the typical and 18 to the so-called atypical group (Table 2). The male:female ratio was about 2:1. The mean age was between 40 (typical HOCM) and 47 years (atypical HOCM) with a range of 6 to 73 years. Most of the patients belonged to clinical class III (NYHA) ($n = 200$). The total hospital mortality rate was 6.6 % ($n = 14$). However, in relation to different periods of progressive experience later this rate could be lowered to 4.5 % during the later years (Table 3).

Table 2. Data of surgical treated patients.

(1963 — Mai 31, 1986; *n* = 208)	Typical HOCM	Atypical HOCM
Patients (*n*)	194	18
Male:female	127:67	12:6
Mean age (years)	40	47
Range (years)	6—73	23—60
Clinical class (NYHA) III	183	17
IV	11	1
Hospital mortality (%)	12 (6.2)	2 (11.1)

Table 3. Hospital mortality in relation to different time periods

Years	HOCM (*n*)	Hospital (*n*)	mortality (%)
1963—1969	12	3	25.0
1970—1980	87	6	5.9
1981—May 31, 1986	113	5	4.6
1963—1986	221	14	6.6

The lowest mortality rate (3.8 %) could be achieved in patients with typical and atypical HOCM and transaortic subvalvular myectomy (TSM) (*n* = 160) and no additional surgical disease and therapy (Table 7). In the group of 52 patients with TSM and additional surgical procedures (including two pts with RV ventriculotomy) the mortality rate was distinctly increased, to 15.4 % (*n* = 8).

Additional surgical procedures

The surgical procedures for all patients (*n* = 208) are listed for the typical and atypical groups (Table 4), also indicating the number of decreased patients. Most of our problems arose from patients with considerable mitral valve incompetence, which is not easy to judge intraoperatively. In 15 patients a primary or secondary mitral valve replacement was necessary and five of these patients died postoperatively resulting in a very high mortality rate of 33.3 %. These results were shocking, especially on the background of contributions from other authors (8—10) in which only a mitral valve replacement (MVR) was performed for relief of HOCM with much better early results. Considerable mitral valve insufficiency is a predictor of a higher surgical risk, in our experience. Only eight of our patients needed coronary revascularization procedures.

Complications

Another aspect of our study was to consider whether intra- and postoperative complications were in close relation to the originating disease (HOCM) or were more related to

Table 4. Surgical treatment of HOCM and additional diseases.

Surgical procedures	Typical HOCM	Atypical HOCM
Transaortic subvalvular myectomy (TSM)	148 (6+)	12 (3.8%)
TSM + splitting of LAD muscle bridge	1 (1+)	—
TSM + WPW-syndrome	1	—
TSM + LV-pseudo diverticle	1	—
TSM + apical LV-ancurysm	1	—
TSM + apical thrombus formation	—	1
TSM + LV ventriculotomy	2	—
TSM + RV ventriculotomy	5 (1+)	—
RV-ventriculotomy	2	—
TSM + aortic valve reconstruction	5	—
TSM + mitral valve reconstruction	2	—
TSM + aortic valve replacement (AVR)	3	—
TSM + mitral valve replacement (MVR)	12 (3+)	3(2+)
TSM + tricuspid valve replacement (TVR)	1	—
TSM + aorto-coronary bypass grafting (ACBG)	7	2
TSM + AVR + ACBG	1	—
TSM + repair of ascending aorta aneurysm (postop. rupture)	1 (1+)	—
	46 (6+)	6 (2+) (15.4%)

general surgical events (Table 5). In the first group there were some injuries to the valves, the septum and the conduction system which needed further partial surgical treatment, such as valve repair or replacement, suturing of the LV wall or septum, or implantation of permanent pacemaker systems. Despite the orientation of the myectomy to the left in nearly half of our cases (n = 94) a postoperative left bundle branch block (LBBB) could be confirmed by repeated ECG tracings. It has not yet been finally decided by postoperative echocardiographic and angiocardiographic controls and by exercise testing whether a permanent LBBB is a real complication or of considerable disadvantage for the HOCM patients during the immediate and late postoperative course.

The problem of postoperative cerebral embolism could be solved, since all patients are anticoagulated using coumadin for 4 to 6 weeks postoperatively. In that time no cerebral complications occurred.

In 20 patients, intraoperative pressure controls indicated an insufficient relief of the obstruction which made an immediate remyectomy necessary, with considerable improvement in the results.

In four patients, a reoperation had to be performed because of insufficient primary myectomy. This occurred in the first patient of our series and she died after reoperation because of myocardial failure.

In a young woman with a HOCM, a prophylactic defibrillator system was implanted after several preoperative ventricular fibrillations with successful resuscitation. Two women died suddenly 10 and 20 days after successful surgery because of ventricular fibrillation and could not be resuscitated in hospital.

Table 5. Intra- and postoperative complications related and non-related to HOCM.

Complications	Procedures		n	Deceased pts
HOCM-related				
Injuries:				
Aortic valve	Repair		2	
Mitral valve	Repair		1	
Mitral valve	Replacement		1	(1+)
Tricuspid valve	Replacement		1	
LV-wall perforation	Repair (suture)		1	(1+)
Muscular septum	Repair (*n* =3)		8	
perfor. (sec. VSD)				
AV-block II, III Pacemaker implantation			7	(1+)
Muscular septum infarction			1	
Left bundle branch block		90		
Cerebral embolism		5		
Intraop. re-myectomy		20		
Reoperation for insufficient primary		4	(1+)	
myectomy				
Late postop. endocarditis AVR + MVR		2		
Defibrillator implantation (prophylactic)		1		
Acute arrhythmias (ventricular fibrillation)		2	(2+)	
Myocardial insufficiency		11	(5+)	
non HOCM-related complications				
Pulmonary embolism		2	(1+)	
Gastro-intestinal bleeding		2	(1+)	
Septicemia		1	(1+)	
Rethoracotomy (bleeding)		9		
Wound dehiscence (sternum)		4		
Pneumothorax		4		
Acute renal insufficiency		2		
Hepatitis B		3		

The complications which were not related to HOCM demonstrate a wide spectrum of postoperatively possible events which, in three cases, were responsible for the unfortunate outcome.

Discussion

It is the purpose of this contribution to report our experience with surgical therapy for HOCM, a disease of unknown etiology and a natural history of slow, but continuing deterioration. In most of the patients this development could be interrupted or alleviated by medical therapy. Only in cases of failing drug therapy is surgical management indicated, which has been evaluated by long-term clinical cardiological experiences in Bethesda, Duesseldorf, or elsewhere (7, 15, 20, 25—27).

In general, this means that the surgeons are at least dealing with the worse group of HOCM patients who demonstrate a continuing progression of the disease despite long-term medical pre-treatment and have reached clinical class III (NYHA) (21, 24, 25, 26).

Aims of surgical treatment

The main aims, of course, optimal relief of the subvalvular (sometimes also an intraventricular) muscular obstruction which is usually indicated by the correction of the
systolic gradient and the paradoxic behavior of the left ventricular and ascending aortic
systolic pressure tracings (Table 6). In about 60 % of the patients with HOCM, a mild,
moderate, or severe mitral valve incompetence can be demonstrated by angiocardiography or by pulsed Doppler echocardiography, only seldom by simultaneous LA and LV
pressure tracings. However, it was an early clinical experience that in most cases after
surgery, mitral incompetence was considerably reduced, completely abolished or no longer visible (9, 35).

The usually asymmetric muscular septal hypertrophy causes a typical angulation of the
left ventricle. The LV longitudinal axis can be partly reconstructed by sufficient subvalvular myectomy.

Another point is that in patients with severe HOCM the diastolic compliance is reduced, due especially to some intramyocardial factors (hypertrophy, increase of fibrotic
tissue, endocardial fibrosis). It is a well-known fact that after verapamil therapy and after
surgery in most patients the diastolic relaxation of the LV or the ventricular filling capacity is improved (31, 38).

There are also intentions to prevent, through surgical treatment, HOCM-related specific complications, such as atrial fibrillation, sudden death, development of mitral incompetence and congestive heart failure. However, today it seems questionable whether
the goal of surgery, to reduce the rate of sudden deaths and to prolong the survival rate,
can be accomplished in reality.

Surgical techniques

The main recommended surgical procedures for relief of HOCM, since 1958, are summarized in Table 7.

Cleland performed the first transaortic subvalvular myotomy for relief of substantial
muscular stenosis in 1958, and this very first patient survived surgery for more than 25
years (3).

This first surgical step was completed to transaortic subvalvular myectomy by Morrow
(29), the now classic surgical procedure. For special indications, the combined transaortic
and LV apical approach with myectomy, begun by Kirklin and Ellis (19), may be of
considerable value for deep midventricular or apical obstruction. However, our primary

Table 6. Aims of surgical treatment.

Considerable relief of systolic LVOT muscular obstruction
Correction of paradoxical pressure behaviour (LV-asc. aorta)
Reduction in accompanying mitral valve incompetence
Geometrical reduction in LV-cavity angulation
Improvement of diastolic relaxation of the LV
Prevention of specific complications (questionable)
(sudden death, long-term survival)

Table 7. Development of surgical techniques.

Cleland, Bentall (3)	1958	Transaortic ventriculo-myotomy
Morrow, Brockenbrough (30)	1961	Transaortic ventriculo-myectomy
Kirklin, Ellis (19)	1961	Transaortic and transapical LV-myectomy
Julian (18)	1963	Fish-mouth type LV-incision and myectomy
Lillehei, Levy (23)	1963	Trans-left-atrial approach and anterior mitral leaflet detachment for myectomy
Dobell, Scott (13)	1964	Trans-left-atrial approach and anterior mitral leaflet incision
Johnson (17)	1964	Trans-left-atrial approach and mitral valve replacement and myectomy
Cooley (12)	1970	MVR without myotomy or myectomy
Stinson, since Shumway (37)	1968	Heart transplantation for end-stage cardiomyopathy
Rastan, Koncz (31) Konno (21)	1975	Aorto-ventriculo plasty
Bernhard (4) Cooley, Norman (11)	1976	Apico-aortic valved conduit
Vouhé (41)	1984	Trans-right-ventricular approach, myectomy
Alvarez-Diaz (2)	1984	Trans-right-ventricular septum resection, patch closure
Bircks, Schulte since	1980	Extended myectomy to commissure between right and left coronary cusps, and to the base of the papillary muscles, to lateral LV-wall; excision of fibrotic endocardium

intention is to avoid any additional injury to the hypertrophied left ventricle. Julian (18) described a fish-mouth type LV incision for this purpose.

All types of primary mitral valve surgery by, e.g., detachment or anterior leaflet incisions (13, 17, 23) have gained no general acceptance. Also, mitral valve replacement as a solution to outflow obstruction (12, 17) has not seemed convincing; however, the Bethesda group (14) has recently started again to gain some experience with this technique.

The therapy of end-stage cardiomyopathies by heart transplantation has to be added as an accepted method today (37).

More complicated surgical techniques for special indications which may be of value in difficult HOCM cases have been reported by Rastan and Koncz (31), Konno et al. (21), Bernhard et al. (4), Cooley and Norman (11).

Recently Vouhé et al. (41) reported a trans-right-ventricular approach with excision of parts of the hypertrophied muscular subvalvular septum and subsequent closure of the divided septum again by sutures, whereas Alvarez-Diaz et al. (2) performed a complete resection of the hypertrophied septum with subsequent closure by a dacron patch.

Advice for surgical treatment

On the background of the known natural history with a slow progression of the disease and in the patient's situation of deterioration despite long-term medical therapy, the advice for surgical treatment may be facilitated by our gained experience, an acceptable operative risk, a low rate of complications, and a close follow-up of the operated and medically treated patients (Table 8). The clinical findings and postoperative hemodynamic data demonstrate a considerable improvement in most patients, including in exercise capacity. Another argument for surgical therapy is the improved prognosis of patients with typical HOCM in clinical classes III and IV (22). These results of a retrospective long-term analysis lead to suggestions of recommending earlier surgery for patients in clinical clas II, for instance. However, this consideration is only acceptable if further reduction in the operative risk can be safely achieved in our view. Up to now there have been no reports of a real recidive of obstruction of a sufficiently performed subvalvular myectomy. There have been reoperations which were caused, however, by a hemodynamically incomplete relief of the left ventricular outflow tract obstruction (LVOTO) during the primary surgical intervention in all cases. Therefore, careful intraoperative simultaneous pressure measurements during normal heart beats and after provocation are absolutely necessary. For instance, a remaining gradient at rest of more than 30 mm HG (more than 50 mm Hg after provocation) is a strict indication for an immediate re-myectomy procedure. However, in patients with a need for intraoperative pacemaker stimulation, the electrodes must be placed near the apex because otherwise a false irregular gradient may be provoked.

Surgical treatment

Surgical therapy was introduced by Cleland by a subvalvular muscular splitting (myotomy) which, in most cases, seemed not to be a sufficient technique. The most efficient procedures was performed by Morrow (transaortic subvalvular myectomy) (29, 30) and evaluated by Braunwald and coworkers (10). This early concept of relief of LVOTO and the early and late clinical and hemodynamic controls, continued to be performed by the cardiological group at Bethesda, who gave us the confidence to continue our own efforts concerning the surgical management of HOCM over some years. With the increasing experience of both our surgeons, the operative risk and the rate of intra- and postoperative complications could be decreased considerably. This improvement was supported by the use of additional technical resources, such as a headlight or special instrumentation. Despite these encouraging early results, there is a continuing operative risk of mortality, especially in patients in need of additional cardiac surgical procedures at the same time. This group of patients demonstrate a distinctly higher mortality, which in our

---

Table 8. Advice for surgical treatment.

Slowly progressive disease
Inadequate response to long-term medical therapy
and clinical deterioration
Acceptable operative risk
Low rate of intra- and postoperative complications
Intraoperative pressure controls for sufficient relief of LVOTO
High probability of subjective and hemodynamic improvement
No reported subvalvular restenosis.

Table 9. Data from literature concerning early mortality.

Authors	Year	Pts (n)	Hosp.-Mort. (%)	Late Mort. total	per year (%) rel. to HOCM
Bigelow (5)	1974	39	7.5	2.4	
Tajik (38)	1974	43	16.0		
Björk (8)	1976	32	6.3		
Agnew (1)	1977	49	4.1		
Maron (27)	1983	240	8.0	2.7	1.6
Binet (6)	1983	75	9.2	2.8	
Rothlin (33)	1983	64	1.6	2.1	1.9
Beahrs (2a)	1983	40	10.0	2.1	1.9
Von der Lohe (40)	1984	33	3.0		
Düsseldorf May, 31	1986	212	6.6	2.2	1.1

experience is about 10 % higher than in patients with transaortic subvalvular myectomy (TSM) alone.

Some data from recent literature (since 1974) from different groups with surgical experience with HOCM patients in the United States, New Zealand and Western Europe (1, 2a, 6, 8, 10, 26, 27, 32—34, 36, 38, 40) demonstrate present results, referring to the numbers of operated patients and the early hospital and late mortality rates (Table 9).

Postoperative prognosis

The most important further question, concerning the total long-term prognosis and a considerable reduction in HOCM-related complications such as further deterioration of the myocardial disease, development of congestive heart failure after surgical treatment and sudden death, is not so easy to answer.

It is our early impression, evaluated by different studies, that nearly all surviving patients feel subjectively better, the complaints are considerably reduced, the work capacity is distinctly increased, and the hemodynamic data indicate a constant improvement over several postoperative controls (22, 24, 25). Similarly good clinical and hemodynamic results have been recently reported by several authors (6, 27, 32, 33, 40).

Concerning late prognosis, our data demonstrate a trend to an improvement after surgery (22). For confirmation of such a trend, all our operated surviving patients will be reinvestigated in the near future and we are waiting for these important results.

In summarizing our surgical experience in patients with clinically advanced HOCM, we recommend transaortic subvalvular myectomy despite a considerable surgical risk concerning early mortality and specific complications. The effectiveness of surgical procedures has to be proven by accurate follow-up of the operated patients in comparison to the medically treated patients and by careful invasive and non-invasive examinations at rest and after exercise.

Summary: The natural history of hypertrophic obstructive cardiomyopathy (HOCM) is usually characterized by development of mitral insufficiency, congestive heart failure

(CHF) and sudden death. In patients (pts) belonging to at least clinical class III (NYHA) after failed medical therapy (β-blocking agents and calcium-antagonists) surgery should be considered (by means of transaortic subvalvular myectomy).

The history and development of different surgical techniques and procedures has been described in detail since 1958, when Cleland performed the first transaortic subvalvular myotomy.

Our surgical series (1963 — May 31, 1986) consists of 212 pts (mean age 40 years, range 6—73 years) with typical and atypical HOCM. The total hospital mortality rate was 6.6 % (n = 14), which was reduced to 3.8 % (n = 6), if only transaortic subvalvular myectomy (TSM) was performed (n = 160). In the group of 52 pts with additional surgical procedures the mortality rate was 15.4 % (n = 8). The main problems occurred in pts with additional mitral valve replacement (MVR) (n = 15, three deaths). The rate of HOCM-related complications (secondary VSD, total AV-block, cerebral embolism, intraoperative re-myectomy) and those related to surgery (bleeding, pulmonary embolism, wound dehiscence, septicemia) was low. Therefore TSM for HOCM is a low-risk surgical procedure with a good long-term prognosis. However, in pts with a need for additional surgical procedures, the risk is considerably increased. Subjective impression of the pts and hemodynamic data indicate a clear clinical improvement postoperatively. Concerning long-term survival and reduction of the sudden death rate, our data do not allow a final judgement at the moment.

References

1. Agnew TM, Barratt-Boyes GB, Brandt PT, Roibe AHG, Loewe JB, O'Brian KP (1977) Surgical resection in idiopathic hypertrophic subaortic stenosis with a combined approach through aorta and left ventricle. A long-term follow-up study in 49 patients. J Thorac Cardiovasc Surg 74: 307—316
2. Alvarez-Diaz F, Cabo J, Cordovilla G, Greco R, Sanz E, Berches D, Alvarado F, Garcia-Aguado A (1984) Surgical correction of diffuse subaortic stenosis by an infundibular septal resection. 33th Congress of the European Society of Cardiovascular Surgery, Madrid, Abstract Book
2a. Beahrs MM, Tajik AJ, Seward JB, Giuliani ER, McGoon DC (1983) Hypertrophic Obstructive Cardiomyopathy: Ten to 21 year follow-up after partial septal myectomy. Am J Cardiol 51: 1160—1166
3. Bentall HH (1966) The place of surgery in hypertrophic bostructive cardiomyopathy (idiopathic hypertrophic subaortic-stenosis). J Thorac Cardiovasc Surg 51: 49—52
4. Bernhard FW, Poirer V, La Farge CG (1975) Relief of congenital obstruction to left ventricular outflow with a ventricular-aortic prosthesis. J Thorac Cardiovasc Surg 69: 223—229
5. Bigelow WG, Trimble AS, Wigle DE, Adelman AG, Felderhof SE (1974) The treatment of muscular subaortic stenosis. J Thorac Cardiovasc Surg 68: 384—390
6. Binet JP, David P, Piot JD (1983) Surgical treatment of hyper trophic obstructive cardiomyopathies. Europ Heart J 4, Suppl F: 191—195
7. Bircks W, Schulte HD (1983) Surgical treatment of hypertrophicobstructive cardiomyopathy with special reference to complications and to atypical hypertrophic obstructive cardiomyopathy. Europ Heart J 4, Suppl F: 187—190
8. Björk VO, Radegran K (1976) Obstructive cardiomyopathy. J Cardiovasc Surg 17: 376—379
9. Bonow R (1986) Effects of verapamil on abnormalities of LV distensibility and relaxation in hypertrophic obstructive cardiomyopathy and relation to improved exercise capacity. 2nd International Workshop on Hypertrophic Cardiomyopathy, Badenweiler, FRG
10. Braunwald E, Lambrew CT, Morrow AG, Pierce EG, Rockoff SD, Ross jr. J (1964) Idiopathic hypertrophic subaortic stenosis. Am Heart Ass Monog 10. Circulation 30, Suppl 4

11. Cooley DA, Norman JC, Mullins CE, Grace RR (1975) Left ventricle to abdominal aorta conduits for relief of aortic stenosis. Cardiovasc Disc 2: 376—381
12. Cooley DA, Wukasch DC, Leachman RD (1976) Mitral valve replacement for idiopathic subaortic stenosis. Results in 27 patients. J Cardiovasc Surg 17: 380—387
13. Dobell ARC, Scott AJ (1964) Hypertrophic subaortic stenosis. Evolution of a surgical technique. J Thorac Cardiovasc Surg 47: 26—31
14. Epstein SE, NIH Cardiology Branch (personal communication)
15. Goodwin JF, Hollman A, Cleland WP, Teare D (1960) Obstructive cardiomyopathy simulating aortic stenosis. Br Heart J 22: 403—408
16. Hopf R (1986) Effects of combined therapy with propranolol and nifedipin. 2nd Intern Workshop on Hypertrophic Cardiomyopathy, Badenweiler, FRG
17. Johnson J (1964) Discussion of Dobell and Scott (13)
18. Julian OC, Dye WS, Javid H, Hunter JA, Muenster JJ, Najafi H (1965) Apical left ventriculotomy in subaortic stenosis due to fibromuscular hypertrophy. Circulation 31, Suppl I: 45
19. Kirklin JW, Ellis FW (1961) Surgical relief of diffuse subvalvular aortic stenosis. Circulation 24: 739—742
20. Kober G (1986) Results of a multicenter study on hypertrophic cardiomyopathy comparing propranolol and verapamil. 2nd Intern Workshop on Hypertrophic Cardiomyopathy, Badenweiler, FRG
21. Konno S, Imai Y, Jida Y, Makajima M, Tetsuno K (1975) A new method for prosthetic valve replacement in congenital aortic stenosis associated with hypoplasie of the aortic ring. J Thorac Cardiovasc Surg 70: 909—917
22. Kuhn H, Gietzen F, Mercier J, Lösse B, Köhler E, Schulte HD, Bircks W, Loogen F (1983) Studies of the clinical picture, course, and prognosis of different forms of hypertrophic cardiomyopathy. Z Kardiol 72: 83—98
23. Lillehei CW, Levy MJ (1963) Transatrial exposure for correction of subaortic stenosis. J Am Med Ass 186: 8—12
24. Lösse B, Kuhn H, Loogen F, Schulte HD (1983) Exercise performance in hypertrophic cardiomyopathies. Europ Heart J 4, Suppl F: 197—208
25. Lösse B (1986) Hemodynamic long-term results after medical andsurgical therapy. 2nd Intern Workshop on Hypertrophic Cardiomyopathy, Badenweiler, FRG
26. Loogen F, Kuhn H, Gietzen F, Lösse B, Schulte HD, Bircks W (1983) Clinical course and prognosis of patients with typical and atypical hypertrophic obstructive and with hypertrophic non-obstructive cardiomyopathy. Europ Heart J 4, Suppl F: 145-153
27. Maron BJ, Epstein SE, Morrow AG (1983) Symptomatic status and prognosis of patients after operation for hypertrophic obstructive cardiomyopathy: efficacy of ventricular septal myotomy and myectomy. Europ Heart J 4, Suppl F: 175—185
28. McKenna W, Borggrefe M, England D, Deanfield J, Oakley CM, Goodwin JF (1981) Prognosis in hypertrophic cardiomyopathy: role of age and clinical, electrocardiographic and haemodynamic features. Am J Cardiol 47: 532—538
29. Morrow AG (1981) Hypertrophic aortic stenosis. Operative methods utilized to relieve left ventricular outflow obstruction. J Thorac Cardiovasc Surg 76: 423-430
30. Morrow AG, Brockenbrough EC (1961) Surgical treatment of idiopathic hypertrophic subaortic stenosis: Technique and hemodynamic results of subaortic ventriculotomy. Ann Surg 154: 181—189
31. Rastan H, Koncz J (1975) Plastische Erweiterung des linken Ausflußtraktes — eine neue Operationsmethode. Thoraxchir 3: 169—175
32. Reis RL, Hannah III H, Carley JE, Pugh DM (1977) Surgical treatment of idiopathic hypertrophic subaortic stenosis (IHSS): postoperative results in 30 patients following ventricular septal myotomy or myectomy (Morrow procedure). Circulation 56, Suppl II, No 3: 128—132
33. Rothlin ME, Gobet D, Haberer T, Krayenbuehl HP, Turina M, Senning A (1983) Surgical treatment versus medical treatmentin hypertrophic obstructive cardiomyopathy. Europ Heart J 4, Suppl F: 215—223
34. Schulte HD, Bircks W, Körfer R, Kuhn H (1981) Surgical aspects of typical subaortic and atypical midventricular hypertrophic obstructive cardiomyopathy (HOCM). Thorac Cardiovasc Surg 29: 375—380

35. Schulte HD, Bircks W, Lösse B (1985) Ursachen und Bedeutung der Mitralklappeninsuffizienz bei der chirurgischen Behandlung der hypertrophischen obstruktiven Kardiomyopathie. Wiener klin Wschr 135: 489—493
36. Schulte HD, Lösse B (1985) Hypertrophische obstruktive Kardiomyopathie: Chirurgische Behandlung und Ergebnisse. Herz 10: 102—111
37. Stinson EB, Shumway NE (1978) Transplantation of the heart. In: Longmore DB: Modern cardiac surgery. MTP-Press Limited, Lancaster, England, pp 3—18
38. Tajik AJ, Guiliani ER, Weidmann WH, Brandenburg RO, McGoon DC (1974) Idiopathic hypertrophic subaortic stenosis, long-term surgical follow-up. Am J. Cardiol 34: 815—822
39. Van der Wall E (1985) Recent views on left ventricular function in hypertrophic cardiomyopathy: Hemodynamic concepts and their clinical implications. In: Van der Wall E, Lie KI (Eds.). Recent views on hypertrophic cardiomyopathy. Martinus Nijhoff Publishers, Boston, Dordrecht Lancester, pp 71—99
40. Von der Lohe E, Müller-Hake C, Minale C, von Essen R, Effert S, Messmer BJ (1984) Septumresektion bei hypertropher obstruktiver Kardiomyopathie. Langzeitergebnisse bei 33 Patienten. Dtsch med Wschr 109: 1749—1753
41. Vouhé PR, Poulain H, Block G, Loisance DY, Gamain J, Lombaer M, Ouiret JC, Lesbre JP, Bernasconi P, Pietri J, Cachera JP (1984) Aortoseptal approach for optimal resection of diffuse subvalvular aortic stenosis. J Thorac Cardiovasc Surg 87: 887—893

Authors' address:
Prof. Hagen D. Schulte, M.D., Department of Surgery B (Thoracic and Cardiovascular Surgery) Moorenstr. 5, D-4000 Düsseldorf, F.R.G.

Capillary density and oxygen supply in human dilated cardiomyopathy

H. R. Figulla[1], F. Vetterlein[2], V. Wiegand[1], S. Schüler[3], H. Kreuzer[1]

[1] Medizinische Klinik, Abteilung für Kardiologie, Universität Göttingen
[2] Institut für Pharmakologie und Toxikologie, Universität Göttingen
[3] Deutsches Herzzentrum, Berlin, F.R.G.

Introduction

Human hearts with dilated cardiomyopathy (DCM) exhibit a hypertrophy of the myocytes (7, 8). Consequently, the intercapillary distance increases, which may impede the diffusable metabolic supply. Factor and Sonnenblick (1) raised the question of whether DCM is caused by microvascular disorders, such as microvascular spasm, which could be demonstrated in cardiomyopathic Syrian hamsters (2, 3).

In the following study, the microvasculature of human hearts with DCM was investigated to answer the following questions:
What is the average capillary density in DCM?
Are the capillaries homogeneously distributed?
How does capillary density and distribution affect myocardial oxygen supply?

Methods

Immediately after death, endothelial swelling affects the microvasculature. Therefore, in this study, living human hearts, excised during cardiac transplantation due to intractable DCM were reperfused via a glass cannula in the ramus circumflexus of the left coronary artery, with 1 l oxygenized, modified Krebs-Henseleit solution containing 1 g fluorescent dye (FITC) bound to dextran (MW 58 000, Sigma). Shortly prior to the end of perfusion, a tissue probe of the beating heart was excised and immediately freeze-stopped. By means of a cryomicrotome frozen sections of the transmural tissue probe were cut perpendicular to the capillaries at the mid-myocardium level. These sections were transferred to slides coated with pure alcohol, precooled in liquid nitrogen. The preparations were kept at − 20 ° until the alcohol impregnated the tissue, which was then embedded in an artificial medium (Entellan, Merck) at room temperature. The FITC dextran complex cannot penetrate the tissue and therefore stains the intravascular space. By means of a fluorescent microscope, the capillaries were detectable precisely and the functional capillary density and distribution could be evaluated. In every patient, four different tissue slices from the mid-myocardium were evaluated and the results averaged. Tissue shrinkage of 3.5 % was considered in the results.

For evaluation of the capillary distribution, a random pattern was superimposed on to the tissue slices and the distances from these test points to the nearest capillary were measured, giving a frequency distribution of the distance tissue to capillary (for further details see ref. [6]).

Results

The average functional capillary density in DCM amounted to 1245 ± 345 capillaries/mm² (n = 8). The average muscle fiber diameter in these hearts was 27.0 ⊥ 6.0 µm. The distribution of the capillaries within the tissue is summarized in Fig. 1. The mean tissue-capillary distance was 14.1 µm. 50% of the tissue was within 12 µm from the nearest capillary.

Discussion

Histomorphometry

The aim of this study was to investigate the functional capillary density and capillary distribution in human myocardium and to consider its effect on oxygen supply in patients with DCM. By means of heart transplantation, living human hearts are now available on which to perform these investigations. Unfortunately, at present there is little data avail-

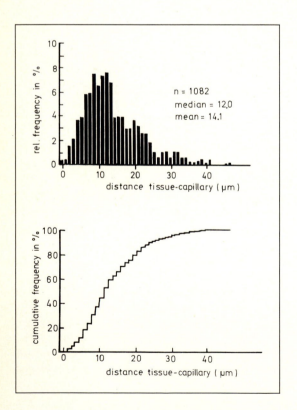

Fig. 1. The distances from 1082 test points (superimposed onto tissue slices from eight human hearts) to the nearest capillary were measured. These data gave a frequency distribution of the tissue-capillary distance (see text).

able on capillary density in human hearts. Rakusan (9) recently reviewed some data and found striking differences in the results, ranging from 1363 to 5734 capillaries/mm² due to different techniques (i.e. dye injection, histochemistry) and different post mortem periods. Probably the most precise data are available from Roberts and Wearn (10) who used a dye injection technique within 1 h after death. They found 3342 capillaries/mm² in normal adult left ventricles and 2483 capillaries/mm² in hypertrophied ventricles

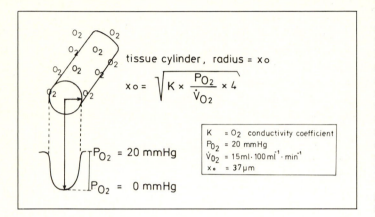

Fig. 2. A simple diffusional model of oxygen transport was assumed. Individual muscle fibers are surrounded by a homogeneous O_2 field of 20 mm Hg. Under the assumption of an oxygen consumption of $\dot{V}_{O_2} = 15$ ml · 100 ml⁻¹ · min⁻¹ and an oxygen conductivity coefficient of $K = 2.5 \cdot 10^{-8}$ ml · cm⁻¹ · min⁻¹ · mm Hg⁻¹ (4), the oxygen pressure will drop to zero within a radius of $x_o = 37$ μm.

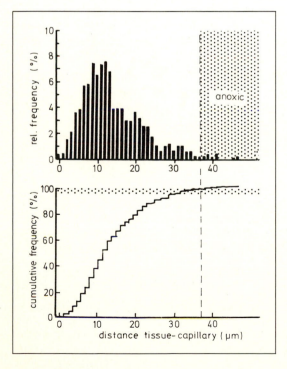

Fig. 3. According to the oxygen supply model in Fig. 2, a small amount of tissue exceeding the distance of 37 μm to the nearest capillary will become anoxic.

(average heart weight 538 g, muscle fiber diameter 19.9 μm). Whether the even lower capillary density that we found in DCM is due to the extreme hypertrophy of the muscle fibers (27.0 μm) or to a specific microvascular disorder in DCM cannot be answered from the present results. Further experiments yielding the capillary-fiber ratio will answer this question, since this ratio is stable even in cardiac hypertrophy, but may decrease if capillaries are temporarily (in spasm) or permanently occluded.

Oxygen supply

If we consider a muscle cylinder surrounded by a homogeneous O_2 field with an oxygen pressure (P_{O_2}) of 20 mm Hg (capillary, venous side) and an oxygen consumption ($\dot{V}_{O_2}$) of 15 ml $\cdot$ 100 ml^{-1} $\cdot$ min^{-1}, oxygen pressure will decrease from 20 to 0 mm Hg within 37 μm (Fig. 2), in accordance with the Hill equation (4). As can be seen from Fig. 1, most of the tissue is within a distance of less than 37 μm from the next capillary. However, if our simple diffusional model is transferred to the measurements of capillary distribution, a small portion of the tissue appears anoxic (Fig. 3) under worsed case conditions.

In conclusion, the results favor the view that: (1) capillary density is low in human DCM, and (2) tissue is on the border of hypoxia. The latter may make therapeutic strategies that cause increased oxygen demand harmful.

Summary: Human hearts with dilated cardiomyopathy (DCM) exhibit a hypertrophy of the myocytes; consequently, the intercapillary distance increases, which may impede the diffusionable metabolic supply. Therefore in the following study the microcirculation of living human hearts with DCM, excised during cardiac transplantation, was investigated. The hearts were reperfused with a FITC-stained salt-solution, this allowed the precise detection of all plasma perfused capillaries. Thus, functional capillary density, capillary distribution and its effect on oxygen supply could be determined.

In eight human hearts, the average functional capillary density amounted to 1245 ± 345 capillaries/mm², while 50% of the tissue was within 12 μm from the nearest capillary. However, a small portion of the tissue (1%) might become anoxic under the assumption of a simple oxygen diffusion model.

The results favor the view that capillary density is low in human DCM and tissue is at the border of hypoxia.

References

1. Factor SM, Sonnenblick EH (1982) Hypothesis: Is congestive cardiomyopathy caused by a hyperreactive myocardial microcirculation (microvascular spasm)? Am J Cardiol 50: 1149—1152
2. Factor SM, Minase T, Cho S, Domnitz R, Sonnenblick EH (1982) Microvascular spasm in the cardiomyopathic Syrian hamster: a preventable cause of focal myocardial necrosis. Circulation 66: 342—354
3. Figulla HR, Vetterlein F, Glaubitz M, Kreuzer H (1987) Inhomogeneous capillary flow and its prevention by verapamil and hydralazine in the cardiomyopathic Syrian hamster. Circulation 76: 208—216
4. Groom AC, Ellis CG, Potter RF (1984) Microvascular architecture and red cell perfusion in skeletal muscle. Prog Appl Microcirc 5: 64—83
5. Grote J, Thews G (1962) Die Bedingungen für die Sauerstoffversorgung des Herzmuskelgewebes. Pflügers Arch 276: 142—165

6. Kayar SR, Archer PG, Lechner AJ, Banchero N (1982) The closest individual method in the analysis of the distribution of capillaries. Microvasc Res 24: 326—341

7. Kunkel B, Lapp H, Kober G, Kaltenbach M (1978) Correlations between clinical and morphologic findings and natural history in congestive cardiomyopathy. In: Kaltenbach M, Loogen F, Olsen EGJ (eds) Cardiomyopathy and myocardial biopsy. Springer, Berlin—Heidelberg—New York, pp 271—283

8. Mall G, Schwarz F, Derks H (1982) Clinicopathologic correlations in congestive cardiomyopathy. Virchows Arch 397: 67—82

9. Rakusan K (1971) Quantitative morphology of capillaries of the heart. In: Bajusz E, Jasmin G (eds) Meth Achievm Exp Pathol. Karger — Basel, pp 272—284

10. Roberts JT, Wearn JT (1941) Quantitative changes in the capillary-muscle relationship in human hearts during normal growth and hypertrophy. Am Heart J 21: 617—633

Authors' address:
Dr. H. R. Figulla, Medizinische Universitätsklinik, Abteilung Kardiologie, Robert-Koch-Str. 40, D-3400 Göttingen, F.R.G.

Long-term observations in mild forms of cardiomyopathy

H. Sievert, B. Kunkel, R. Maier, and M. Kaltenbach

Department of Cardiology, Center of Internal Medicine, J. W. Goethe-University, University Hospital Frankfurt, F.R.G.

Introduction

The syndrome of chest pain with normal coronary arteries is well known from the literature. It has also been named syndrome X or latent cardiomyopathy (7, 12). Ejection

Table 1. 24 patients, suffering from histologically confirmed mild form of cardiomyopathy, followed-up over a period of 5.5 ± 1.9 years.

Patient No.	Age (years)	Symptoms	Heart volume (ml/1.73 m²)	Ejection fraction (3)	Followup (years)
1	34	A.p., D.	680	68	6
2	43	A.p., D., Palp.	680	64	6
3	38	D., Palp.	820	63	8
4	63	A.p., D., Palp.	1300	64	4
5	47	D., Palp.	1350	71	5
6	53	A.p., D.	950	70	9
7	39	A.p., D., Palp.	860	80	5
8	37	A.p., D., Palp.	1060	58	7
9	55	A.p., D.	780	55	2
10	53	A.p., D., Palp.	1000	61	7
11	50	A.p., D., Palp.	1010	65	6
12	57	A.p., D., Palp.	770	83	4
13	56	A.p., D., Palp.	1090	76	5
14	47	A.p., D.	700	60	8
15	43	A.p., D., Palp.	1100	71	4
16	47	A.p., D.	580	76	6
17	47	A.p., D.	810	74	5
18	32	D., Palp.	980	65	9
19	53	A.p., D.	1280	69	5
20	35	A.p., D., Palp.	770	56	4
21	43	A.p., D.	910	69	6
22	35	A.p., D., Palp.	590	65	2
23	46	A.p., D., Palp.	770	70	5
24	49	A.p., D.	590	66	3
Mean	48		893	68	5.5
±1SD	± 8		±224	± 7	±1.9

SD = standard deviation; A.p. = angina pectoris; D. = dyspnea; Palp. = palpitations.

fraction and left ventricle wall thickness are normal. In a previous study, many of these patients had shown a moderate hypertrophy of myocardial cells and several ultrastructural changes seen in left ventricle biopsy, e.g., nuclear abnormalities, degeneration of mitochondria, loss of myofibrils (15). According to this, a cardiomyopathic process (nondilative and nonhypertrophic) was documented in this subgroup of patients. We followed 24 patients with this histologically confirmed mild form of cardiomyopathy over a period of 5.5 ± 1.9 years.

Patients and Methods

We investigated 24 consecutive patients (six women and 18 men) with a mean age of 46 ± 8 years at the time of left ventricle biopsy and then followed them up for 5.5 ± 1.9 years. They suffered from a histologically confirmed mild form of cardiomyopathy with normal or nearly normal ejection fraction (Table 1). The initial and the follow-up investigation included a detailed clinical history, standard 12-lead electrocardiogram, exercise testing, determination of the heart volume by X-ray (10), M-mode echocardiography and right heart catheterization. The results of both studies were compared.

Results

History

Patients predominantly complained about dyspnea (100%), angina (88%) or palpitations (63%) (Fig. 1). Dyspnea was experienced mainly on effort whereas angina often

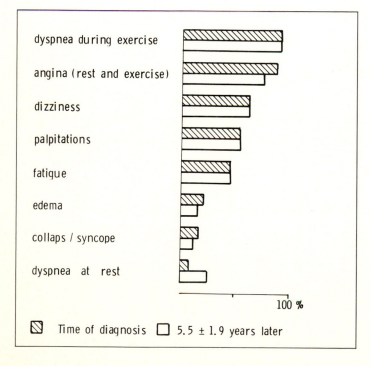

Fig. 1. Clinical symptoms of 24 patients with histologically confirmed mild cardiomyopathy.

occurred at rest, too. Nitroglycerin did not usually lead to prompt relief of the symptoms and in many cases no relief at all was observed. Within the 5.5 years, symptoms had remained the same in most patients. They had slightly increased in severity or frequency in eight patients, decreased in two patients, and remained constant in 14.

Electrocardiogram

The electrocardiogram was abnormal in 20 out of 24 patients. The most common disorders were atrial fibrillation (21%) or paroxysmal atrial tachycardia (13%) and premature ventricular beats (unifocal in 25%, multifocal in 8%). A I°, II° or III° AV block was seen in three patients, a left anterior hemiblock or a complete left bundle branch block was observed for each in three others, and a right bundle branch block in four patients. Most patients showed non-specific changes of ST-segment and T-waves.

During the 5.5 years, the electrocardiographic pattern had remained unchanged in 16 patients, while eight patients displayed a different pattern. Four of these developed an

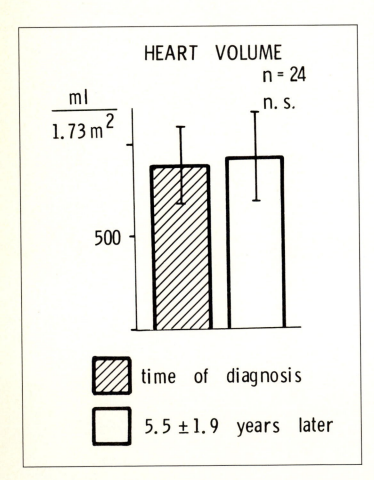

Fig. 2. Heart volume determined by X-ray 5.5 years after myocardial biopsy.

intermittent III° AV-block — three of them treated by pacemaker — two a left or right heart hypertrophy, one a left anterior hemiblock and one a complete left bundle branch block.

Exercise test

The exercise test of the first and second investigation could be compared in 15 patients. The exercise capacity had decreased in nine patients, remained unchanged in three and increased in three. The mean workload had decreased insignificantly from 608 ± 214 W·min/1.73 m² to 545 ± 149 W·min/1.73 m², and the exercise heart rate from 125 ± 26 min⁻¹ to 115 ± 23 min⁻¹ (N.S.).

Heart volume (Fig. 2)

At the time of diagnosis, the heart volume was normal (below 800 ml/1.73 m² in men and below 700 ml/1.73 m² in women) in ten out of 24 patients, and 5.5 years later in nine out of 24 patients. The mean heart volume increased nonsignificantly ($p < 0.05$) from 893 ± 224 ml/1.73 m² to 933 ± 245 ml/1.73 m².

Echocardiogram (Fig. 3)

The echocardiogram of the first and second investigation could be compared in six patients. The enddiastolic (EDD) and endsystolic diameter (ESD) of the left ventricle showed no significant change (EDD 5.5 ± 1.1 to 5.6 ± 0.6 cm, ESD 3.9 ± 1.2 to 3.7 ± 0.7 cm).

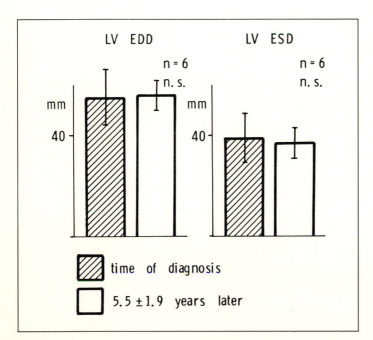

Fig. 3. Left ventricular enddiastolic (EDD) and endsystolic (ESD) diameter determined by echocardiography after 5.5 years.

Hemodynamics (Fig. 4)

At rest the pulmonary artery pressure was normal in ten patients and moderately elevated (> 15 mm Hg) in 14 out of 24 patients. After 5.5 years, the pulmonary artery pressure was normal in 12 patients. The mean value had remained constant (18 ± 5.9 to 17.8 ± 4 mm Hg). Mean cardiac output had decreased significantly from 5.6 ± 1.6 to 4.5 ± 0.7 l/min/1.73 m² ($p < 0.01$) and the stroke volume from 89.5 ± 40.8 to 62.3 ± 17.3 ml/1.73 m² ($p < 0.01$; $n = 18$). The heart rate had remained constant (70.8 ± 18.3 vs. 76.8 ± 13.1 min⁻¹; N.S.; $n = 18$). During initial and follow-up exercise testing with identical workload, mean pulmonary artery pressure remained unchanged (40.5 ± 9.5 vs. 37.4 ± 7.8 mm Hg; N.S.) cardiac output decreased from 13 ± 4.1 to 10.4 ± 2.3 l/min/1.73 m² ($p < 0.05$). Mean blood pressure was normal in all patients when first investigated and was normal in all, except for three, when followed up (95.6 ± 11.2 mm Hg vs. 101.0 ± 11.3 mm Hg; N.S.).

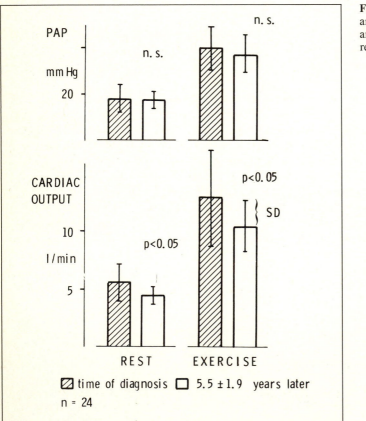

Fig. 4. Mean pulmonary artery pressure (PAP) and cardiac output at rest and during exercise.

Discussion

Syndrome X or the syndrome of angina or dyspnea with normal coronary arteries and no other known heart disease is well known from the literature (7, 9, 16, 17). Some of these patients may have a non-cardiac cause of their pain, such as esophageal spasm (4) or psychosomatic causes (2). However, many have an elevation of left ventricular end-diastolic pressure at rest or during exercise (3, 14), a limited coronary flow reserve (17) and an abnormal lactate production (1, 8, 17). Several investigators have found histological abnormalities — a moderate hypertrophy of the myocardial cells and ultrastructural changes — which identify a cardiomyopathic process (13, 15, 17). We followed a group of 24 patients with this histologically proven "mild form of cardiomyopathy" over 5.5 ± 1.9 years.

Subjective parameters showed only minor changes. Four patients had developed an intermittent III° AV-block (three of them treated by pacemaker) and cardiac output at rest and during exercise had decreased considerably. The mean pulmonary artery pressure as well as the heart volume and the left ventricle diameter remained unchanged. There was no serious clinical course, the prognosis of this mild form of cardiomyopathy being therefore rather promising. Several investigators have also reported a comparably good prognosis in patients with angina and normal coronary arteries (3, 9, 18) and even in mild dilative cardiomyopathy (5).

A marked deterioration seems to be unusual, and patients must not be considered as suffering from an early stage of congestive cardiomyopathy (6, 11) with poor prognosis.

Summary: 24 patients suffering from a mild cardiomyopathy with normal or nearly normal ejection fraction and histologic evidence of cardiac fiber hypertrophy were followed-up over 5.5 ± 1.9 years. Patients presented predominantly with dyspnea, angina and palpitations. During the observation period, the severity of symptoms increased only slightly. The ECG showed atrial arrhythmias in 34% and premature ventricular beats or conduction disturbances in the majority. During the 5.5 year follow-up period four patients had developed an intermittent III° AV-block and two patients a bundle branch block. The heart volume determined by X-ray increased insignificantly (893 ± 224 to 933 ± 245 ml/1.73 m²; n.s.), while left ventricle enddiastolic (5.5 ± 1.1 to 5.6 ± 0.6 cm) and endsystolic (3.9 ± 1.2 to 3.7 ± 0.7 cm) diameter remained nearly constant. Pulmonary artery pressure at rest (18 ± 5.9 to 17.8 ± 4 mm Hg) and during exercise (40.5 ± 9.5 to 37.4 ± 7.8 mm Hg) showed no significant change. However, cardiac output decreased significantly at rest from 5.6 ± 1.6 l/min/1.73 m² to 4.5 ± 0.7 l/min/1.73 m² ($p < 0.01$) and during exercise from 13 ± 4.1 l/min/1.73 m² to 10.4 ± 2.3 l/min/1.73 m² ($p < 0.05$).

It is concluded that patients with this mild cardiomyopathy show only minor changes over a period of 5.5 years. The prognosis seems to be promising in most cases.

References

1. Arbogast R, Bourassa M G (1973) Myocardial function during pacing in patients with angina pectoris and normal coronary arteriograms. Comparison with patients having significant coronary artery disease. Am J Cardiol 32: 257—263

2. Bass C, Wade C, Hand D, Jackson G (1983) Patients with angina with normal and nearly normal coronary arteries: clinical and psychosocial state 12 months after angiography. Br Med J 287: 1505—1514
3. Bemiller C R, Pepine C J, Rogers A K (1973) Long-term observations in patients with angina and normal coronary arteriograms. Circulation 47: 36—43
4. Benjamin S B, Castell D O (1983) Chest pain of esophageal origin. Arch Intern Med 143: 772—779
5. Curtius J M, Welslau K, Breuer H-W M, Loogen F (1985) Verlaufsbeobachtungen bei Patienten mit geringen Graden einer dilatativen Kardiomyopathie. Z Kardiol 74: 369—373
6. Hess O M, Turina J, Krayenbühl H P (1981) Latente Kardiomyopathie — Frühform der kongestiven Kardiomyopathie. Schweiz Med Wschr 111: 1959—1961
7. Kemp H G (1973) Left ventricular function in patients with the anginal syndrome and normal coronary arteriograms. Am J Cardiol 32: 375—376
8. Kemp H G, Elliot W C, Gorlin R (1967) The anginal syndrome with normal coronary arteriography. Trans Assoc Am Physician 80: 59—63
9. Kemp H G, Vokonas P S, Cohn P F, Gorlin R (1973) The anginal syndrome associated with normal coronary arteriograms. An J Med 54: 735—742
10. Klepzig H, Frisch P (Hrsg.) (1965) Röntgenologische Herzvolumenbestimmung. Thieme, Stuttgart
11. Kübler W, Kuhn H, Loogen F (1972) Die Kardiomyopathien. Z Kardiol 62: 2—22
12. Kuhn H (1980) Die latente Kardiomyopathie (LCM). Intern Welt 10: 373—377
13. Kuhn H, Breithard G, Knieriem H J, Loogen F (1978) Endomyocardial catheter biopsy in heart disease of unknown etiology. In: Kaltenbach M, Loogen F, Olsen E G J (eds) Cardiomyopathy and myocardial biopsy. Springer Berlin—Heidelberg—New York, pp 121—137
14. Kuhn H, Knieriem H J, Lösse B, Breithard G, Köhler E, Seipel L, Loogen F (1978) Prognosis and possible presymptomatic manifestations of congestive cardiomyopathy. Postgrad Med J 54: 451—459
15. Kunkel B, Schneider M, Kober G, Bussmann W-D, Hopf R, Kaltenbach M (1982) Die Morphologie der Myokardbiopsie und ihre klinische Bedeutung. Z Kardiol 71: 787—794
16. Likoff W, Segal B L, Kasparian H (1967) Paradox of normal selective coronary arteriograms in patients considered to have unmistakable coronary heart disease. N Engl J Med 276: 1063—1067
17. Opherk D, Zebe H, Weihe E, Mall G, Durr C, Gravert B, Mehmel H C, Schwarz F, Kübler W (1981) Reduced coronary dilatory capacity and ultrastructural changes of the myocardium in patients with angina pectoris and normal coronary arteriograms. Circulation 63: 817—825
18. Pasternak R C, Thibault G E, Savoia M, De Sanctis R W, Hutter A M (1980) Chest pain with angiographically insignificant coronary arterial obstruction. Am J Med 68: 813—817

Authors' address:
Dr. med. H. Sievert, Abteilung für Kardiologie, Zentrum der Inneren Medizin, Klinikum der Universität, Theodor-Stern-Kai 7, D-6000 Frankfurt am Main, F.R.G.

Comparison of verapamil and bepridil in the therapy of familiar cardiomyopathy of the Syrian hamster

B. Kunkel, U. Hofmann, M. Mutschler

Medizinische Poliklinik der Universität Erlangen und Institut für Pharmakologie der Universität Frankfurt, F.R.G.

Introduction

The effect of verapamil on the cardiomyopathic hamster is wellknown from the basic works of Loßnitzer (6—9). It is not known, however, whether different calcium-antagonists have the same cardioprotective potency. In this study we analyzed the effect of bepridil, on the cardiomyopathic hamster. Bepridil is shown to be a calcium antagonistic drug (10) with documented antianginal (1) in humans efficacy.

Material and Methods

The study was designed according to the works of Loßnitzer (6—9). Five untreated hamsters (strain BIO 8262) were sacrificed at the age of 30 days, to define the prenecrotic phase of the animals. Five hamsters were kept on bepridil for 15 days (life-days 30—45), five others for 30 days (life-days 30—60). A dose of 10 mg/kg was injected subcutaneously twice daily. This dose was derived from experiences of clinical efficacy. Seven animals were treated with verapamil, 10 mg/kg twice daily for 30 days (life-days 30—60), to compare the effects of bepridil and verapamil. Another ten animals treated with NaCl served as controls.

The animals were sacrificed under ether anesthesia. The hearts were excised and fixed in formalin. One section of the basal region and one apical section of the hearts were analyzed. The area of necrosis was measured morphometricly according to the principles of Weibel (11). The sections were divided into adjacent areas, upon which a square grid consisting of 100 test points was superimposed. For analysis of the total circumference of the right and left ventricle, between eight (apical region in young animals) and 22 areas (basal region in 60-days-old animals) had to be investigated. In this manner, 800—2200 points per section were counted. The area of necrosis was calculated using the formula

$$\frac{p_n}{p_t} \times 100$$

= volume density of necrotic myocardium (percentage of total myocardium); p_n = number of points falling on necrosis; p_t = total number of points falling on myocardium. The mean volume density of necrosis of the basal and apical region is given in the figures and table. In the peripheral muscles (m. quadriceps femoris and diaphragm) eight test areas (800 test points) were analyzed.

The tissue contents of calcium, magnesium, potassium and sodium of the heart and m. quadriceps femoris and the diaphragm were measured by atomic absorption spectrophotometry (for method see 6). The hamsters included were: seven at the age of 30 days, seven treated with bepridil for 30 days, seven treated with verapamil for 30 days and seven control animals treated with NaCl for 30 days.

Results

Histology

In accordance with the literature, no myocardial necrosis was observed on day 30. In contrast, the peripheral muscles (quadriceps femoris and diaphragm) already showed myocytolysis with calcification during that early phase (Table 1). On day 45, two out of five animals of the control group had myocardial necrosis. The development of necrosis could not be prevented by bepridil (four out of five cases with myocytolysis after 15 days treatment). A few of the control animals (one out of five) exhibited small calcifications, which were also seen in the bepridil group (three in five). After 1 month of treatment (life-day 60), nearly all control animals (nine out of ten) showed necrosis and calcifications. Cell damage was seen to the same extent in the controls and bepridil-treated animals. On the other hand, myocardial cell necrosis could be completely prevented by verapamil. In contrast to the superior protective effect of verapamil in the heart, there was no difference in the peripheral muscles between controls and bepridil or verapamil treated hearts.

The necrotic lesions showed typical distributions and localizations. Areas with cell damage were predominantly localized in the left ventricle while the right ventricle was affected in a few cases only. Within the left ventricle, the free wall was clearly more affected than the septal area (Fig. 1). The necrotic lesions could be observed in all parts of the ventricular wall with a clear preponderance of the mid-ventricular central area, whereas a minority of myocytic lesions were seen in the subendocardial or subepicardial region (Fig. 2).

Table 1. Incidence of myocardial necrosis and calcification.

	C_{30}	C_{45}	B_{45}	C_{60}	B_{60}	V_{60}
Myocardium						
Necrosis	0/5	2/5	4/5	9/10	10/10	0/7
Calcification	0/5	1/5	3/5	9/10	7/10	0/7
Diaphragm						
Necrosis	5/5	2/5	5/5	0/10	10/10	7/7
Calcification	0/5	2/3	1/5	2/10	1/10	0/7
M. quadriceps femoris						
Necrosis	5/5	4/5	3/5	7/10	8/10	7/7
Calcification	0/5	1/5	0/5	1/10	1/10	0/7

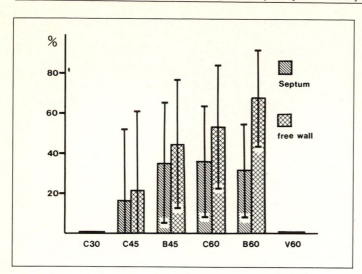

Fig. 1: Distribution of necrotic lesions within the left ventricle. (C) control, (B) bepridil treatment, (V) verapamil treatment. Numbers indicate life-day. The areas of necrosis were predominantly localized in the left ventricular free wall.

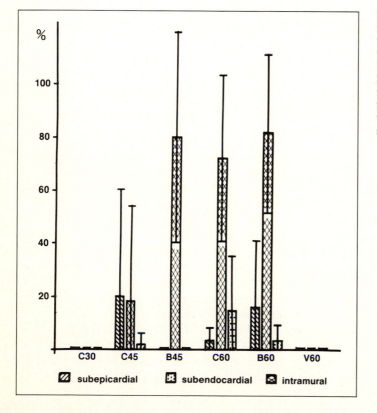

Fig. 2. Localization of necrotic lesions in the ventricular wall. (Abbreviations: see Fig. 1). Most necrotic areas were located in the mid-ventricular wall, while only a few lesions were found in the subendocardial or subepicardial region.

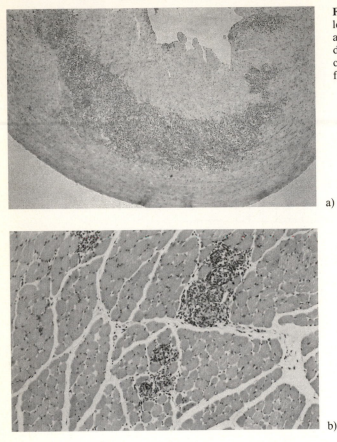

Fig. 3. (a) Infarct-like necrotic lesion within the left ventricle of a bepridil-treated animal (Life-day 60). (b) Small group of necrotic cells in the m. quadriceps femoris (control, life-day 45).

a)

b)

In the model of a disease due to an error of metabolism, it should be assumed that cell necrosis predominantly affects single cells or small groups of cells. This could be confirmed for the quadriceps femoris and the diaphragm. In the peripheral muscles, small foci of necrosis were the predominant lesions. In the heart, we observed infarct-like lesions or large groups of necrotic cells in all cases, whereas single cell necroses were found only in a very few cases (Fig. 3). During the course of the disease, the necrotic areas were invaded with macrophages and subsequently organized. Other foci developed calcifications. Calcifications in these animals usually occurred without previous cellular infiltrations.

The total area of necrosis was measured morphometricly. On day 45 (after 15 days of treatment) less than 1% of the total left ventricular myocardium was affected in the control group. In the bepridil-treated animals, about 2% of the myocardium was involved. After 1 month of treatment, 3—4% of the left ventricular myocardium showed myocytolysis of various stages in the controls as well as in the bepridil-treated animals. There was a significant variation within the different groups. Under verapamil no necrosis occurred until life-day 60 (Fig. 4).

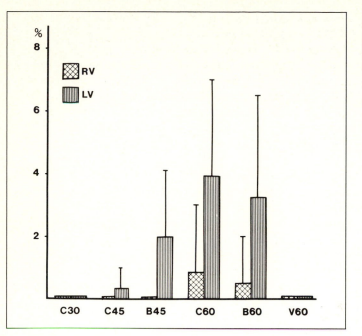

Fig. 4. Area of necrosis in the right and left ventricle. The maximal area of necrosis was observed on day 60 (4%) in the left ventricle. Necrosis was not influenced by bepridil but could be prevented by verapamil.

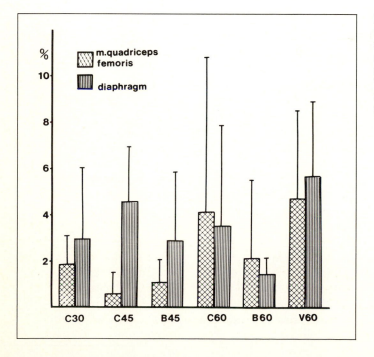

Fig. 5. Area of necrosis in the skeletal muscle and diaphragm. The maximal area of necrosis was observed on day 60 (6%). The necroses were influenced neither by bepridil nor by verapamil.

In the right ventricle, dystrophic lesions were not observed before day 45 and the area involved was less than 1% of the total right ventricular myocardium (Fig. 4). In conclusion, the total amount of myocardial necrosis and fibrosis was not very high.

Figure 5 demonstrates the area of necrosis in skeletal muscle. It can be seen that in the peripheral muscle fiber damage is already present on day 30, before the heart muscle is involved. On the day 60, the mean necrotic area is 5—6% of the total muscle volume, both in the quadriceps femoris and the diaphragm. The myocytolytic lesions in the verapamil group were more widespread than in the bepridil group. There was, however, a marked variation within the various groups and this observation did not reach significance.

The changes in the calcium content of the myocardium and peripheral muscle during the experiment are shown in Fig. 6. There is a low normal calcium content in the heart in the prenecrotic phase (16.8 ± 3.2 mVal/kg). A ten-fold increase is observed during the next month (152 ± 111 mVal/kg). The calcium overload of the heart is not influenced by bepridil (Ca content 126 ± 108 mVal/kg). The verapamil-treated animals have normal, low calcium values in the heart (12.3 ± 5.9 mVal/kg).

In the periphery, the calcium content of the muscles shows a maximum as early as day 30 (110.6 ± 82.6 mVal/kg). On day 60, the calcium concentrations are lower than in the early phase (47.0 ± 27.5 mVal/kg). The calcium concentrations were not influenced by calcium antagonist treatment, either bepridil (66.3 ± 51.3 mVal/kg) or verapamil (63.3 ± 51 mVal/kg). Identical values were found under control conditions and calcium antagonist treatment.

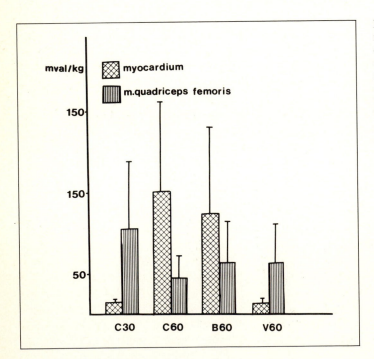

Fig. 6. Ca content of the myocardium and the m. quadriceps femoris in controls and under treatment. The myocardial calcium overload could be completely prevented by verapamil and was not influenced by bepridil. Both drugs were ineffective in peripheral muscles.

Discussion

According to the basic investigations of Fleckenstein, calcium overload causes myocardial cell death (3—5). Various mechanisms such as ischemia, or catecholamines, etc. may give rise to increased cellular calcium concentrations. In the cardiomyopathic hamster, an inherited mechanism leading to myocardial calcium accumulation forms the basis of the disease (8). The nature of this genetic defect is not completely understood. Loßnitzer postulates a progressive membrane defect to explain normal calcium concentrations in the prenecrotic phase of the animal's life and development of calcium accumulation and cell necrosis after about 1 month (8).

Our results confirm the studies of Mohr and Loßnitzer (9), that the necrotizing process of the myocardium begins after the first month of life. In the peripheral muscles necrotic and calcified fibers were found even before that time. In addition to a few lesions with focal myocytolysis, large infarct-like necrotic areas were observed in the myocardium in our experiments. These areas formed the predominant pathologic lesion. In this respect, our findings are different from the observations of Mohr and Loßnitzer who described small multifocal necrotic areas (9). While small groups of necrotic cells are typical lesions for metabolic disorders, the infarct-like lesions observed in our animals point rather to a vascular genesis of the necrosis. In a perfusion experiment, Factor et al. observed numerous areas of microvascular constriction, diffuse vessel narrowing and luminal irregularities, while fixed structural lesions of the vessels could not be demonstrated (2). The authors conclude that focal transient spasm of the small blood vessels, probably secondary to vasoactive substances, might cause myocytolic lesions. Mohr (9) describes two types of cell damage in the Syrian hamster: coagulative necrosis and cellular calcification inducing the formation of the slowly degenerating myocardial giant cells. The latter finding can be attributed to the disturbance of calcium metabolism, while the infarct-like areas with coagulative necrosis may be regarded as being of vascular origin. Both mechanisms obviously coexist in the animal model of the Syrian hamster. The occurrence of vascular spasm in the presence of high cellular calcium concentrations is not surprising. In human cardiomyopathies, small vessel disease has often been postulated but has never been confirmed by morphologic bioptic investigations. The assumption of microvascular spasm, however, would be a reasonable pathogenetic mechanism for various forms of human cardiomyopathies. The existence of atypical angina in many patients with various types of cardiomyopathies points to that mechanism. Also, the positive effects of calcium antagonistic drugs on angina in the hypertrophic cardiomyopathy and many patients with mild cardiomyopathy support that concept.

Myocardial calcium accumulation and cell necrosis can be completely prevented by verapamil (6—9). In addition, magnesium aspartate and beta-blocking agents with unspecific membrane effects also prevent or reduce myocardial necrosis in the Syrian hamster (7). On the other hand, selective beta-blockers without nonspecific membrane effects do not influence the necrotizing process (7). In this study, the myocardial calcium content and extent of myocardial necrosis were not influenced by bepridil. It may be speculated that this drug is not a classic calcium antagonist. Secondly, the well-documented antianginal effect (1) might be different from the metabolic effects on the cellular calcium influx. It is also possible that the substance is not effective only in this particular animal species, or the doses administered, derived from clinical experiences, were not. No definite answer to this problem can be drawn from our study.

The calcium content of the peripheral muscles and the area of necrosis could not be influenced either by verapamil or by bepridil. This might be due to the fact that peripheral muscle cell necrosis starts as early as in the first week of life and reaches its maximum after 30 days. Furthermore, the question arises of whether the cellular receptors for calcium antagonistic substances of myocardial and peripheral striated muscle are identical.

Summary: The effect of bepridil compared to verapamil on the cardiomyopathic hamster (Strain Bio 8262) was evaluated. Bepridil (10 mg/kg) was injected twice daily for 15 and 30 days. Verapamil (10 mg/kg) was injected twice daily for 30 days. Control animals were treated with NaCl. After life-day 30, large infarct-like lesions predominantly located in the central portion of the left ventricular walls were observed, while single cell necrosis occurred only in a few cases. In peripheral muscles, the necrotizing process started even before life-day 30.

In the skeletal muscles, small foci of cell necrosis were the predomiant type of lesion. Myocardial calcium accumulation and cell necrosis could be completely prevented by verapamil and were not influenced by bepridil. Both drugs were ineffective in the skeletal muscles. The infarct-like lesions of the myocardium demonstrate that a vascular component is involved in the pathogenesis of necrosis, in addition to the inherited disturbance of calcium metabolism. The results demonstrate that not all drugs with calcium antagonistic potencies have identical cardioprotective effects in the cardiomyopathic hamster.

References

1. Canicave JC, Den J, Jacq Z, Paillet R (1980) Therapie 35: 607
2. Factor S, Minase T, Cho S, Dominitz R, Sonnenblick E (1985) Microvascular spasm in the cardiomyopathic Syrian hamster: A preventable cause of focal myocardial necrosis. Circulation 66: 342—354
3. Fleckenstein A, Janke J, Döring HJ, Leder O (1971) Die intracelluläre Überladung mit Calcium als entscheidender Kausalfaktor bei der Entstehung nicht coronarogener Myokardnekrosen. Verh Dtsch Ges Kreislaufforsch 37: 345—353
4. Fleckenstein A, Janke J, Döring HJ, Pachinger O (1973) Ca overload the determinant factor in the production of catecholamine-induced myocardial lesion. In: Bajusz E, Rona G (eds) Cardiomyopathies. Recent in the Study of Cardiac Structural Metabolism. Advances Vol 2. University Park Press, Baltimore—London—Tokyo, pp 455—466
5. Fleckenstein A, Frey M, Keidel JJ (1982) Prevention by Verapamil of Isoproterenol-induced hypertrophic cardiomyopathy in rats. In: M Kaltenbach, S Epstein (eds) Hypertrophic cardiomyopathy. Springer Verlag, Berlin—Heidelberg-New York, pp 113—120
6. Loßnitzer K, Steinhard B, Grewe N, Stauch M (1975) Charakteristische Elektrolytveränderungen bei der erblichen Kardiomyopathie des Syrischen Goldhamsters (Stamm Bio 8262). Basic Res Cardiol 70: 508—520
7. Loßnitzer K, Konrad A, Zeger D, Mohr W (1982) Prevention of myocardial cell necrosis in the Syrian hamster. Results of long-term treatment. In: M Kaltenbach, S Epstein (eds) Hypertrophic Cardiomyopathy. Springer Verlag, Berlin—Heidelberg—New York, pp 99—114
8. Loßnitzer K (1975) Genetic Induction of a Cardiomyopathy. In: Born GVR, Eichler O, Farah A, Herken H, Welch AD (eds) Handbuch der experimentellen Pharmakologie. Vol XVI/3, Springer Verlag, Berlin—Heidelberg—New York, pp 309—344

9. Mohr W, Loßnitzer K (1974) Morphologische Untersuchungen an Hamstern des Stammes Bio 8262 mit erblicher Myopathie und Kardiomyopathie. Beitr Path 153: 178—193
10. Murphy KMM; Gould RJ, Largent BJ, Snyder SH (1983) Proc Natl Acad Sci USA 80: 860
11. Weibel E, Kistler GS, Scherle WF (1966) Practical stereological methods for morphometric cytology. J Cell Biol 30: 23—38

Authors' address:

Prof. Dr. B. Kunkel, Medizinische Poliklinik der Universität Erlangen, Östliche Stadtmauerstraße 29, 8520 Erlangen, F.R.G.

Calcium antagonist treatment in mild forms of cardiomyopathy

H. Sievert, B. Kunkel, M. Wirtz, R. Hopf, and M. Kaltenbach

Department of Cardiology, Center of Internal Medicine, J. W. Goethe-University, University Hospital Frankfurt, F.R.G.

Introduction

The syndrome of angina with normal coronary arteries (14, 15), also referred to as syndrome X (14), is well known from medical literature. Many patients with this disease also complain about dyspnea or palpitations. The electrocardiogram may show various abnormalities. Ventricular systolic function is normal at rest. The enddiastoic filling pressure is elevated (3) during exercise or even at rest reflecting a disturbance in diastolic ventricular function. This has also been demonstrated by gated blood pool scintigraphy (3). An increase in myocardial lactate production (19) and a reduction in coronary flow reserve (4, 5, 6, 19) have been found. Several investigators have presented histologic evidence of a cardiomyopathic process (10, 17—19). A hypertrophy of myocardial cells is the most common.

Medical treatment of these patients has always been unsatisfactory; however, recent investigations have shown that the use of calcium antagonists has improved clinical symptoms (7). In an open randomized cross-over study we therefore investigated the clinical efficacy and especially the hemodynamic response of verapamil in these mild forms of cardiomyopathy, also called latent cardiomyopathy (16).

Patients and Methods

21 patients (12 men and 9 women with a mean age of 51 ± 6.9 years) were included. They mainly complained about angina (19 patients) and/or dyspnea (16 patients). Hypertrophy of myocardial cells was identified in all of those patients who were subjected to left ventricular biopsy. Where biopsy had not been performed, as was the case with seven patients, a rise in diastolic pulmonary artery pressure during exercise or even at rest served as an inclusion criterion. The ejection fraction was normal. Patients with other known heart diseases or arterial hypertension were not included in this study.

Patients received either 120 mg verapamil, three times a day, or no therapy at all for a period of 2 months, followed then the by the cross-over. A history was obtained and right heart catheterization was performed after each period, i.e. after 2 and 4 months, respectively. The pulmonary artery pressure and cardiac output (thermodilution), as well as blood pressure and heart rate, were recorded at rest and during exercise with subma-ximal work load (50—100 W, mean: 64 ± 23 W).

All data are reported as means ± SD and were tested for significance using the Wil-coxon matched-pairs signed rank test ($a = 0.05$).

Results

History

In 14 out of 21 patients, clinical symptoms improved by at least one grade (NYHA) during verapamil treatment (Fig. 1). Six patients remained unchanged and only one pa-tient's condition deteriorated. This beneficial effect of verapamil proved significant ($p < 0.05$).

Hemodynamics

At rest (Fig. 2), all hemodynamic data — cardiac output, blood pressure, heart rate, diastolic pulmonary artery pressure (PADP) and peripheral resistance, showed no sig-nificant changes (cardiac output: 5.7 ± 1.4 to 5.9 ± 1.5 l/min; mean blood pressure: 96.6 ± 7.0 to 93.4 ± 4.9 mm Hg; heart rate: 71.7 ± 9.8 to 70 ± 9.7 min^{-1}; diastolic pulmonary artery pressure: 10.7 ± 5.2 to 9.0 ± 4.5 mm Hg; peripheral resistance: 1220 ± 216 to 1224 ± 352 dyn · s · cm^{-5}). In those nine patients (Fig. 3) with elevated

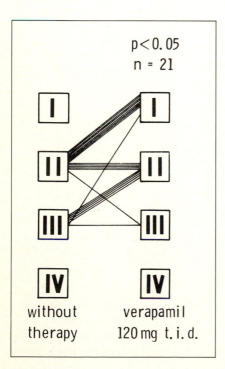

Fig. 1. NYHA classification of 21 patients taking ver-apamil for a period of 2 months.

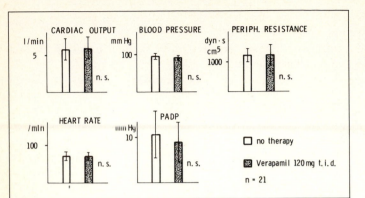

Fig. 2. Hemodynamic data at rest with and without verapamil treatment.

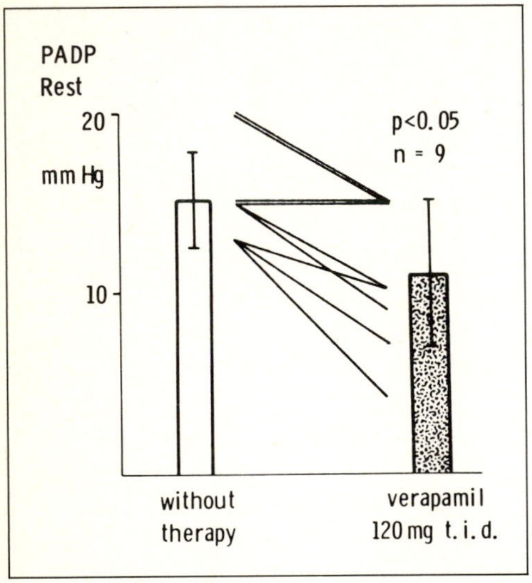

Fig. 3. Patients with elevated diastolic pulmonary artery pressure at rest with and without verapamil ($n = 9$).

diastolic pulmonary artery pressure at rest (> 12 mm Hg) PADP decreased slightly after verapamil treatment (15.4 ± 2.7 to 11.1 ± 4.1, $p < 0.05$).

During exercise, PADP decreased in 14 patients, remained constant in five and increased in two after verapamil treatment (Fig. 4). The mean PADP decreased significantly from 25.3 ± 7.6 to 20.1 ± 6.6 mm Hg ($p < 0.05$). Cardiac output during exercise displayed no significant change (10.5 ± 2.2 to 11.1 ± 2.8 l/min, N.S.), as did blood pressure (121 ± 13 to 115 ± 11 mm Hg; $n = 12$; N.S.) and peripheral resistance (836 ± 178 to 801 ± 208 dyn $\cdot$ s $\cdot$ cm^{-5}; $n = 12$; N.S.).

Discussion

Patients with angina and normal coronary arteries, as well as the subgroup with histologically-confirmed cardiomyopathy, are usually known to have a good prognosis (1, 15,

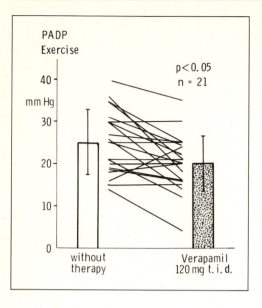

Fig. 4. Mean diastolic pulmonary artery pressure during exercise, with and without verapamil.

20). Clinical symptoms, on the other hand, may be severe and disabling (20). To date treatment of these symptoms has been disappointing (9). Nitrates and beta-blockers are often referred to as ineffective; however, systematic studies on the effectiveness of these agents have not yet been carried out. Calcium antagonist treatment, however, has shown beneficial effects in patients with abnormal vasodilator reserve (7) but has not bee so far reported in patients with these histologically-proven mild forms of cardiomyopathy.

In some of our patients, verapamil achieved favourable results. Therefore, we investigated the long-term efficacy of verapamil in this cross-over study.

Because elevation of left ventricular filling pressure and of diastolic pulmonary artery pressure is a characteristic finding in these patients during exercise of even at rest, right heart catheterization was performed before and after treatment with verapamil.

In most patients, the clinical symptoms (dyspnea and angina) improved after verapamil therapy. As a consequence it was possible to assign 14 out of 21 patients to a lower NYHA class. The diastolic pulmonary artery pressure at rest showed no significant change in the whole group, possibly because it was normal in many of them from the very beginning. The nine patients with elevated diastolic pulmonary artery pressure at rest demonstrated a significant decrease after taking verapamil. During exercise, the diastolic pulmonary artery pressure rose in most patients and decreased significantly after verapamil.

All other hemodynamic data remained constant (blood pressure, heart rate, cardiac output, peripheral resistance). Therefore a reduction in afterload or preload of the left ventricle cannot explain the beneficial effect of verapamil on the diastolic pulmonary artery pressure which, likewise, reflects the left ventricular filling pressure. Verapamil taken orally has either no, or only slight, negative influence on left ventricular contraction (8, 13). The predominant mechanism of this treatment may thus be attributed to an improvement in diastolic ventricular function. A similar action has been ascribed to verapamil treatment in hypertrophic cardiomyopathy (2, 11, 12).

Our results might therefore indicate that diastolic ventricular dysfunction is an important aspect in the above described mild form of cardiomyopathy.

Summary: Twenty-one patients with a mild form of cardiomyopathy (with normal ejection fraction but histologically-confirmed hypertrophy of myocardial cells and/or elevated diastolic pulmonary artery pressure during exercise) received 120 mg verapamil t.i.d. or no therapy at all for a period of 2 months in an open randomized cross-over study.

Out of the 21 patients, 14 improved clinically, one patient's condition deteriorated and six remained unchanged ($p < 0.05$). The mean diastolic pulmonary artery pressure during exercise decreased (25.3 ± 7.6 to 20.1 ± 6.6 mm Hg, $n = 21$, $p < 0.05$). At rest, the decrease was only significant in the subgroup with pressures above 12 mm Hg (15.4 ± 2.7 to 11.1 ± 4.1 mm Hg, $n = 9$, $p < 0.05$). All other hemodynamic data displayed no significant change.

The benefits of verapamil therapy may be attributed to an improvement in diastolic ventricular function. The disturbance in diastolic relaxation might be of greater importance than the disturbance in systolic function in patients with mild forms of cardiomyopathy.

References

1. Bemiller CR, Pepine CJ, Rogers AK (1973) Long-term observations in patients with angina and normal coronary arteriograms. Circulation 47: 36—43
2. Bonow RO, Rosing DR, Bacharach SL, Green MV, Kent KM, Lipson LC, Maron BJ, Leon MB, Epstein SE (1981) Effects of verapamil on left ventricular systolic function and diastolic filling in patients with hypertrophic cardiomyopathy. Circulaton 64: 787—796
3. Bush CA, Fanning W, Kolibash AJ, Leier CV (1982) Elevated left ventricular filling pressure as a cause of angina in patients with normal coronary arteries. Am J Cardiol 49: 950
4. Cannon RO, Bonow RO, Bacharach SL, Green MV, Rosing DR, Leon MB, Watson RM, Epstein SE (1985) Left ventricular dysfunction in patients with angina pectoris, normal epicardial coronary arteries, and abnormal vasodilator reserve. Circulation 71: 218—226
5. Cannon RO, Leon MB, Watson RM, Rosing DR, Epstein SE (1985) Chest pain and "normal" coronary arteries — role of small coronary arteries. Am J Cardiol 55: 50 B-60 B
6. Cannon RO, Watson RM, Rosing DR, Epstein SE (1983) Angina caused by reduced vasodilator reserve of the small coronary arteries. J Am Coll Cardiol 1: 1359—1373
7. Cannon RO, Watson RM, Rosing DR, Epstein SE (1984) Efficacy of calcium antagonist therapy in patients with angina pectoris, normal epicardial coronary arteries and abnormal vasodilator reserve. J Am Coll Cardiol 3: 550
8. D'Agostino HJ, Pritchett ELC, Shand DG, Jones RH (1983) Effect of verapamil on left ventricular function at rest and during exercise in normal men. J Cardiovasc Pharmacol 5: 812—817
9. Day LJ, Sowton E (1976) Clinical features and follow-up of patients with angina and normal coronary arteries. Lancet 334—355
10. Frenzel H, Kasper M, Kuhn H, Lösse B, Reifschneider G, Hort W (1985) Licht- und elektronenmikroskopische Befunde in Früh- und Spätstadien der Herzinsuffizienz. Untersuchungen an Endomyokardbiopsien von Patienten mit latenter (LCM) und dilatativer (DCM) Kardiomyopathie. Z Kardiol 74: 135—143

11. Hanrath P, Mathey DG, Kremer P, Sonntag F, Bleifeld W (1980) Effect of verapamil on left ventricular isovolumic relaxation time and regional left ventricular filling in hypertrophic cardiomyopathy. Am J Cardiol 45: 1258—1264
12. Kaltenbach M, Hopf R (1985) Treatment of hypertrophic cardiomyopathy: Relation to pathological mechanisms. J Mol Cell Cardiol 17 (Suppl 2): 59—68
13. Kaltenbach M, Hopf R, Kober G, Bussmann W-D, Keller M, Petersen Y (1979) Treatment of hypertrophic obstructive cardiomyopathy with verapamil. Br Heart J 42: 35—42
14. Kemp HG (1973) Left ventricular function in patients with the anginal syndrome and normal coronary arteriograms. Am J Cardiol 32: 375—376
15. Kemp HG, Vokonas PS, Cohn PF, Gorlin R (1973) The anginal syndrome associated with normal coronary arteriograms. Am J Med 54: 735—742
16. Kuhn H (1980) Die latente Kardiomyopathie (LCM). Intern Welt 10: 373—377
17. Kuhn H, Breithard G, Knieriem HJ, Loogen F (1978) Endomyocardial catheter biopsy in heart disease of unknown etiology. In: Kaltenbach M, Loogen F, Olsen EGJ (eds) Cardiomyopathy and myocardial biopsy. Springer Berlin—Heidelberg–New York, pp 121—137
18. Kunkel B, Schneider M, Kober G, Bussmann W-D, Hopf R, Kaltenbach M (1982) Die Morphologie der Myokardbiopsie und ihre klinische Bedeutung. Z Kardiol 71: 787—794
19. Opherk D, Zebe H, Weihe E, Mall G, Durr C, Gravert B, Mehmel HC, Schwarz F, Kübler W (1981) Reduced coronary dilatory capacity and ultrastructural changes of the myocardium in patients with angina pectoris and normal coronary arteriograms. Circulaton 63: 817—825
20. Pasternak RC, Thibault GE, Savoia M, De Sanctis RW, Hutter AM (1980) Chest pain with angiographically insignificant coronary arterial obstruction. Am J Med 68: 813—817

Authors' address:
Dr. med. H. Sievert, Abteilung für Kardiologie, Zentrum der Inneren Medizin, Klinikum der Universität, Theodor-Stern-Kai 7, D-6000 Frankfurt am Main, F.R.G.

Subject Index